2915 Geneseo Rd
Paso Robles CA
238-4937
1982

TAKE CHARGE OF YOUR HEALTH

Take Charge of Your Health

THE COMPLETE NUTRITION BOOK

Gladys Lindberg and Judy Lindberg McFarland

1817

Harper & Row, Publishers, San Francisco

New York, Grand Rapids, Philadelphia, St. Louis
London, Singapore, Sydney, Tokyo, Toronto

Designer: Jim Mennick

Library of Congress Cataloging in Publication Data

Lindberg, Gladys.
   TAKE CHARGE OF YOUR HEALTH.

   Bibliography: p. 251
   Includes index.
   1. Naturopathy. 2. Food, Natural. 3. Health.
I. McFarland, Judy Lindberg. II. Title.
RZ440.L57   613.2   81-47836
ISBN 0-06-250519-X   AACR2

94 95 96   15 14 13 12

I want to dedicate this work to my father,
WALTER HAROLD LINDBERG,
for without his vision, love, brilliance, and hard work,
Mother would not have had a platform from which to teach.

Contents

Preface   ix
Acknowledgments   xi

 1. "Healthy People Don't Have That, So Let's
    Make You Healthy"   1
 2. The Wheat Germ Lady   7
 3. What Did Our Ancestors Do Right That We Are
    Doing Wrong?   17
 4. Understanding Stress   23
 5. Hypoglycemia: A Much Misunderstood Health
    Problem   41
 6. The Protein Story   59
 7. Protecting the Heart   76
 8. Digestion and Elimination   99
 9. The Immune System: Helping Your Body's
    Defense Mechanism   115
10. Lively Longevity: Aging Without Growing Old   134
11. Take Charge of Your Health: A Comprehensive
    Program   149

Appendix A. Meal Suggestions   170
Appendix B. Vitamins and Minerals   174
Bibliography   251
Index   255

Preface

We often do not appreciate our health until we become ill. Then all the money in the world may not enable us to regain it.

Take Charge of Your Health is meant to provide practical, easy-to-follow suggestions for maintaining good health and the sense of well-being, physical and mental, that is your birthright. We want to help you prevent degenerative diseases, illness, and the heartaches that come with a loss of one's health. We hope to teach you how to prevent some of the suffering that characterizes so many lives.

If you use this information to diagnose any illness, or try to treat your own disease, you have missed the point. This book is to help those who are well to prevent subclinical disease—the "I just don't have any energy" syndrome. If you are ill, you should be under the care of a physician, one who understands nutrition and will work with you. There are many fine doctors who are trained and believe in the use of vitamins and minerals.

My immediate family, as well as other relatives and friends, have appealed to me to record Mother's personal story and the nutrition program she has lived and taught these past forty years. She has a vast store of knowledge and an easy, understandable way of relating it to others, but she can only reach a few people at a time. I knew I would be sorry indeed if I did not make her knowledge more widely available. Thus I assumed the task of gathering the background information, recording the nutritional teaching, and confirming the data—all with the help and support of my family.

Gladys Lindberg is a fine example of what she teaches. A vivacious great-grandmother who long ago passed her seventieth birthday, she has an amazing energy level and a schedule to match; she puts in a full day's work every day. For years she has counseled clients, helping them establish a dietary routine to satisfy their particular needs, and she knows what works. She is not a doctor and does not prescribe, but she is eager to share her cumulative knowledge of nutrition. I cannot tell you how many times I have heard people tell Mother how grateful they are for her help. Often they say their loved ones wouldn't be alive today if it were not for Mother's advice.

Growing up in a family interested in nutrition was unique many years ago. When we were young, we were considered "health nuts," but times have changed. People today are interested in nutrition and realize its significance. Through the years, my family has come to know the pioneers in the field, and we have learned from them. I attended many a lecture, seminar, and convention with Mother. Now I take my own children, in order to preserve our heritage.

Nutrition alone is no guarantee of good health, of course. All the food in the world cannot make us healthy and energetic if we fail to exercise adequately. Nutrition and exercise work together to maintain the marvelous machine that is the human body.

The emphasis in our family was on the physical care of the body until that day when I was born again. Then I recognized that each of us is a trinity—body, soul (mind), and spirit—and that each of these aspects of our being requires nourishment. Our faith is centered in Jesus Christ, and we use the Bible as our handbook for living. Now we know both spiritual and physical well-being. While this book does not address itself to our spiritual needs, we would be remiss if we neglected to convey our belief that a whole person is one who is alive spiritually as well as physically and emotionally.

We have written this book with a continual prayer in our hearts that you will be motivated to take charge of your health and the health of family members and those dear to you. Regardless of your age, now is the time to take charge.

JUDY LINDBERG McFARLAND
January 1982

Acknowledgments

Thanks must first go to my family: my husband, Don, my sons, Gary, Dan, and Doug, and my daughter, Laura. It was Don who motivated me to write this book, always patiently and understandingly pitching in whenever he was needed. From footnotes to household chores, his love was manifested throughout the project. Doug and Laura kept the house running, while their mother labored on for seemingly endless months. Laura and Gary typed and retyped, a monumental task requiring patience and endurance, especially toward the end. Dan deserves special thanks for organizing and researching Appendix B: Vitamins and Minerals. His positive spirit, keen mind, and desire for accuracy inspired us all. I'll always be grateful.

To Helen Koiman Hosier I extend many thanks for her work on the manuscript, her love for the project, and her belief in what we were trying to communicate.

Kathy Reigstad, production editor at Harper & Row, also deserves special thanks for her conscientious attention to the manuscript.

This whole project, from start to finish, was an answer to many prayers. We believe that an answer came in the person of Roy Carlisle, our editor at Harper & Row. He believed in the project, patiently pulled it all together, and worked day and night with us to make our deadlines. We all experienced a wonderful sense of unity in that endeavor.

Finally, I have to praise God for sustaining us throughout the writing and editing of the book. We experienced his guidance in many ways, especially in the fine people who helped along the way.

NOTICE

The material in this book is intended solely to report the experiences Gladys Lindberg has had over the past forty years in the field of nutrition and what she has learned in her work. There is no intention on her part to diagnose any medical condition or to prescribe medication or suggest treatment for any ailment or disease condition. Gladys Lindberg is not a physician and does not purport to act as one. It is recommended that any reader suffering from any medical condition consult his or her physician.

❧ 1. "Healthy People Don't Have That, So Let's Make You Healthy"

> Frequently I hear the wishful remark, "Maybe some day they'll find cures for degenerative diseases." Let us stop waiting for cures and practice prevention by applying to our own lives, *right now*, the wonderful discoveries of nutrition.
> —GAYELORD HAUSER

When people come to one of the Lindberg Nutrition stores for a consultation with my mother, Gladys Lindberg, it is often because they have some specific health problem. "They are looking for health," she explains. Although she reminds such visitors that she is not a doctor, she patiently listens to their complaints and symptoms. "I cannot treat disease," she responds, "but healthy people don't have that. So let's make you healthy."

As she listens to those desperately searching for health, she often shares her own experiences. She too had to search for that which would contribute to and help maintain good health, and she understands how difficult it can be.

When people first meet the energetic and attractive Gladys Lindberg, dressed in pink in keeping with her motto, "Keep in the Pink," they probably think she knows an easier life than their own. No doubt there are even some who suspect that she doesn't know what it is to struggle, what it's like to worry about where the next meal is coming from.

On the contrary! Her name is over the door today only because of struggle, hard work, and sacrifice. Before World War II, when my father's salary was minimal, Mother started taking in laundry. She kept that up for over ten years, working herself to exhaustion, some weeks doing washing and ironing for fifteen to twenty families so there could be food on the table. I never heard her complain, but I can tell she hasn't forgotten those days. Because of her own ill health and her family's early battles with disease, her compassion and understanding are genuine. She understands what it is to live on this side of disease.

The Twilight Zone of Health

What do I mean when I speak of "living on this side of disease"? An overwhelming number of people simply don't feel well. Although they do not have an obvious illness, these people live in the twilight zone of health—what Mother calls "this side of disease." Their ill health has not become a real problem yet; they intend to get to the bottom of it—eventually—before it does. Others, less health-conscious, or unwilling to admit that their life-style needs changing, will endure the unpredictable pattern of feeling fairly good one day and not so good the next until serious, life-threatening disease does result. These people need help. They could, in fact, help themselves.

Perhaps you are such an individual. Even if you are not now in this twilight state of health, the day may come when you will be, for none of us is immune from the stresses of life and those factors that contribute to the breakdown of health.

"Healthy people don't have that." But just what is it that healthy people don't have? Anything from major degenerative diseases—cancer, heart trouble, crippling arthritis, mental illness, diabetes—to minor health problems that mar one's enjoyment of life. Individuals with these problems know that their prospect of a long life is diminished unless their illness is arrested and their health is restored. If statistics can be relied on, degenerative diseases are responsible for more than 70 percent of all deaths in this country. Drugs will not conquer such diseases; only a life-style change can prevent or correct them.

People who are healthy feel well in body and mind. Free from aches and pains, they have robust energy, a spring to their step, bright eyes, good color, and a pleasant outlook on life. That is not to say healthy people don't have their share of situations that try their patience and temper. But when circumstances *are* difficult, healthy people are much more likely to cope in a calm, capable manner. They are usually fit in body, soul, and spirit.

What Is Optimum Health?

People are often confused about what constitutes good health. The confusion stems, in part, from our individuality. We all get old, but we get there by different routes: we may develop various diseases through different means, because no two individuals have any two cells alike. Nonetheless, there are a number of general indicators of good health.

If you get up in the morning feeling great—happy; full of pep, and hungry, your nose and head clear—you are probably in good health.

Tongue color is another significant health indicator, since it sometimes reveals what is happening within your digestive tract. It used to be that the first thing doctors would say when you consulted them was, "Stick out your tongue." If it was nice and pink, chances were that you were in good health.

Your health is reflected in the way you look. Smooth skin, free from blemishes; good color; a shiny, full head of hair; straight teeth, free from decay; good posture; firm muscle tone—all these are "symptoms" of good health.

When your digestion is good, the utilization and elimination of food are so natural that you don't stop to worry about digestion or elimination. Everything is functioning properly and you feel good.

Your outlook on life and your disposition are also directly related to the proper functioning of your entire system. Because you are healthy and energetic, you are able to resist infections and withstand the stresses of life. You age with grace and charm, your faculties remain alert, and you stay active. You look forward to the adventures of each new day.

But you must understand that good, abundant health is not simply the absence of disease. The body is always trying to make you well; it is constantly in the process of making trillions of cells. These cells have to reach into your blood stream for as many as forty chemicals: amino acids (the building blocks of protein), fatty acids, minerals, trace elements, vitamins, and enzymes. These chemicals have to come from the food we eat, the water we drink, and the air we breathe. When our food is hydrogenated, homogenized, refined, preserved, emulsified, pasteurized, chemicalized, colored, bleached, and sterilized, something is lost. As a result, we have health problems.

Dr. Roger Williams, a noted biochemical researcher, says that if our body cells are ailing, as they must certainly be in disease, then chances are excellent it is because they are being inadequately provisioned.[1] The nutritional value of the foods you consume is perhaps the major factor in your state of health. You can do all the wrong things nutritionally for twenty or thirty years with little obvious ill effect, but you will eventually have problems. And not everyone can get away with it for that long.

People often fail to recognize the relationship of poor nutrition to poor health. They have symptoms—fatigue and a variety of aches and pains—that indicate their health is below par. But instead of learning what they can do to reverse the situation, they run to the doctor with a list of complaints. The physician often writes out a prescription, but, if poor nutrition is the root of the problem, the drug may mask the symptoms without eliminating the problem.

In fact, as Dr. Williams and Dr. Dwight Kalita explain, drugs can "contaminate the internal environment, create dependence on the part of the patient, and often complicate the physician's job by erasing valuable clues as to the real source of the trouble."[2] Williams and Kalita provide a helpful analogy: "Like the ecology of our natural environment, man's inner physiological ecology can be easily upset by 'alien chemical' [i.e., drug] interference of natural processes. We have had to learn a painful lesson about introducing, for example, DDT and other contaminating chemicals into our natural environment. Similarly, there is concern among 'medical ecologists' that alien chemicals [that is, chemicals not normally occurring in the human body] introduced into man's biochemical-physiological environment can also contaminate and do damage to important processes within the body."[3]

Because so many people fail to understand this delicate "ecological balance" within their bodies, they fail also to understand the role of nutrition. They unknowingly deprive themselves of optimum health. Their minor abnormalities, left uncorrected, frequently lead to more serious disease. Recognizing subtle deviations from good health and taking steps to correct them early is preventative medicine at its best; this is *taking charge of your health*. We ourselves often hold the key to the prevention of serious illness.

Perhaps an illustration will help. Back in the early 1940s, a young boy and his mother came to our home. He had been seeing his physician on a regular basis for a variety of problems but was not responding well. Today that young boy, Richard Ryder, is a practicing physician in Long Beach, California. He describes what happened on that first visit with Mother, and what happened in succeeding years:

I remember spending an evening in the Lindberg home discussing with Gladys and my mother what an adequate nutritional program was, and foods that we had to eat, and the dietary supplements that could be helpful in the restoration of good health. The foods were not some obscure foods that were not readily available, but everyday foods that were available in the grocery store. She also had some dietary supplements and vitamins, such as yeast, blackstrap molasses, and wheat germ, which she carried in her home as a convenience for people like us. I went on what has now become a very famous Lindberg nutritional program. Within a matter of weeks, I was feeling much better. I was no longer seeing my physician on a regular basis, and I was restored to complete health. . . .

This was a very wonderful and truly miraculous experience for a fifteen-year-old boy. It changed the entire course of my life. . . . All through high school I began to direct my career towards the field of either biochemistry or into the field of medicine, which I eventually fell into. I can remember during the years coming home from high school, many many times passing the Lindberg home, and there were always plenty of cars parked out in front. Mrs. Lindberg was talking to people about nutrition and her nutritional approach to health. . . . I don't think she ever hung out a sign, or ever ran an ad in the newspaper. It was strictly one person saying to another something like, "I think Gladys Lindberg has an answer and I think you should go listen to her. I think it will help you in your day-to-day living and make you a much healthier person." . . .

Over the years in talking with her, and during my years in medical school and college, I used to share with her some of my textbooks; and even though she didn't have any advanced degrees or post-graduate work, she was able to read that very complicated material and translate it into simple lay terms so that the ordinary person could understand it. This is really a gift, something very few people have. . . .

I am sure there are members of the scientific community who would criticize the Gladys Lindberg "shotgun" approach to human nutrition. It has never been studied in any great university center. Gladys Lindberg has never ever promised to cure anybody of anything. All she has ever done was show or teach them how to eat properly and how to supplement their diet in order that the human organism could thrive in its present environment. The fact that she has been successful, the fact that many people have obtained results from her dietary methods, is proof enough.[4]

All of us (including those in the medical profession) would like to believe that there is a single "magic" cure—some one vitamin, mineral, or "X" factor—for every condition or disease. For example, if a doctor diagnoses anemia, he or she will probably recommend iron tablets—"magic bullets." However, a person may become anemic not only from an iron deficiency, but from simultaneous deficiencies of vitamins B-1, B-2, B-12, niacin, folic acid, copper, protein, and other nutrients.[5] Thus we believe in the "shotgun" approach—taking *all* the known minerals and vitamins as well as the unknown factors in foods such as brewer's yeast, alfalfa, acidophilus, and so on—to be sure you are on the road to good health.

NOTES

1. Roger J. Williams and Dwight K. Kalita, *A Physician's Handbook on Orthomolecular Medicine* (New York: Pergamon Press, 1977), p. 2.
2. Ibid., p. 1.
3. Ibid.
4. Personal communication from Richard C. Ryder, M.D., F.A.A.F.P., to Judy Lindberg McFarland, 31 December 1980.
5. Adelle Davis, *Let's Get Well* (New York: Harcourt, Brace, & World, 1965), pp. 280–285.

2. The Wheat Germ Lady

> It seems weird that devastating, even fatal, illness can be produced by the absence of something. Microbes are murderers, visible assassins. How can the absence of anything be murderous? It's mentally tougher to deal with negatives than with positives, to think of sickness as caused by what is *not* there than by what *is* there.
>
> —PAUL DE KRUIF

The study of nutrition is a relatively new science. Only in the last century have we recognized the major role good nutrition plays in overall health and sought to understand it.

Just as the science as a whole has evolved, so too have individual nutritionists. The development of my mother's theories about nutrition are an interesting example of such evolution. Mother's interest in nutrition became a passion when she had three children of her own to care for. It seems we kids were always coming down with something. Every month Mother took us to the "well baby clinic" of a Los Angeles hospital, where she was given a diet sheet recommending such foods as cream of wheat, pasteurized milk, and white bread with margarine. She faithfully followed the outline, but still we were never healthy.

Finally she appealed to the doctor: "Can't you help me? Look at these pale, skinny, sniffly children. Can't you see what is happening? They're just never well. They always have fevers, colds, croup, or upset stomachs. They catch every sickness that comes along. Can't we do *something* to *prevent* this?"

The doctor impatiently replied, "Go on home, Mrs. Lindberg. You're just looking for trouble."

Mother was so shocked at the doctor's response—"to think I was 'looking for trouble' because I wanted to *prevent* the children from being sick!"—that she never took us to the clinic again.

What happened next was to change drastically the course of all our lives. My sister had a very high fever one night. It seemed there was nothing Mother could do to help Janice, who had these fevers frequently. That night, while Janice's body fought the fever, Mother did a lot of praying. She prayed specifically for knowledge on how to keep this child well.

In the morning, Janice's body was cool, and Mother knew her prayers had been answered. "I came to the realization that everything I'd been doing for my family all those years was wrong. Almost everything we ate had been tampered with in some way." She had realized the hard way that good nutrition is essential to good health.

After it became clear to Mother that everything she had been doing for her family was wrong, she wasted no time in getting to work. World War II was raging, and citizens were being urged to plant "victory gardens," but it was more than patriotic fervor that sent Mother into our backyard. She knew from her past and from the way her ancestors lived that garden-grown foods and raw milk were necessary. Resolute, she dug up the backyard with a zeal that would have made her ancestors proud. Soon her composted garden had produced so much beautiful chard, greens, and vegetables of all kinds that she was able to supply food for the neighbors as well as her family.

Next, she convinced my father to drive her out to a dairy farm to purchase raw milk, cream, and fertile eggs. She began to churn her own butter. She discovered the virtues of wheat germ, soy flour, and other supplements and introduced them to us gradually. At the end of that first season, she felt an immense sense of satisfaction. She had taken the first step toward preventing future illness from overtaking us again.

Father supported her efforts to educate us kids and change our eating habits, and slowly his habits changed also. Through the years, Mother has encountered many women who complain, "If only I could get my husband to understand what I'm trying to do." She tells them, "Never stop trying. Just make sure it tastes good."

Mother's reading convinced her that she should provide those vitamins that had been discovered by then (some of them not well known or generally accepted), minerals, and cod liver oil for her family. The B-vitamins were making the news those days; she immediately put this information into practice.

Although health food stores were still a novelty, she found one in Los Angeles and became a regular patron. When she learned that many vitamins and trace elements were to be found in brewer's yeast, she purchased a bag. Dismayed to discover that the mixture had a bitter taste—one she knew we kids would never tolerate—she put it on the top shelf of her cupboard.

Then she came down with a bad bout of flu herself and was

forced to remain in bed for several days. The dishes stacked up in the sink; housework went undone. Remembering the brewer's yeast, she decided to give it a try. She took it with milk and miraculously felt the strength come back first into her hands and then into the rest of her body. "Yeast always tasted good after that!" she remembers.

Discovering a New Vitamin

Mother began to read the accounts of pioneering nutritionists. Sir Robert McCarrison's book, *Studies in Deficiency Disease,* was a gold mine of information. He described, among other things, the seven years he spent in the Himalayas among the Hunzas, a race of people "unsurpassed in perfection of physique and in freedom from disease in general, whose sole food consists of grains, vegetables, and fruits, with a certain amount of milk and butter." He concluded that "the enforced restriction to the unsophisticated foodstuffs of nature is compatible with long life, continued vigour, and perfect physique."

McCarrison, a noted English physician and dedicated researcher in the early 1920s, believed a deficient and ill-balanced diet to be the major contributing factor in disease. Whether the person he treated lived in the lap of luxury or in poverty made little difference, he observed. "Some there are, living in luxury, whom ignorance or fancy debars from choosing their food aright; others for whom poverty combines with ignorance to place an impassable barrier in the way of discriminating choice. . . . With increasing knowledge of nutritional problems, it has become apparent that our dietetic habits need remodelling, and that education of the people as to what to eat and why they eat it is urgently necessary."[1]

She read, too, of the amazing work of Dr. Joseph Goldberger of the United States Public Health Service, who tackled the pellagra epidemic in poverty-stricken areas of the deep South in the spring of 1913. Pellagra, characterized by diarrhea, dermatitis (skin eruptions), and dementia (insanity), was considered an infectious disease, but to Goldberger it seemed significant that the patients had no vegetable gardens, nor did they eat chicken, eggs, or meat. Their diet consisted largely of fat pork, cornbread, corn syrup, dried beans and peas, sweet potatoes, and yams.

Goldberger further observed that in hospitals where the nurses and doctors ate superior food, they did not contract the disease. He arranged for meat, milk, eggs, yeast, and liver, along

with fresh fruits and vegetables, to be fed to children in an orphanage where pellagra ran rampant. To the intense astonish-
ment of the orphanage's director, the epidemic abated. It seemed
that Goldberger had proof that pellagra was a disease caused by
diet deficiencies.

Yet a scientific commission that investigated Goldberger's
findings concluded that, on the contrary, there was *no* connection
between nutrition and pellagra. They reaffirmed the theory that
pellagra was an infectious disease and claimed that it could be
traced to the sting of a certain fly. Goldberger was horrified. To
prove his theory, he made a number of tests on himself, while
other physicians controlled the experiment.

Into his own body he injected mucous from the nasal passages
of the sick, and scales from their diseased skin. If pellagra were
really an infectious disease, then surely he would succumb. He
did not! So encouraged by his fearless example were his col-
laborators that they repeated his tests. The results were negative, in every instance, and the old infection theory was swept
aside. A momentous step had been taken.

The problem was far from solved, however. Goldberger was
convinced it was the absence of something that was causing the
problem, but the absence of what? He discovered that yeast and
liver extracts brought about a cure, but, at the time of his death
in 1929, he had not succeeded in isolating the mysterious substance in these foods that prevented the disease and hastened
the cure.

Mother also read of young Dr. Tom Spies, a crusader against
human misery in a campaign that would, in time, benefit millions. I heard so much about this great man of medicine as I was
growing up that I almost felt he was a family friend.

Tom Spies was just out of Harvard Medical School when he
was confronted by his first desperately sick pellagra victim. He
gave the patient Dr. Goldberger's diet, but the patient died.
Spies was frustrated but intrigued.

He needed pellagrins on whom he could experiment, so he devised an unorthodox method of herding pellagrous drunks into a
hospital for testing: he bribed them with the promise of liquor. If
they would just eat what he gave them, they could have all the
liquor they wanted.

He threw the nutrition book at his research subjects. He
coaxed and bribed them into eating enormous meals of beef,

eggs, milk, yeast, wheat germ, and liver. After weeks of his superfeedings, the flaming redness faded from their faces, the rawness vanished from their tongues, and clearheadedness replaced their mental symptoms. By the end of 1934, Spies had treated 125 severely diseased pellagrins and had cut the death rate from 54 percent to 6 percent. He was sent to Hillman Hospital in Birmingham, Alabama, to see if he could duplicate his results. In the spring and summer of 1936, Spies tested his intensive feedings on 50 pellagrins, all of whom were very sick, most at the point of death. Only three of them died. And even in those three, postmortems revealed no evidence of pellagra; their pellagra had been cured, but they had succumbed to other diseases.

Tom spent months in private rooms feeding his patients around the clock, and actually saw these dying patients come back to life through a slow resurrection. Spies's approach was obviously successful, but impractical and costly. There had to be a faster and less expensive treatment. He heard of a substance called nicotinic acid amide (extracted from liver) that had been used on a dog dying from a dietary deficiency disease called black tongue. The morning after he had been given the substance, the dog was jumping about in his cage. Spies wondered, was black tongue the canine replica of human pellagra? When a family had pellagra, so did the dog, because the dog ate the scraps from the table! Might nicotinic acid amide provide the cure for pellagra in humans?

Nicotinic acid is the chemical child of nicotine, a potent human poison. Would it be deadly to humans? Pharmacologists were not sure; there was only one thing to do: Spies would make nicotinic acid in the lab and try it on himself. First a few milligrams orally, then up to a thousand milligrams a day—it did nothing more than flush his face and make his arms and legs itch and tingle. He concluded that it was safe to use on humans. (Later nicotinic acid was renamed niacin (B-3) to avoid confusing it with the deadly nicotine.)

Tom Spies groped and tested his way. Like Louis Pasteur and Robert Koch sixty years before, Spies had to adjust his thinking—it wasn't the presence of microbes that drove pellagra victims crazy or killed them; it was the absence, over a period of years, of a fraction of a millionth of an ounce of niacin from the cells of their brains that finally made them ill and crazy (the dementia of pellagra). It was chemical insanity!

Lean meat is one of the richest sources of niacin, but the beef from a trainload of cattle yields hardly more than a spoonful of the natural crystals of this vitamin.[2] Spies knew poor people couldn't afford that type of food, so he administered the synthesized vitamin, produced in the laboratory at low cost. Patients who had been raging mad, severely psychotic, or deeply depressed became clear-headed within a few days. Their other symptoms also vanished. In the cheap crystals of this comparatively simple chemical lay the difference between life and death, between mental clarity and utter insanity. These human beings were chemically imperfect or broken down, and he was out to fix them.[3]

After years of additional research, Spies realized that niacin alone was no panacea; the idea of a single vitamin deficiency had been too simple. Pellagra seemed now to be a spectrum of diseases caused by a variety of chemical deficiencies. He asked himself, does our lack of vitamins and other essential chemicals lower our resistance to microbic disease? Does it cause enfeeblement and even signs of premature old age in children? Does chemical starvation explain not only nervous and mental diseases in grownups, but also the great degenerative sicknesses of the blood vessels that strike at the heart, kidneys, and brains of millions of us in our prime?[4]

Spies's research into chemical deficiencies continued. When organic chemists crystallized a complex of new vitamins, the B-complex, in the late 1930s, Spies began trying them on people who had vague, chronic complaints, people who didn't have pellagra—yet.

The following account is an example of how Spies used the new B-complex chemicals to fit the deficiency:

A 50-year-old white man ... came to Tom at Hillman Hospital. For months he'd lost weight. He didn't want to eat. He complained of indigestion—cramps and diarrhea alternating with constipation. His tongue and mouth burned. He couldn't sleep. He could hardly remember. He had cramps in the soles of his feet and muscles of his legs. His gait was bad and he could walk just a few steps at a time. For years he had noticed that this general breakdown waxed in the spring and waned towards winter. Now at last ... he had come to Tom with all these miseries plus the first actual sore-tongue sign of early pellagra.

In the hospital Tom for some days held this man on the terribly deficient diet on which he had lived for years. Then nicotinic acid [was given] and away went the signs of pellagra, yet the man remained miserable. Then injections of thiamine (B-1), and his neuritis got better. Then the yellow vitamin, riboflavin (B-2), and the little sore cracks disappeared from the corners of his mouth and he felt much stronger. Then huge doses of ascorbic acid, vitamin C—and the signs of scurvy disappeared from his gums. He couldn't see well in the dark; and this defect was conquered by vitamin A. His gait and his walking still bothered him. Vitamin B-6, pyridoxin, and in a few days he could walk two miles. He was still anemic. For this there was as yet no pure chemical bullet—but his blood grew thicker after injections of extract of crude liver....[5]

Mother was fascinated by the research of Tom Spies and by his ability to give new life to victims of a hidden hunger. His combination of B-complex vitamins and good foods—meat, eggs, fruits, vegetables, yeast, and liver—seemed to work. Tom Spies knew it was the combination that was all important. As Mother says, it is the known in the vitamins and the known and the unknown in the yeast and liver and nutritious foods that make the difference and get results.

Pioneer in Applied Nutrition

Mother herself now began to experiment. She was determined to make a nutritious regimen palatable, even tasty. The more she experimented, the more palatable her concoctions became. She would add bananas, concentrated orange juice, and an apple or other seasonal fruit to the milk. Then in would go the brewer's yeast and raw liver powder. Even we children became convinced that Mother was doing the right things for us. And why not? We changed from sickly kids to energetic youngsters. Teachers at Normandie Avenue Elementary School were the first to comment about the change. At a neighbor's urging, Mother became involved with the PTA. As a result, teachers started sending mothers to our house to learn what they could about nutrition and keeping their children healthy. They came again and again —bringing friends with them. Mother, full of missionary zeal, was overjoyed. Today she smilingly recalls, "That's what started the whole thing. It was just one person telling another."

When Mother was asked to become nutrition chairman for the PTA, she gladly accepted the responsibility as another way in which she could help other mothers with their children's health. She was even able to convince the Board of Education to allow a mid-morning nutrition break each day, since the time span from eight o'clock until lunch time was too long for children. "I would like to make a wheat germ candy and offer it with a glass of milk to the children," she suggested. From that time on, for twenty-five cents each week, children could participate in the program.

Because Mother did not drive, she convinced my father that she could handle the program with a homemade wheelbarrow. My brother Bob painted the wheelbarrow white, and on Monday mornings, Mother could be seen walking down the busy streets near the school, picking up the supplies. She ordered fresh wheat germ in hundred-pound sacks and each week took twenty-five pounds to school, along with blackstrap molasses, peanut butter, and raisins. She made hundreds upon hundreds of pieces of the nutritious treat each Monday morning—enough to last a week—and the school children affectionately called her the "Wheat Germ Lady." Teachers begged Mother for the recipe so they could send it home with the children. And to this day, some of those children, now grown and with children of their own, call Mother to ask for the recipe.

Perhaps one of the most significant events in my mother's early years of searching occurred when she heard Adelle Davis lecture at a department store in downtown Los Angeles. Adelle was giving a series of lectures while promoting her book, *Vitality Through Planned Nutrition.*

After the lecture, Mother introduced herself and enthusiastically shared with Adelle her own experiences, subsequent findings, and the results in her children's lives. She ended with, "I've been doing all the things you're talking about with my family."

Thus began a lifelong friendship with Adelle. She and Mother got together frequently for discussions on what was new in the field of health. They were both pioneers in applied nutrition and learned much from each other. Their commitment to raising people's consciousness about nutrition and good health became even more intense for Mother after Adelle's death of bone cancer. Adelle herself had attributed her cancer to the bad habit of heavy smoking (though she had quit two years before her death), her diet, her heavy work schedule, and an overexposure to X rays required for insurance reasons. During her illness, I visited her frequently, and she, knowing of my relationship with God, asked many penetrating questions. At last, she asked to be taken to a special religious service, and that day I saw this great lady surrender her life to Jesus Christ.

Adelle was quite controversial, but—criticism notwithstanding—more people around the world have been turned on to nutrition by reading Adelle's books than any other writings on the subject. Mutual affection and admiration characterized our family's relationship with Adelle.

Mother was an avid reader of scientific journals, and she attended scientific lectures and conventions on all aspects of nutrition. Incorporating such research into her own experience, she developed a successful program for our family, relatives, neighbors, friends, and others. Word of her accomplishments spread throughout the Los Angeles area.

She was constantly being asked for the vitamins and minerals that she was giving to us; she bought them a thousand at a time. She continued to hold classes around the dining room table as friends stopped in for advice and vitamins. People counted out their own vitamins and put them in white envelopes and paid mother exactly what it had cost her. She wasn't making any money, but she had the satisfaction of seeing people's health improve from week to week.

One blind woman couldn't distinguish the different vitamin and mineral tablets, so mother spread out a hundred small squares of wax paper on the table, added the daily supply of minerals and vitamins, and twisted them into packets. Only after trying many variations of doing this by hand did we finally have a machine to accomplish the task. As fast as she replenished her stock of vitamins, they ran out. My father said, half-jokingly, "Gladys, this has become a business. You're going to end up in jail if we don't get this out of the house."

Finally, several years later, my father, with his unique business ability, perseverance, and hard work, took the initiative and found the location for their first store. It was his idea that it be called the Lindberg Nutrition Service. "Our services will be Gladys giving her time to help people become nutrition-wise, and it will be free advice," he stated.

We were the first tenants in a new building in southwest Los Angeles, unaware that this modest beginning was the forerunner of a chain of such stores in southern California. The business grew so quickly that my father left his management position in a steel company.

Mother likes to tell people who consult her in the stores that if they commit themselves to a well-balanced diet, supplemented by vitamins, minerals, and other supplemental foods, they will be providing for themselves and their families a form of health insurance that cannot be equaled. I have often heard her say,

"Our best life insurance is our investment in health. It is the most valuable insurance we can buy. Because when we lose our health, all the money in the world can't return us to an active life."

NOTES

1. Sir Robert McCarrison, *Studies in Deficiency Disease* (London: Henry Frowde and Hodder & Stoughton; reproduced by photo-lithography, 1945, Lee Foundation for Nutritional Research, Milwaukee, Wisconsin), pp. 8, 9.
2. Paul de Kruif, *Life Among the Doctors* (New York: Harcourt, Brace and Company, 1949), p. 75.
3. Ibid., p. 52.
4. Ibid., p. 90.
5. Ibid., p. 77.

3. What Did Our Ancestors Do Right That We Are Doing Wrong?

> If primitive races have been more efficient than modernized groups in the matter of preventing degenerative processes, physical, mental, and moral, it is only because they have been more efficient in complying with Nature's laws.
>
> —DR. WESTON A. PRICE

Mother's South Dakota ancestors lived to be ninety-five years old; they had twelve healthy children, almost all of whom lived into their nineties; and they went to their graves with perfect teeth. What did they do right that we are doing wrong?

With all of our hospitals, research laboratories, universities, and drugs, you'd think we would have conquered most disease by now. It is true that the germ and viral diseases that claimed the lives of so many of our ancestors—diseases such as tuberculosis, smallpox, plagues, and diphtheria—have almost been conquered, thanks in large part to the discovery of antibiotics, and modern refrigeration and sanitation.

But the diseases rampant today are what are known as *degenerative diseases,* diseases hardly known before the Industrial Revolution brought masses of people from farms into the cities. *Degeneration,* according to the *American Medical Dictionary,* is "deterioration; change from a higher to a lower form; especially change of tissue to a lower or less functionally active form. When there is chemical change of the tissue itself, it is *true degeneration.*"[1]

It is generally recognized that degenerative diseases are not caused by viruses, bacteria, or parasites. The real killer is malnutrition—more commonly referred to as diabetes, cancer, arthritis, emphysema, arteriosclerosis (hardening of arteries) and atherosclerosis (fatty deposits in arteries), and other degenerative maladies. These are diseases usually caused by the absence of some substance (vitamin, mineral, or trace element), as Drs. Goldberger, Spies, and many others have found. In the meantime, there is a growing awareness on the part of the public that we need to get back to what God has provided: the wisdom, the knowledge, and the substance to maintain healthy bodies.

There is much confusion about what constitutes an adequate diet, a diet that promotes total health and a feeling of well-being, strength, and vitality. One nutritionist says one thing, another contradicts those statements. One book reports certain findings, another book, magazine article, or health column refutes those claims. While nutritional controversy rages among the "experts" —those who should be paving the way for a better understanding of that which contributes to health and longevity—the public is left to decide what they will believe and whose advice they will follow.

Dr. Richard Kunin, a medical doctor who spent years in a conventional practice before exploring nutrition, describes as "micro-malnutrition" the phenomenon of poor eating habits that masquerade as a well-balanced diet. He berates the myth that good nutrition is a fact of life in America or is at least within the grasp of anyone on a "normal American diet." Nothing could be further from the truth. Most so-called balanced diets are woefully *out* of balance, because of the nutrient depletion that begins with modern cultivation and continues through the transportation, storage, processing, and cooking of foods.

"A balanced diet is a practical impossibility in the society in which we live," argues Kunin, "even though it's an ideal at which to aim."[2] He projects a subclinical "walking" malnutrition for millions of Americans, a way of life that will eventually result in overt illness and a shortening of life unless they heed the warning and take steps to improve their diet and take vitamin and mineral supplements.

We pay a high price for our poor eating habits. Dr. Tom Spies claims that *all* disease, of whatever origin, ultimately involves nutrition. Fifty percent of the American diet is composed of nonessential foods (soft drinks, pastries, potato chips, and so on), according to Dr. George Briggs, professor of nutrition at the University of California at Berkeley, who warns that when our diet is diluted by even 25 percent nonessential foods, we can expect health problems. People who ignore the threat of micro-malnutrition are "likely to suffer the consequences of disease unless they remedy their eating habits," he warns.[3]

Many choose to ignore all advice, preferring to eat and do as they please. These are the people who, for the most part, are digging early graves with their fork, knife, and spoon; they are the most likely candidates for chronic degenerative diseases.

Others believe that good health is our birthright and should not be squandered. They note the correspondence between the decline in American eating habits in the last century and the increased incidence of degenerative diseases, and they take heed. They look to history for a lesson in health.

Down on the Farm

Our ancestors knew long days of arduous physical labor. They consumed and burned thousands of calories a day, often eating five meals a day. The quality and quantity of the foods they ate provided them with all the vitamins and minerals they needed. The sedentary life-style so common today was unknown to most of them. And they were healthy.

Some of my ancestors worked the fertile farmlands of South Dakota. What vegetables they did not grow themselves they were able to purchase from local farmers; in either case, the vegetables were fresh. Their produce, unlike ours, was not picked green and then stored or transported across the country, losing valuable vitamins in the process. And although they probably did not use the term *organic gardening,* the manure that had accumulated in the barns and barnyards during the long winter months provided fertilizer that produced crops and vegetables superior in every way.

My grandparents and their parents canned their own fruits and vegetables in glass jars. Rarely did they have white sugar for canning or use at the table; it was simply too costly. This was a blessing in disguise. Their low intake of sugar in all likelihood spared them many of the degenerative diseases we suffer today and contributed to their longevity. They did have beehives and enjoyed honey that was unprocessed, uncooked, and unfiltered. And they sun-dried naturally sweet fruits for later use.

They did their own baking, using stone-ground wheat rich in the all-important B vitamins, vitamin E, and valuable trace minerals. (Vitamins and minerals are concentrated in the bran and germ portions of cereal grains.) Cornmeal, too, was home-grown and ground fresh.

Farm families consumed dozens of eggs weekly. Old-time doctors knew that eggs helped prevent and treat both tuberculosis and rheumatic fever, among other things, and that when people were sick, soft-boiled eggs or an eggnog were good medicine. The eggs they ate were fertile—that is, had they not been eaten, they could have hatched—so they contained RNA and DNA, which nourish our living cells. Eggs, a near-perfect food rich in B vitamins, vitamins A and D, protein, and minerals (especially phosphorus), have received a lot of bad press lately. Millions of Americans have been scared into thinking that by eating eggs they are contributing to their risk of heart disease. Ironically, the cholesterol scare has deprived them of lecithin, abundant in eggs—the very substance they need to keep cholesterol moving through their blood. Humans have been eating eggs for thousands of years, and heart attacks were rarely diagnosed or found in autopsies until early in the present century. Strange, isn't it, that it took researchers living in this era to tell us that eggs should be eliminated from our diets as a public enemy!

Our ancestors used roots and herbs in abundance. Garlic and onions, particularly, were staples. Germs do not like garlic; in fact, they cannot live in its presence. Ancient civilizations relied heavily on this bulb as a medication for indigestion, diarrhea, worms, skin diseases, dizziness, headaches, bronchitis, pneumonia, influenza, tuberculosis, infections and wounds, heart problems, arthritis, aging, and even cancer. In recent years, people have rediscovered the medicinal merits of garlic in warding off colds and in the treatment of high blood pressure, strokes, and cardiovascular disease. Interestingly, countries where garlic is consumed in large quantities—Italy and Spain, for example—have a lower death rate from heart disease than America does.[4]

My grandparents lived on reservation land in South Dakota that had been opened up to white settlers who wished to homestead. The old Indian squaws taught my grandmother how to make many Indian remedies, including a spring tonic using bark, roots, and herbs. It was a black and bitter substance, but it gave them a pickup after the hard South Dakota winters.

Milk was important to our forebears, not only for itself but for what it could be made into. Theirs was raw milk, produced by cows raised on green feed, and superior nutritionally in almost every way to our pasteurized milk.[5] Both clabbered milk (similar to yogurt) and cottage cheese were often homemade. Cottage cheese contains just the proteins of milk, not the minerals, which "escape" into the whey. Our ancesters saved the whey and it was used in cooking and breadmaking or given to the hogs and chickens. It is a very rich source of natural minerals, especially calcium.

The farm families ate a lot of meat and poultry. Their livestock roamed the fields and ranges and ate green grass. As a result, the meat had a low fat content. But it was also tough. So today we confine our animals to feedlots, fill them full of hormones to fatten them and antibiotics to keep them from spreading diseases, and then pass on those chemicals in one form or another to our dinner table. Although there have been some successful attempts to return to the natural way of raising animals, it is still not a widespread practice, because of the time, effort, and cost involved.

The water my forebears drank was spring or well water, fresh-tasting, cold, and very hard. It was pure, uncontaminated by industrial wastes and agricultural chemicals. Around the turn of the century our water supplies began to be treated with chlorine. Even in the minute quantities needed to kill germs, chlorine undermines the body's defenses against heart disease. Regrettably, most of us in cities and suburban towns have little choice; we are *dependent* on a chlorinated municipal water supply. Chlorine not only smells and tastes bad; research indicates that it is bad for us.[6]

Isolated peoples throughout the world who have continued to live as our ancestors did bear witness to the correlation between diet and disease. In the 1930s Dr. Weston Price observed primitive racial stocks in northern Italy, the Swiss Alps, the New Hebrides, the islands of the South Pacific, eastern and central Africa, Australia, New Zealand, South America, Alaska, the north of Canada, and other remote regions of the world. There he discovered a high immunity to many of mankind's serious illnesses. Dr. Price concluded that diet made the difference:

The writer is fully aware that his message is not orthodox; but since our orthodox theories have not saved us we may have to readjust them to bring them into harmony with Nature's laws. Nature must be obeyed, not orthodoxy. Apparently many primitive races have understood her language better than have our modernized groups. Even the primitive races share our blights when they adopt our conception of nutrition. . . . No era in the long journey of mankind reveals in the skeletal remains such a terrible degeneration of teeth and bones as this brief modern period records. Must Nature reject our vaunted culture and call back the more obedient primitives? The alternative seems to be a complete readjustment in accordance with the controlling forces of Nature.[7]

So long as these "primitives" lived in accordance with the nutritional programs that were directed by the accumulated wisdom of the group, they were free from the degenerative diseases that afflict modern humanity. They were free, too, from tooth decay, although the toothbrush was unheard of among them. In every instance, however, where individuals of these same racial stocks lost their isolation and adopted the food habits of our modern civilization (such as white sugar and white flour), there was an early loss of the high-immunity characteristics of the original groups.

Mother and her family never used a toothbrush when she was growing up, but they didn't have tooth decay. In fact, she had her first cavity in young adulthood, after she moved to Los Angeles.

These illustrations are not intended to glorify the romance of the "good old days." There is much to learn from our ancestors and from studies of primitives, but most of us would not care to return to those days—the long hours of hard work, the lack of modern conveniences. Nor would many of us want to live in a primitive setting just because we wanted to be healthy. But we pay a high price for the conveniences of modern living—air pollution, water pollution, harmful chemical preservatives in our foods, and decreased food values from processing—some of which is the result of having moved off the farm into the city.

We must protect ourselves against the contaminants in the environment and in our food. We must begin to understand how best to provide the necessary nutrients for maintaining healthy bodies.

NOTES

1. W. A. Newman Dorland, *The American Illustrated Medical Dictionary, Twenty-Fifth Edition* (Philadelphia and London: W. B. Saunders Company, 1974).
2. Richard A. Kunin, M.D., *Mega-Nutrition* (New York: McGraw-Hill, 1980), pp. 7, 12.
3. Ibid., p. 23.
4. Paavo Airola, M.D., Ph.D., *Every Woman's Book* (Phoenix: Health Plus, Publishers, 1979), pp. 440–442.
5. The International College of Applied Nutrition, "Nutrition—Applied Personally," ed. Michael Walczak, M.D. (La Habra, Calif.: ICAN Publications, 1973), pp. 18–19.
6. Kunin, *Mega-Nutrition*, pp. 61–63.
7. Weston A. Price, M.D., *Nutrition and Physical Degeneration* (Los Angeles: The American Academy of Applied Nutrition, 1950), pp. 6, 7.

✃ 4. Understanding Stress

> How can a person know that he is experiencing undue stress
> before he suffers evident damage, with obvious diseases ...
> such as a nervous breakdown, peptic ulcers, or a heart at-
> tack? A certain amount of stress is needed to tune you up for
> action and keep you on your toes.... On the other hand, we
> must learn the limits of our endurance before we exceed
> them dangerously.
>
> —DR. HANS SELYE

Simply put, stress is the wear and tear on our bodies caused by
life. The dictionary defines it as "a physical, chemical, or emotional factor that causes bodily or mental tension and may be a
factor in disease causation."[1] There is considerable agreement, in
fact, that the stress of modern life is *the* greatest contributing
factor in today's killer diseases.

Each and every one of us is under some degree of stress from
the day we are born until the day we die. It need not be debilitating, however. The same stress that makes one person sick is an
invigorating experience for someone whose system is prepared
for it.

We tend to think of certain stereotypical situations as stressful: the high-powered executive facing a crucial decision, the surgeon and those assisting in a long surgical procedure, the lawyer
pleading a difficult case, the teacher trying to control unruly
students, the college student striving for good grades.

What we may fail to recognize is that stress wears many faces.
The mother agonizing over a child's misbehavior is under stress,
as is that same child, facing peer pressure and temptation. The
driver pulling onto the freeway is in a stressful situation. Husbands and wives caught in marital discord know only too well
the meaning of stress; and their children also are caught in the
vicious web of stress. Even our enjoyable pursuits—watching or
participating in a fast-paced ball game, playing bridge or chess,
taking part in a spirited conversation, or a passionate embrace—
place us under stress.

Here is a list of stressors you may never have considered: allergies, antibiotics, bright blinking lights, chemical preserva-

tives, chemotherapy, dietary deficiencies, excesses of sugar, drugs, hormones, alcohol, caffeine or nicotine, fasting, extremes of cold or heat, exercise, injections of toxic agents, insecticides, intense noise, pregnancy, and X-rays.

It is our adrenal glands, perched atop the kidneys, that come to our aid in times of stress. They manufacture cortical hormones, the substances that prepare us for "flight or fight." The body must be supplied with adequate protein, vitamins A and C, vitamin E, pantothenic acid, and the B-complex vitamins; we cannot make the vital secretions of hormones without these nutrients, vitamin C in particular. It is precisely at such times of stress that most people fail to eat properly. That is one of the reasons why we emphasize that we must fortify the body.

During acute periods of stress, adrenaline, the stress hormone, is pumped into the blood stream, setting off the alarm reaction that stimulates the central nervous system. Then the thalamus and the hypothalamus react on the pituitary, triggering production of a hormone called ACTH (adrenolcorticaltropic hormone) that stimulates the adrenal cortex to produce cortical hormones. These hormones set off catabolism, a destructive metabolic process in which there is tissue change and the body, as Mother puts it, cannibalizes itself.

These cortical hormones pull calcium and minerals out of the bones, sugar out of the liver, and protein out of the muscles. After the emergency situation is over, the thyroid and the male and female hormones put the calcium back in the bones, the protein back in the muscles, and sugar back into the liver. This process of rebuilding is called anabolism. But when the destructive and deteriorative processes of catabolism predominate over the body's anabolic processes, we become ill and/or we age. When the glands are adequately nourished, however, and a metabolic *balance* is maintained, we enjoy good health.

Actually, a whole series of physiological functions have to be rapidly coordinated: blood pressure has to rise, heart rate has to increase, the nervous system and the muscles have to be put on alert for action, and the body's mechanism for supplying energy has to be stepped up. Carbohydrate, protein, and fat metabolism have to be mobilized for energy and tissue repair.

A Medical Student's Introduction to Stress

Years ago, Mother first came across a newspaper article on stress in which Viennese-born Hans Selye, a young medical doctor, talked about how stress could lead to various diseases. His identification of the stress concept of illness was a new and revolutionary tenet that met with objections from and aroused disagreement within the scientific community. When his book, *The Story of the Adaptation Syndrome* (1952), was finally published, Mother found it fascinating. Later the book would be revised and expanded, and become a classic under the title *The Stress of Life*.[2] But as Mother read the original work, she saw not only how stress could be harmful, but how the stress that pervaded all of life could be handled positively.

Selye first began to investigate stress in 1925 when he was a student at the medical school in Prague. Students were shown patients in the early stages of various infectious diseases. As each patient came in, the professor would carefully question and examine him. Each patient felt and looked ill, had a coated tongue, and complained of diffused aches and pains in the joints and intestinal disturbance with loss of appetite. Most of the patients also had fever, and some showed mental confusion. Some had an enlarged spleen or liver, inflamed tonsils, skin rash, and other symptoms of illness. But it was evident to Selye that the professor attached very little significance to any of this.[3]

The professor was looking for secondary symptoms that would tell him whether the patient had measles, mumps, chicken pox, or some other disease. Until these characteristic signs of a specific disease appeared, not much could be done. Meanwhile, the many general features of illness that were already manifest were labeled "nonspecific" and considered "of no use" diagnostically to the physician.

Selye could understand that the professor had to find specific disease manifestations in order to identify a particular disease and prescribe a suitable drug for treatment. However, he also began to realize that there was a "general syndrome of just being sick," the condition of pre-sickness that he later came to call the "General Adaptation Syndrome."[4] In the years to come Selye would revolutionize medical thinking by proving that the body reacts to *every* variety of stress in the same way.

Selye experimented with rats, binding the animals to a board for twenty-four hours and depriving them of food. Though the rats were not injured in any way, an autopsy of their bodies revealed that even the mental stress of fear, worry, and anxiety caused the adrenal glands to swell to twice their normal size, change in color, and hemorrhage. We know that when hemorrhage occurs, it indicates a lack of vitamin C, and Selye was later able to show that this all-important vitamin is stored in the adrenals.

In addition, the thymus, the spleen, and the lymph nodes of the rats under stress had atrophied and were full of lipids—the proteins and carbohydrates and related compounds that constitute the principal structural component of all living cells. When Selye saw how these nodes had shriveled, he realized that the thymus was the gland that makes antibodies (white blood cells called leukocytes). He also realized that, had he given these animals another stressor—such as a draft—they would have developed pneumonia and died because they would have had no antibodies to fight the infection.

Selye reasoned that what had happened to these rats represented their bodies' nonspecific reaction to general damage, *regardless of what caused the damage.* And he reasoned that other types of acute stress should produce similar results. He subjected other animals to numerous types of nonchemical stress—excessive muscular exercise, cold, fasting, emotional excitement, and intense sound and light—and found that *all* these nonchemical types of stress produced the same unmistakable "alarm reaction" in the animals.

The "alarm reaction" is the first of three stages in what Selye called the "General Adaptation Syndrome." The other two stages he called the "stage of resistance" and the "stage of exhaustion."

THE ALARM REACTION   In his animal experiments, Selye found that the stomachs of his normal control rats did not change. In contrast, after a twenty-four hour period of stress, his alarmed rats, which had no food in their stomachs, developed acute gastric, bleeding ulcers. For when there is no food in the stomach, the digestive juices digest the protein lining of the stomach. This process begins because the adrenals, under stress, swell up and throw out cortical hormones. The production of cortisone, in turn, causes hydrochloric acid to pour into the stomach. When the body is adequately fed, tissues remain unharmed. Thus, Mother concluded, the individual who, instead of eating breakfast, downs a cup of coffee or two and smokes a couple of cigarettes before getting on the freeway is going to get his breakfast from the lining of his stomach. This led Mother to realize the importance of small, frequent meals.

In addition, Selye's rat experiments showed bleeding in the

STRESS RESPONSE

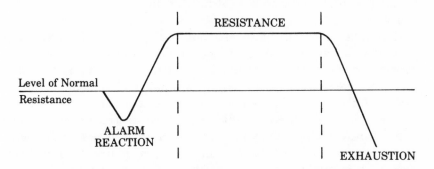

Stage I: ALARM REACTION	The body is subjected to a stress and its level of resistance drops significantly.
Stage II: RESISTANCE	The body adapts to the stress. It works overtime and raises its level of resistance considerably above normal.
Stage III: EXHAUSTION	The above-normal level of resistance runs out and drops below normal. Exhaustion sets in and sickness or even death may result.

SOURCE: Hans Selye, M.D., *The Stress of Life,* p. 111.[5]

kidneys and hemorrhage in the heart. The little broken capillaries in the kidneys and tubes would indicate a vitamin C deficiency. This area may then fill up with scar tissue. If this went on for years, it could be a contributing factor in bringing on hardening of the arteries and kidneys. Every time your heart beats, your blood goes through the kidneys. When scar tissue impedes the flow of blood, blood pressure goes up. The same thing happens in the blood vessels that feed the heart.

THE STAGE OF RESISTANCE   Selye continued his experiments to ascertain what would happen if he exposed his rats to continuous, prolonged stress that was strong enough to strain their defenses almost to their limits, but not of sufficient intensity to overwhelm the animals in a relatively short time. The animals were subsequently subjected to sublethal daily stress for several weeks, a situation comparable to that of a cancer patient receiving chemotherapy and radiation over an extended period of time.

During the first few days of the experiment, the rats responded with the usual alarm reaction, but as the stress continued unabated, the animals that survived the alarm reaction began to recover.

They had in some way accomplished an adaptation to the continuing stress and entered what Selye called the "stage of resistance."

It should be noted, however, that their resistance increased only against the *one* type of stress employed from the beginning of the experiment. If, in the middle of this recovery period, a different stress was substituted, the animals succumbed immediately. While the rats' specific resistance to the initial stress increased, their resistance to any other stress decreased.

In your own life, when you are under a great stress and there is no way out for a while, you must protect yourself. Take the necessary nutrients, fortify yourself with extra vitamin C, and eat a high protein diet five times a day (more frequent but smaller feedings). Also, keep out of drafts, avoid getting chilled, and rest when you feel tired. Take it easy; pamper yourself a little. Give your body all that it needs, and then some, to help it withstand what is stressing you.

THE STAGE OF EXHAUSTION   Continued experimentation by Selye showed that the second stage, adaptation by the rats to the original stress, was not permanent. As stress continued after the recovery period, the animals became progressively weaker. Their adrenals enlarged again and discharged their lipids; the thymus lost the mass it had recovered; sugar and chlorides fell to dangerous levels. After a few weeks, all defenses collapsed and life ceased. This last "stage of exhaustion" was similar to the initial alarm reaction. The end was like the beginning.

How can we fortify ourselves against such an enemy as stress? First of all, we can learn to control our emotional reactions to stressful situations; second, we can properly nourish and care for our bodies. Let's look at each of these protective strategies in turn.

Learn to Control Your Emotional Reactions to Stressful Situations

We are living in what has been described as "an age of anxiety." We are anxious, tense, fearful people; we harbor unforgiveness. Such unresolved conflicts can set up a host of destructive chemical changes—stress—in the body. The effects of stress on Selye's rats were similar whether emotional or physical. In his infinite wisdom, God has given us the means to care for our bodies: he has provided food and told us how to handle emotional stress. The Bible reminds us to "let all bitterness and wrath and anger be put away from you, ... and be kind to one another, tenderhearted, forgiving one another, as God in Christ forgave you."[6]

The disease-producing factors of envy, self-centeredness, resentment, hatred, an unforgiving spirit, jealousy, and anger are all dealt with in the Bible. (I call it the Manufacturer's Handbook.) Obedience to God's word can free us from that which contributes to disease and poor health. All kinds of magazine articles and books have been written about handling stress. Psychiatrists and psychologists have many answers, good and bad, about how people can express their hostilities and thereby drain off their pent-up emotions. But God has given instructions that, when followed, give inner peace and make you the master of your circumstances, not the victim.

The Apostle Paul repeatedly stressed the need to replace our destructive emotions with positive ones. His thirteenth chapter of First Corinthians, often called the "love chapter," is strong testimony indeed.

Love is very patient and kind, never jealous or envious, never boastful or proud, never haughty or selfish or rude. Love does not demand its own way. It is not irritable or touchy. It does not hold grudges and will hardly even notice when others do it wrong. It is never glad about injustice, but rejoices whenever truth wins out. If you love someone you will be loyal to him no matter what the cost. You will always believe in him, always expect the best of him, and always stand your ground in defending him. . . . There are three things that remain—faith, hope, and love— and the greatest of these is love. Let love be your greatest aim. . . .[7]

There are other very specific remarks in the Bible about emotional reactions to stressful situations. God created us as emotional beings and knows we experience anger, but he admonishes, "Do not let the sun go down on your anger,"[8] lest we suffer the consequences: "Surely vexation kills the fool, and jealousy slays the simple."[9] We are advised: "Repay no one evil for evil, but take thought for what is noble in the sight of all. . . . Do not be overcome by evil, but overcome evil with good."[10] When I feel angry and betrayed in a personal or business relationship, I remember Jesus' words, "Love your enemies, do good to them which hate you. Bless . . . and pray for them which despitefully use you. . . ."[11] Seemingly unaware of the baser side of human nature, these words give me strength to do that which they advise; they are an antidote to disease- and stress-producing emotions. The Bible's counsel to us in worrisome and stressful situations is capsulized in this passage:

Finally, brethren, whatever is true, whatever is honorable, whatever is just, whatever is pure, whatever is lovely, whatever is gracious, if there is any excellence, if there is anything worthy of praise, think about these things. What you have learned and received and heard and seen in me, do; and the God of peace will be with you.[12]

God gave us a spirit of power and love, not of fear; he gave us a sound mind.[13] If we are willing to make a conscious effort to control our thoughts, we can overcome our negative feelings.

We need joy and laughter in our lives. *Saturday Review* editor Norman Cousins found that regular belly laughter worked as an anesthetic that gave him painless sleep for up to two hours at a time. In 1964, he was diagnosed as having a crippling spinal disease with a one in 500 chance for survival.

Cousins began to search for the cause of his illness and for a cure. "I felt a compulsion to get into the act. . . . It seemed clear to me that if I was to be that one in five hundred, I had better be something more than a passive observer."[14] He was fortunate in that he had read Walter B. Cannon's famous book, *The Wisdom of the Body,* and Hans Selye's classic, *The Stress of Life.* He recognized that his was a severe case of adrenal exhaustion, possibly caused by, among other things, emotional tension and negative emotions. He asked himself, if negative emotions produce negative chemical changes in the body, would positive emotions produce positive chemical changes? Is it possible that love, faith, laughter, confidence, and the will to live have therapeutic value? Do chemical changes occur only on the downside?[15]

Cousins's doctor shared his excitement over this realization and cooperated with him. Cousins checked out of the hospital and booked himself into a hotel room. He methodically read humorous books and watched funny movies. He requested of his doctor that he be given massive intravenous feedings of vitamin C over a period of three or four hours daily. By the end of one week, he was receiving 25 grams of vitamin C per day. At the end of the eighth day, he was able to move his thumbs without pain; his sedimentation rate was somewhere in the 80s and dropping fast.* "There was no doubt in my mind that I was going to

---

* Sedimentation rate readings measure signs of inflammation in the body, a major characteristic of Cousins's illness.

make it back all the way.... The feeling was indescribably beautiful."[16]

Cousins speculates that laughter may increase the production of endorphins, the body's own natural painkiller. "I have learned never to underestimate the capacity of the human mind and body to regenerate—even when the prospects seem most wretched ...," he said. "What was significant about the laughter ... [was] that it creates a mood in which the other positive emotions can be put to work, too. In short, it helps make it possible for good things to happen."[17]

We have to work at finding things worth laughing about, just as we have to work at anything else that is worthwhile. We all know individuals who use sarcasm and cynicism to pump themselves up at the expense of others. But, according to more than one psychologist, *why* you laugh is just as important as *how* you laugh.

What Cousins discovered was known all along by those who read the Bible. The Psalms and Proverbs, in particular, are full of references pointing up the importance of having a merry heart and a hopeful, fun-loving outlook on life. The Bible says, "A cheerful heart does good like medicine: but a broken spirit makes one sick,"[18] and "the joy of the Lord is your strength."[19]

On the other hand, while laughter is a great tension release, so is crying. We have all been equipped with a natural valve to let off steam—the kind of crying that gives expression to one's emotions. There is a beautiful therapy in the crying that comes from deep within one's soul. The Bible assures us that God takes notice of our tears, and we are even told that he records them in his book of life.[20] David, who wrote so many of the Psalms, cried to express his pain, his need for forgiveness, his desire for deliverance from his enemies, his bewilderment at what was happening, and his innermost longings. His grief spilled over in tears as he acknowledged his failures both to God and others. But David could say that while weeping may endure for a night, joy comes in the morning.[21]

You may have heard people say, "I feel so much better after a good cry!" Unfortunately, in our American culture, from the time a boy is old enough to understand, he is told, "Big boys don't cry." Boys *and* men should have the same freedom to cry as girls and women. Crying is not a sign of weakness, but a sign of release.

And Remember to Exercise

Tranquilizers are commonly prescribed for those who complain of the side effects of stress. Every year, an estimated 50 million prescriptions are written for Valium. It quickly became a best-selling (legal) drug, and this would seem to indicate there are an awful lot of people who haven't learned how to handle stress.[22]

Studies show that exercise is far more effective than tranquilizers in reducing tension. Dr. Herbert de Vries, of the University of Southern California's School of Medicine, tested volunteers, age 52 to 70, from Leisure World, a retirement community in Laguna Hills, California. Without exception, they all admitted to experiencing symptoms associated with stress—nervous tension, irritability, anxiety, perpetual worry, and feelings of panic. Some of these participants were given tranquilizers; others exercised moderately for fifteen minutes a day. By comparing the two groups, de Vries was able to establish that, when people are tense and unable to relax, exercise is a highly effective tension-release. Many of the volunteers in his study had suffered from migraine headaches for years. After a few weeks of the exercise program, their headaches stopped.[23]

It is an established fact that exercise is one of the necessary ingredients for optimum, vibrant health. Human beings were designed and created for movement. It is becoming increasingly clear that we have not adapted well to the reduced level of activity that our life-style has imposed upon us.

Basically, the body has four fundamental requirements: food, water, rest, and movement. Deterioration sets in when we do not keep our bodies limber and use our muscles. Every organ in the body benefits from exercise—the heart, the circulatory system, the respiratory system, the digestive and eliminative organs, and the bones.

Measure Your Stress Quotient

Before moving on to look at the nutrients you need to help your body deal with stress, a stress rating chart is provided to enable you to see too many stressful situations with which we cope. This chart was designed by Dr. Thomas H. Holmes and Dr. Richard H. Rahe to measure the level of stress an individual is enduring. Check the events that have occurred in your life during the past year and then add the point values assigned to those events. If your total score is less than 150, your chance of becoming sick in the next two years is only 37 percent. With a score of more than 300 points, your chance of illness rises to 80 percent, and the odds continue to increase as your score goes up.

Event	Value	Event	Value
Death of spouse	100	Trouble with in-laws	29
Divorce	73	Outstanding personal	
Marital separation	65	achievement	28
Jail term	63	Spouse begins or stops work	26
Death of close family member	63	Starting or finishing school	26
Personal injury or illness	53	Change in living conditions	25
Marriage	50	Revision of personal habits	24
Dismissal from work	47	Trouble with boss	23
Marital reconciliation	45	Change in work hours, conditions	20
Retirement	45	Change in residence	20
Change in family member's		Change in schools	20
health	44	Change in recreational habits	19
Pregnancy	40	Change in church activities	19
Sex difficulties	39	Change in social activities	18
Addition to family	39	*Mortgage or loan under $40,000	17
Business readjustment	39	Change in sleeping habits	16
Change in financial status	38	Change in number of family	
Death of close friend	37	gatherings	15
Change to different line of work	36	Change in eating habits	15
Change in number of marital		Vacation	13
arguments	35	Christmas season	12
*Mortgage or loan over $40,000	31	Minor violation of the law	11
Foreclosure of mortgage or loan	30		
Change in work responsibilities	29		
Son or daughter leaving home	29		

SOURCE: Thomas H. Holmes and Richard H. Rahe, "Social Readjustment Rating Scale," from *Journal of Psychosomatic Research,* 2 (1967), pp. 213–218.
 * Updated to a present relative value from a $10,000 figure in 1967.

Holmes and Rahe emphasize that these figures are indicators of possible illness only. Furthermore, the events listed on this chart measure only what would be considered acute stress. Chronic stress, such as that experienced by the workaholic or activity addict, is not measured here. Most people are startled by their high stress quotient. This does mean that we must be prepared emotionally and physically for the onslaught of stress. We can combat this common modern problem by taking charge of our diet, and using appropriate nutritional supplements.

Good Nutrition Protects Against Stress

We can alleviate stress by choosing to deal with it in positive ways, but we cannot abolish stress. And even low-grade stress, particularly when it is chronic, depletes the body's stores of available nutrients. If we do not take care to replenish those stores, our bodies will not be able to withstand the onslaught, and disease will result.

Let's look at the relationship between specific nutrients and stress.

Vitamin A is known to boost the body's immune defense system, and it has a beneficial effect upon human healing. It is also necessary for the proper structure and function of the adrenal glands, which, as has been shown, control our response to stress. When the body is under stress, the adrenal glands secrete hormones that orchestrate the activities of various organs. And remember: our stress response evolved out of the threat of physical danger, that is the danger our body prepares for, even when we are threatened by *emotional* danger. "Our heart rate speeds up, the blood pressure rises, and the conversion of fat and proteins to energy increases in order to make more energy available for the muscles."[24]

The *B-complex vitamins* may be the single most important factor for the health of your nerves. It is important to remember that all the B-complex vitamins need to be taken together, since each B-vitamin affects all the others. For example, high doses of B-1 can bring on a B-6 and B-2 deficiency. Although we do not know how many such specific interactions exist, we do know that *all* the B-vitamins are necessary for normal functioning of the nervous system. And the need for the B-complex vitamins increases during times of stress. The B-vitamins have a profound effect on our emotions and our overall mental stability.

The adrenal cortex needs *pantothenic acid* (vitamin B-5), which is an essential part of coenzyme A, for cellular metabolism. Every cell in the body depends on pantothenic acid. Pantothenic acid is known as "the antistress vitamin." Any form of stress exhausts the body's supply of pantothenic acid.

Linda Clark, in *Know Your Nutrition,* writes that pantothenic acid's greatest known contribution is its effects on the adrenal cortex. A pantothenic acid deficiency can result in allergies, low resistance to stress, and some forms of arthritis. "This vitamin can be used instead of cortisone without the side effects," Clark emphasizes.[25]

In one experiment, four healthy young men were fed a diet free of pantothenic acid and injected with known antagonists of the vitamin. Symptoms of deficiency started to appear during the second week of the experiment and in the following two weeks, the four men exhibited all of the symptoms of adrenal exhaustion—constipation, loss of appetite, personality changes, numbness and tingling in the hands and feet, diminished balance, coordination, and reflexes, and respiratory infections. One man even developed pneumonia. The severity of the symptoms required that the men be given pantothenic acid supplements to overcome the effects of the vitamin antagonists. But the symptoms grew so much worse and the men became so fatigued and lethargic that the doctors, alarmed by these developments, stopped the experiment. These men had entered the stage of stress exhaustion. They were treated with cortisone to aid their adrenal glands, their regular diet was restored, and they were given multivitamins and injections of the B-complex vitamins and pantothenic acid.[26]

These results strongly suggest that ingesting extra amounts of pantothenic acid may help us deal better with the stresses that we encounter in our lives.

The body's *vitamin C* concentrations are usually highest in the adrenal glands, and when these glands are stressed in any way, vitamin C must be mobilized from them, as well as from other tissues. Many animals are capable of producing their own supply of vitamin C. Humans, however, along with guinea pigs, monkeys, and some bats, have somehow lost their ability to make this vitamin. Vitamin C is easily destroyed by the process of cooking, so our main, natural source of the vitamin is from such foods as citrus fruits, berries, greens, cabbages, peppers, and other vegetables eaten raw.

Vitamin C in huge amounts has been shown to protect animals from every form of stress. The body's need for this nutrient increases tremendously in times of stress; if the body is undersupplied, the glands quickly hemorrhage and the output of hormones markedly decreases. Since the body uses vitamin C to detoxify harmful substances formed in the body during stress, greater than normal quantities of the nutrient are lost in the urine at this time. Experiments with monkeys showed that if they were given more than three times their normal daily requirement of vitamin C, they remained healthy when subjected to the stress of severe cold. Translated into human terms, this would be approximately 4,000 milligrams—a large amount, but not excessive during severe stress.[27]

Accumulating evidence points to stress as a factor in the development of cancer. Dr. Linus Pauling believes that an individual's daily intake of vitamin C should be from 1 gram to 10 grams (1000–10,000 mg.) per day to stay in the best of health.[28]

In his book *The Healing Factor: Vitamin C Against Disease,* Dr. Irwin Stone explains why we need so much vitamin C:

There are no large storage depots for ascorbic acid [vitamin C] in the body and any excess is rapidly excreted. When saturated, the whole body may only contain 5 grams. This means that the body requires a continuous supply to replenish losses and depletions. The livers of nearly all mammals are constantly making and pouring ascorbic acid into their bloodstreams, but man's liver is unable to do this. He needs a constant, large, outside supply to make up for this genetic defect.[29]

Stone points out that vitamin C tends to concentrate in the organs and tissues that have high metabolic activity—such as the adrenal cortex, the pituitary gland, the brain, the ovaries, the eyes, and other vital tissues. Any form of biochemical stress or physical trauma will cause a precipitous drop in the body's vitamin C levels, but the affected organs or tissues in particular will lose this vitamin. Since your body cannot replace what vitamin C has been destroyed or utilized in combating the ravages of stress, you have to supply it.

Vitamin E is one of the most versatile of all the vitamins. Experiments with animals show that their ability to cope with stress depends to a considerable degree on their ability to produce pituitary and adrenal hormones. Vitamin E, which is concentrated in the pituitary gland more than in any other part of the body, is essential to the pituitary and adrenal hormones to keep them from being destroyed by oxygen.[30]

Vitamin E protects against some of the damaging stress of oxidation during exercise (remember, excessive exercise is considered a stress), and this may help explain why vitamin E has been reported to alleviate muscle cramps.

Everybody should keep vitamin E ointment or cream on hand as first aid for burns that can happen in the home and for sunburn, cuts, and abrasions. The relief is quick and there is a minimum of blistering. If you don't have the ointment or cream, reach for your vitamin E capsules and use them locally as well as orally.

Surgery, accidents, and burns damage blood vessels and thereby reduce the body's oxygen supply. Vitamin E decreases the need for oxygen, thus increasing stamina and endurance in cellular respiration. The oxygen-saving effects and the antithrombin (blood-clot dissolving) activity of vitamin E makes it the best possible nutritional protection against heart attacks. It also helps to heal a damaged heart. The importance of vitamin E in the treatment and prevention of heart disease, and in minimizing the damaging effects of stress on the heart, is recognized.[31] Indeed, this essential nutrient performs so many tasks, and guards the body against so many diseases and health problems, that its significance can scarcely be overstated.

Like many vitamins and minerals, *zinc* seems to be involved in the body's response to stress. In animal experiments, zinc supplements markedly reduced the number of stress ulcers produced during extreme stress.

Dr. Carl Pfeiffer, of the Brain Bio Center in Princeton, New Jersey, reports that stress of any kind depletes the body's supply of zinc. As one example, burn patients often end up with only one-third of the normal amount of zinc in their bodies, and most burn centers use zinc supplements in treating their patients.[32]

In human studies, blood levels of zinc have been found to rise considerably when stress is anxiously anticipated, as well as when actual stress (such as surgery) is experienced. Anesthetic drugs were found to depress zinc levels in the blood, however. Excretion of zinc has been found to increase by a factor of three to five during stress—another indication that the body prepares to deal with stress by increasing the amount of zinc available to tissues for healing and any other purpose zinc has in the body.[33]

Dr. Hans Selye, in his experiments with rats, investigated the effects of stress on the heart. He gave special attention to cardiac failures and learned much of the role that *potassium* and *magnesium* play in protecting the body in times of stress.

Selye found that healthy animals could take stress in stride, but those whose hormones had been upset soon succumbed. And if sodium salts were given to the animals, the end came more quickly. Under severe stress, their adrenals went into high gear, and their bodies retained sodium and lost potassium and magnesium.

The changes that appeared in those animals parallel what happens to adult human beings who live through years of stress. Selye's theory was that a person who is weakened by an imbalance of hormones and various chemicals, and then subjected to additional outside stresses, may develop a sudden heart attack and die quite unexpectedly from cardiac arrest. The blood supply to a portion of the heart muscle is blocked because, without potassium and magnesium, the heart muscle cannot contract. The muscle cannot get the oxygen it needs to continue its job of pumping blood to the rest of the body and, thus starved, it dies. Selye found serious heart disease in all the animals given stress tests, with the exception of those that had been given doses of potassium and magnesium. Since sodium salts speeded up the heart damage, Selye had attempted to counteract this salt by giving the other two salts—potassium and magnesium. His strategy worked against the sodium and saved the animals.[34]

Stress places a heavy physiological demand on the body's store of *protein,* draining it from the muscles. Advocates of a low-protein diet seem to forget this. For instance, an individual who is dieting is under tremendous emotional and physical stress. Since proteins are the "building blocks" of the body, our nutritional needs escalate when we are under stress, especially our need for protein.

In short, any severe stress—including illness, injury, trauma, or extraordinary energy expenditure—boosts the body's requirements for protein.

The combination of *nutrients found in liver* makes it a truly extraordinary food. No one has yet succeeded in identifying the factor in raw liver that guards against stress. However, there is overwhelming evidence that liver is most effective in protecting us against this number-one threat to health.

It was in 1947 that Dr. Benjamin Ershoff's much-publicized studies proved the amazing benefits of liver in helping the body to withstand stress. In one study, Ershoff selected a number of rats and divided them into three groups. All three groups received a typical diet fed to experimental animals, but supplemented with vitamins. One of the groups, however, was given extra doses of B vitamins, while another group had liver powder added to the diet.

After three months of such feedings, all three groups of rats were tested to the limits of their endurance. Ershoff placed the rats in a barrel of chilly water. The rats that had been fed the regular diet were able to swim an average of about thirteen minutes before surrendering to fatigue. Those rats that had received the extra B vitamins also swam for about thirteen minutes; but the rats on the liver diet swam for an amazing two hours! And they were still going strong when the test was stopped. The test was repeated after four and seven days and the results were almost identical.[35]

Similar studies have shown that rats fed liver were able to resist the toxic effects of massive doses of drugs and of extremes of cold. Also, liver prolonged the lives of rats subjected to one of the most intense forms of stress—radiation.[36]

We have always emphasized that liver is a potent source of unknown and known nutrients. Until researchers can isolate these unknown factors, all we can do is supplement our diet with liver.

Since liver is not regularly on most family menus, the best and easiest way to get it into yourself and your family is in the form of dessicated liver tablets or powdered liver. Thirty raw, defatted liver tablets or one rounded tablespoon of raw, defatted liver powder equals 2.25 ounces of fresh raw liver. A tablespoonful of the powdered defatted raw liver can be blended in four ounces of tomato juice, with an ounce of water and a squeeze of lemon. If taken daily, it will equal eating a pound of raw liver by the end of the week. Another recipe is given on page 152 which describes the use of liver powder in Mother's fortified protein drink called the Serenity Cocktail.

Regardless of how you take liver, the increase in your endurance and ability to withstand stress will amaze you. Moreover, taking liver is a good way to build your hemoglobin, which is the oxygen carrying pigment of the red blood cells.

Stress cannot be avoided; it is here to stay. It can be a positive force in our lives, however, if we learn to work with it. It is nutritional factors, in part, that determine whether we overcome the inevitable stress or are overcome by it. And the Bible speaks to our human condition of stress with words of strength, comfort, and encouragement: "Cast all your anxieties on him, for he cares about you."[37]

NOTES

1. *Webster's Seventh New Collegiate Dictionary* (Springfield, Mass.: G. & C. Merriam Co., 1971), p. 868.
2. Hans Selye, M.D., *The Stress of Life* (New York: McGraw-Hill, 1956), p. 76.
3. Ibid., p. 171.
4. Ibid., pp. 34–38.
5. Ibid., p. 111.
6. Ephesians 4:31–32, RSV.
7. I Corinthians 13:4–7, 13; 14:1a, The Living Bible.

8. Ephesians 4:26, RSV.
9. Job 5:2, RSV.
10. Romans 12:17, 21, RSV.
11. Matthew 5:44, KJV.
12. Philippians 4:8, 9, RSV.
13. II Timothy 1:7, KJV.
14. Norman Cousins, *The Anatomy of an Illness* (New York: Bantam, 1979), p. 31.
15. Ibid., pp. 34, 35.
16. Ibid., p. 43.
17. Ibid., p. 48.
18. Proverbs 17:22, The Living Bible.
19. Nehemiah 8:10, RSV.
20. Psalm 56:8, KJV.
21. Psalm 30:5, KJV.
22. Milton Moskowitz, Michael Katz, and Robert Levering, eds., *Everybody's Business: An Almanac* (San Francisco: Harper & Row, 1980), p. 219.
23. Herbert de Vries, *Vigor Regained* (Englewood Cliffs, N.J.: Prentice-Hall, 1974).
24. Dominick Bosco, *The People's Guide to Vitamins and Minerals* (Chicago: Contemporary Books, 1980), p. 21.
25. Linda Clark, *Know Your Nutrition* (New Canaan, Conn.: Keats Publishing, 1973), p. 116.
26. Bosco, *The People's Guide*, p. 108.
27. Irwin Stone, *The Healing Factor* (New York: Grosset & Dunlap, 1972), pp. 166–167.
28. Linus Pauling, "Recent Developments on Vitamin C," interview by Jack J. Challem in *Let's Live*, March 1981, p. 14.
29. Stone, *The Healing Factor*, p. 47.
30. Adelle Davis, *Let's Get Well* (New York: Harcourt, Brace & World, 1965), pp. 17–18.
31. Evan V. Shute, *The Heart and Vitamin E* (New Canaan, Conn.: Keats Publishing, 1956), pp. 69, 76.
32. Carl C. Pfeiffer, Ph.D., M.D., *Zinc and Other Micro-Nutrients* (Connecticut: Keats Publishing, 1978), p. 13.
33. Bosco, *The People's Guide*, p. 259.
34. Selye, *The Stress of Life*, pp. 209–211.
35. Emory W. Thurston, Ph.D., Sc.D., *Nutrition for Tots to Teens (And All Other Ages)* (Encino, Calif.: Argold Press, 1976), pp. 54–55.
36. Adelle Davis, *Let's Get Well* (New York: Harcourt, Brace & World, 1965), p. 22.
37. I Peter 5:7, RSV.

✂ 5. Hypoglycemia: A Much Misunderstood Health Problem

The sugar-laden American diet has led to a national epidemic of hypoglycemia, an ailment characterized by irrational behavior, emotional instability, distorted judgment, and nasty personality defects.

—DR. EMMANUEL CHERASKIN

Irritability, nervousness, "the shakes," weakness, headaches—do these complaints sound familiar? How about fatigue, dizziness, tremors, cold sweats, rapid heartbeat, and heart palpitations? These are just some of the many symptoms of a highly controversial and much misunderstood condition, hypoglycemia. Not an incurable or debilitating disease, but a problem of epidemic proportions nonetheless, hypoglycemia is a metabolic dysfunction related to our sugar intake.

In the form of glucose, sugar is a normal and necessary blood constituent. The body converts it from carbohydrates, protein, fats, and sugar into energy. Maintaining the proper level of sugar in your blood is crucial for the efficient operation of the body. The right level is moderated by insulin, a hormone produced in the pancreas, which takes extra sugar out of the blood and stores it (in the form of glycogen) in the liver and muscles. Then, when additional energy is needed, adrenaline releases this stored glycogen back into the blood.

Like body temperature, our blood sugar level fluctuates within a "normal" range, often cited as from 80 to 120 milligrams per 100 cubic centimeter. During active periods of the day, however, our blood sugar level is actually about 140 on the same scale.

Protein is the best nutrient to eat in order to maintain an even blood sugar level, because it is metabolized over a long period of time. An impressive 58 percent of protein can be converted to glucose if need be. Carbohydrates, on the other hand—particularly refined carbohydrates, such as sugar—are quickly metabolized, causing a rapid rise in blood sugar level. When refined sugar enters the bloodstream, insulin must flood to the rescue, to keep the glucose at its proper level.

A person whose blood sugar drops rapidly is suffering from hypoglycemia (meaning "below normal blood sugar": hypo—below or under; glycemia—glucose in the blood stream). Insufficient insulin, on the other hand, characterizes diabetes. The blood sugar of a diabetic is too high; the pancreas cannot produce enough insulin to moderate the glucose.

Both of these extreme conditions can develop from *overconsumption of sugar*. When the pancreas is constantly bombarded by requests for insulin, it can become desensitized and respond with too much or too little insulin. The symptoms of low blood sugar (hypoglycemia) can occur in the case of too much insulin. Excess insulin takes too much sugar (or glucose—which provides instant energy) out of the blood and converts it to glycogen (stored energy). This happens when the adrenal glands have been overtaxed by stress and stimulants and cannot produce enough of the hormone cortisone, which normally prevents insulin levels from going too high.

Sugar: Its Many Guises

Sugar appears in many forms, some of which are beneficial. *Glucose* is a sugar usually found with the other sugars in fruits and vegetables. It is a key material in the metabolism of all plants. Many of our principal foods are converted into glucose (often called blood sugar) in our bodies.

Fructose is a fruit sugar, found naturally in fruit and honey. It is metabolized in the liver by the enzyme fructokinase, which requires insulin in very small amounts, if at all. Fructose is absorbed into the blood stream more slowly than refined sugar (sucrose). Because it requires a lower level of insulin and has a slower rate of absorption, fructose is much less likely to set off wide fluctuations in blood sugar levels than sucrose.

The malting of grain with natural enzymes breaks the grain's starch molecules down into a sugar known as *maltose*. The two most popular forms of maltose are barley malt and rice syrup. They are also absorbed more slowly and evenly than sucrose and do not create fluctuations in the blood sugar level.

Honey, sweeter than most sugars, consists of equal parts fructose and glucose. It is absorbed quickly and can raise blood sugar levels.

Lactose, or milk sugar, occurs only in milk and is not eaten as a sugar to sweeten foods. It is only one-sixth as sweet as sucrose.

Sucrose is refined sugar made from sugar cane or the sugar beet. The white sugar everyone is so familiar with is 99.95 percent sucrose. Brown sugar, turbinado sugar, and molasses are all from this family. For sucrose to be used by the body, it must be broken down into its constituent sugars—glucose and fructose. Sucrose sugars are broken down quickly. If a large amount of sucrose is taken in, too much insulin may be triggered. The result is a low blood sugar letdown.

Molasses is about 50 percent sucrose. It's a residue left behind when sugar is refined from sugar cane. Blackstrap molasses is the thickest and blackest of the liquids left behind and is very rich in the trace minerals and the B-complex vitamins (with the exception of B-1 and folic acid, which are destroyed in the cooking process). The blacker the molasses, the more concentrated the minerals iron, calcium, copper, magnesium, potassium, zinc, and chromium.

Brown sugar and turbinado sugar contain about 96 percent and 99 percent sucrose, respectively. The body handles them the same as it handles white sugar, but they have a little molasses added back. Turbinado sugar has skipped the final stage of white sugar purification.

Maple syrup is about 65 percent sucrose. Sap is drawn from maple trees and then heated to concentrate the liquid. Thirty-eight gallons of sap produce only one gallon of maple syrup.

Sucrose Addiction

Sucrose addiction may be a comparatively new phenomenon in the history of mankind, but it is widespread. We create confusion by using the word *sugar* to describe two substances that are far from identical: they have different chemical structures and affect the body in profoundly different ways. Sugar pushers tell us how important sugar is as an essential component of the human body, how it is oxidized to produce energy, how it is metabolized to produce warmth, and so on. The sugar they are talking about is glucose, which is manufactured in our bodies. However, we may be led to believe that they are talking about sucrose, which is made in their refineries and used for candy, sweets of all kinds, and soft drinks. In fact, refined sugar is a starvation food that has been stripped of its nourishment. Sugar-laden foods can temporarily satisfy your desire for food, but they leave your hungry cells in trouble, misbehaving and dying.

Nonetheless, sucrose addiction is widespread. So many people assume that eating sugar is the only way to get sugar into our blood. They excuse themselves for eating candy or some sweet by saying, "I need quick energy." That's a myth. The energy is quick, all right—a sweet-induced pickup that is gone in minutes, leaving you worse off than when you began. The healthy body has an adequate supply of glycogen in the liver and muscles, ready to be converted into glucose when that extra boost is needed.

The Sneak Thief of Health

If you saw your child or grandchild eating fifteen teaspoons of sugar out of the sugar bowl, you would probably have a fit. Yet you might not think twice about giving that same child a piece of chocolate cake. The amount of refined sugar hidden in common foods may surprise you. The following chart will help you determine how many teaspoons of hidden sugar you have been getting.

The average American consumes something like 120 pounds of sugar a year, or about one-third of a pound a day. The craving for sweets gets its start in infancy, when we have no control over what we eat. Unknowing parents predispose their children to a lifetime addiction to sweets. Many children get their first sugar in their bottle of formula. You even see punch and artificial juices in baby bottles. By the time the child is old enough to hold a spoon, he is given a sugary cereal and soon he graduates to the other dietary sins that "grace" the table at mealtime.

A number of years ago, Dr. John Yudkin, distinguished British physician, biochemist, and researcher, raised a storm in the scientific world that spread into the sugar industry. His best-selling book, *Sweet and Dangerous,* is still causing rage. In a shocking indictment, Yudkin pointed to ordinary table sugar as a principal cause of heart disease, diabetes, and other killers. It was Yudkin who first suspected that sugar was the cause of deposits on the inside walls of the arteries which lead to the eventual risky stage of atherosclerosis. Around these plaques forms a buildup of fatty material that includes a fairly high proportion of cholesterol. Yudkin drew his conclusions from the re-

**Approximate Refined Carbohydrate Content of Popular Foods
Expressed in Amounts Equivalent to Teaspoonfuls of Sugar**

100 gm. = 20 teaspoonfuls = 3½ oz. = 400 calories

Food	Amount	Serving	Sugar Equivalent
Candy			
Hershey Bar	60 gm.		7 tsp.
Chocolate cream	13 gm.	(35 pieces to 1 lb.)	2 tsp.
Chocolate fudge	30 gm.	1½ inches square	4 tsp.
Chewing gum		1 stick	⅓ tsp.
Life saver		1	⅓ tsp.
Marshmallow	7.6 gm.	1 (60 to 1 lb.)	1½ tsp.
Cake			
Chocolate cake (iced)	100 gm.	1/12 of 2-layer cake	15 tsp.
Angel cake	45 gm.	1/12 of cake	6 tsp.
Sponge cake	50 gm.	1/10 of cake	6 tsp.
Cream puff (iced)	80 gm.	1 average custard-filled	5 tsp.
Doughnut plain	40 gm.	3-inch	4 tsp.
Cookies			
Macaroons	25 gm.	1 large or 2 small	3 tsp.
Gingersnaps	6 gm.	1 medium	1 tsp.
Brownies	20 gm.	2 x 2 x ¾ inches	3 tsp.
Custards			
Baked custard		½ cup	4 tsp.
Gelatin		½ cup	4 tsp.
Junket		⅛ quart	3 tsp.
Ice Cream			
Ice cream		⅛ quart	5 to 6 tsp.
Water ice		⅛ quart	6 to 8 tsp.
Pie			
Apple pie		⅙ of pie	12 tsp.
Cherry pie		⅙ of pie	14 tsp.
Custard, coconut pie		⅙ of pie	10 tsp.
Pumpkin pie		⅙ of pie	10 tsp.
Spreads			
Jam	20 gm.	1 level tbsp.	3 tsp.
Jelly	20 gm.	1 level tbsp.	2½ tsp.
Marmalade	20 gm.	1 level tbsp.	3 tsp.
Honey	20 gm.	1 level tbsp.	3 tsp.
Chocolate sauce	30 gm.	1 tsp. thick	4½ tsp.
Milk Drinks			
Chocolate		5 oz. glass	6 tsp.
Cocoa		5 oz. glass	4 tsp.
Soft Drinks			
Coca Cola	180 gm.	6 oz. glass	4⅓ tsp.
Ginger Ale	180 gm.	6 oz. glass	4⅓ tsp.
Cooked Fruits			
Peaches, canned in syrup	10 gm.	2 halves, 1 tbsp. juice	3½ tsp.
Rhubarb, stewed, sweetened	100 gm.	½ cup	8 tsp.
Apple sauce, unsweetened	100 gm.	½ cup	2 tsp.

**Approximate Refined Carbohydrate Content of Popular Foods
Expressed in Amounts Equivalent to Teaspoonfuls of Sugar**

100 gm. = 20 teaspoonfuls = 3½ oz. = 400 calories

Food	Amount	Serving	Sugar Equivalent
Prunes, stewed, sweetened	100 gm.	4 – 5, 2 tbsp. juice	8 tsp.
Fruit cocktail	120 gm.	½ cup	5 tsp.
Dried Fruits			
Apricots, dried	30 gm.	4 – 6 halves	4 tsp.
Prunes, dried	30 gm.	3 – 4	4 tsp.
Dates, dried	30 gm.	3 – 4	4½ tsp.
Figs, dried	30 gm.	1½ – 2 small	4 tsp.
Raisins	30 gm.	¼ cup	4 tsp.
Fruit Juices			
Orange juice	100 gm.	½ cup	2 tsp.
Pineapple juice, unsweetened	100 gm.	½ cup	2⅕ tsp.
Grapefruit juice, unsweetened	100 gm.	½ cup	2⅗ tsp.
Grape juice, sweetened	100 gm.	½ cup	3⅔ tsp.

SOURCE: Carlton Fredericks, *Low Blood Sugar and You* (New York: Grossett and Dunlap, 1969), pp. 12 – 13.

sults of control studies performed over a period of time. And he is quick to point out that sugar is not the *only* cause of these degenerative diseases—in particular, heart disease—but is a *major* contributing factor.

Sugar cane in its natural form is a grass, rich in nutrients, vitamins, and trace elements. But we do not get sugar in its natural form; we eat "refined" sugar that not only fails to provide nutrients, but actually robs the body of the nutrients it vitally needs. In particular, the valuable B-vitamins, especially thiamine, are destroyed. Thiamine, a member of the B-complex, is one of the most important vitamins for good health, contributing to growth, good appetite, and the smooth functioning of the digestive tract. For good reason, it is called "the morale vitamin."

When you eat white sugar, you are presenting your digestive tract with something that contains no thiamine or other B-vitamins to aid in the process of digestion. In order to handle this sugar, the body must draw thiamine from its storage places in the liver, kidneys, and heart, and divert it from other processes. Applying Mother's formula *blood sugar + B-vitamins = energy* to our intake of refined sugar, we come up short.

The milling of grain, the process by which the outer bran coating and the wheat germ are removed in the production of white flour, further compounds the problem. Of the rich store of vitamins and minerals to be found in grains, milling depletes 90 percent of the vitamins, 86 percent of the manganese, 85 percent of the magnesium, 78 percent of the zinc and other trace minerals, as well as fiber and essential amino acids. (The milling process was developed to combat weevils and rodents. Everything that promoted life was removed so the grains could be stored for years.) Though many of our flours and breads are "enriched," in fact only three of the many B-vitamins are added back, plus inorganic iron. Ordinary white bread is so low in nutritional value that laboratory rats fed it for 90 days died of malnutrition.[1]

The list of major ailments caused directly or indirectly by refined sugar consumption includes almost everything from obesity and diabetes to common colds. It is clearly understood that sugar weakens the immune system as it replaces the natural foods that would supply the body with the vitamins, minerals, and protein it needs.

After Christmas and the New Year holiday each year, the news reports another flu epidemic. Each year the epidemic is given a new name, but it has the same cause. What happens is that, during these busy holidays, people become more easily fatigued. They have indulged in large amounts of sweet foods, chocolate, and alcohol and their immune systems are depressed. Their cells have been sabotaged, so they end up with the flu or a cold.

Our systems simply weren't designed to function at their best while overloaded with the refined carbohydrates of most breakfast cereals, cakes, candies, and other sweet foods. Therefore Mother urges people to get off sugar as quickly as possible. She recommends:

Don't even have sugar, sugar-coated cereals, soft drinks, or anything containing sugar in the house. After you are on a good diet, with small, frequent feedings, you won't even crave sweets. If you do want something sweet, enjoy fruit. Once you have made the break with sugar-loaded foods, you will begin to notice how much better foods taste, that there are flavors you had forgotten or never appreciated before. The sensitivity of your palate has been blunted by sugar; you ought to give it an opportunity to return to what it was meant to be.

Hypoglycemia

Of the specific illnesses related to sugar, hypoglycemia is perhaps the most common. The hypoglycemic's problems can be caused by inborn errors of metabolism (babies can be born with exhausted adrenals); may be acquired as a result of overindulgence in refined carbohydrates or other substances, such as alcohol, stimulants,* and drugs; or may be triggered by stresses that exhaust the adrenal glands. And the physical problems have psychological manifestations.

Many years ago Mother began seeing individuals suffering from what was later to be classified as hypoglycemia. They had tried drugs, but the problem persisted. Hearing their complaints and learning of their dietary habits she was prompted to study the problem. She reached the conclusion that there was too much sugar and devitalized refined carbohydrates (white rice, white flour products, white sugar) in their diets.

The problem has not changed through the years. Almost everyone she sees shows some evidence of one or many symptoms commonly associated with low blood sugar.

These symptoms are so multiple that Dr. Stephan Gyland, himself a victim of low blood sugar, treated 600 patients and compiled a long list of symptoms, along with the percentage of hypoglycemic patients in which each of the symptoms occurred. Here is his list:[2]

Nervousness	94%	Insomnia	62%
Irritability	89%	Constant worrying,	
Exhaustion	87%	unprovoked anxieties	62%
Faintness, dizziness, tremor,		Mental confusion	57%
cold sweats, and/or weak		Internal trembling	57%
spells	86%	Palpitation of heart and/or	
Depressions	77%	rapid pulse	54%
Vertigo, dizziness	73%	Muscle pains	53%
Drowsiness	72%	Numbness	51%
Headaches	71%	Indecisiveness	50%
Digestive disturbances	69%	Unsocial, asocial, or	
Forgetfulness	67%	antisocial behavior	47%

---

* The adrenal glands are stimulated when anything toxic enters the body. Fear, worry, anxiety, coffee, caffeine, nicotine, alcohol, drugs and medications—all of these substances stimulate the production of adrenaline, which triggers the alarm reaction in the body. This alarm reaction stimulates the central nervous system through the thalamus and the hypothalamus to the pituitary gland, which manufactures a hormone called ACTH. The ACTH works on the outside core (adrenal cortex) of the adrenal gland to produce cortisone and about 55 other hormones.

Cortisone raises the blood sugar by pulling glycogen out of the liver, calcium out of the bones, and protein out of the muscles. In effect, you "cannibalize" yourself. When this alarm reaction becomes exhausted by years of overuse and runs out of material to make cortical hormones, then we may suffer from arthritis, asthma, and other degenerative conditions.

Crying spells	46%	Smothering spells	34%
Lack of sex drive in female	44%	Staggering	34%
Allergies	43%	Sighing and yawning	30%
Incoordination	43%	Impotence in males	29%
Leg cramps	43%	Unconsciousness	27%
Lack of concentration	42%	Night terrors, nightmares	27%
Blurred vision	40%	Rheumatoid arthritis	24%
Twitching and jerking of		Phobias, fears	23%
muscles	40%	Neurodermatitis	21%
Itching and crawling		Suicidal intent	20%
sensations of the skin	39%	Nervous breakdown	17%
Gasping for breath	37%	Convulsions	2%

Thousands of hypoglycemics have been misdiagnosed. Here is a partial listing, compiled from the reports of Drs. Gyland, Salzer, Fredericks, Martin, Weller, Cheraskin, and others, of such incorrectly diagnosed hypoglycemia:[3] mental retardation, diabetes, alcoholism, menopause, neurosis, Parkinson's Syndrome, chronic bronchial asthma, allergy, psycho-neuroticism, cerebral arteriosclerosis, Meniere's Syndrome (loss of hearing, dizziness associated with it, and noises in the ears), neurodermatitis (nervous skin disorders), chronic urticaria (hives), autonomic nervous system disorders, brain tumor, senility, migraine, epilepsy, and schizophrenia. Is it any wonder that low blood sugar is considered by many doctors and nutritionists to be one of the most difficult and thought-provoking problems known? It has been nicknamed "the great impersonator." And no wonder, since its symptoms include just about every imaginable complaint.

Often individuals who suffer from low blood sugar will think their problem is just "nerves." Or they will think they have "an emotional problem" or a "psychosomatic illness." Although the hypoglycemic's problems are not psychological *in origin,* psychological problems are often part of the hypoglycemic's symptoms. A typical hypoglycemic victim is, in fact, an emotional yo-yo, strung out on a chemical reaction he cannot control, with reactions so severe they frequently resemble insanity.

THE GLUCOSE TOLERANCE TEST The glucose tolerance test will reveal if a person's problems are due to low blood sugar. The test must be administered by a physician specially trained to interpret the glucose tolerance curve, and it is a long procedure that can take five to six hours. For this test to be accurate, the blood should be analyzed every half hour, which frightens some people, although some of the trauma can be alleviated by a ma-

GLUCOSE TOLERANCE TEST (I)

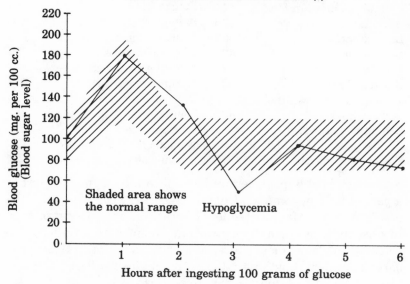

Hours after ingesting 100 grams of glucose

I. Typical hypoglycemic curve. This curve is almost normal, except for at the three hour mark, where the blood sugar level drops sharply to about 55. This is the point at which the symptoms of hypoglycemia occur, and the body loses sodium, glucose, calcium, and oxygen.

chine that tests the blood by a prick of the finger. Mother does not recommend that people go through this procedure unless their symptoms are severe. It is unnatural to take the large glass of sugar water—100 grams of glucose—which is required, and Mother feels that if you have the symptoms of low blood sugar, then it is best to assume you have it and change your diet. But first, ask your physician and follow his advice.

What Happens When Your Blood Sugar Falls

The blood sugar drops when the adrenal glands become exhausted. They run out of the material needed to make the cortical hormones that would prevent this from happening.

When the blood sugar falls rapidly to 60 or 70 milligrams, the symptoms are comparatively mild and may consist of slight headaches, faintness, muscular weakness, hunger, irritability, and perhaps a feeling of nervousness or tension. If it falls still lower, the symptoms become more severe, including headaches (even migraines), dizziness, fatigue, sweating, tremors, heart palpitations, marked irritability, and general nervousness. If the blood sugar continues to fall to 40 milligrams or lower, the suf-

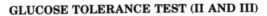

GLUCOSE TOLERANCE TEST (II AND III)

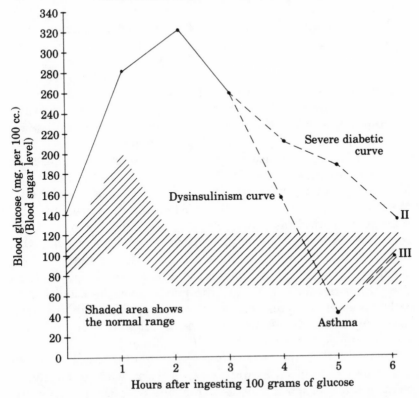

II. Severe diabetic curve. This subject's pancreas cannot produce enough insulin to bring the blood sugar level down to normal.

III. Dysinsulinism curve. If the glucose tolerance test had been conducted for only three hours, the subject would have been considered a diabetic. But notice that in the last three hours, blood sugar level drops down to that of a hypoglycemic. The pancreas finally secretes insulin, but too much; the blood sugar drops below normal. This is the point at which asthma occurs.

ferer can experience palpitations of the heart (a feeble but rapid pulse), and pallor will be more pronounced, until unconsciousness and convulsions occur.

Not only does your blood sugar level drop as your adrenals become exhausted, but the amount of calcium in the blood is affected as well. When the adrenals are stimulated by stress, drugs, and other stimulants, they go into high gear and pull calcium out of your bones. The big muscles at the side of your neck and head go into contraction, fluid gathers in the brain, and you feel like the top of your head is going to come off. You feel shaky, trembly inside. You have "restless legs," and your back aches.

When blood sugar goes low so does your supply of oxygen. You yawn (gasping for oxygen). You cannot concentrate. You doze off at meetings and find it hard to stay alert.

Your blood carries oxygen to every cell in your body. Glucose is almost the only fuel used by the brain and central nervous system. The combination of glucose with oxygen keeps the brain functioning. A drop of glucose in the blood stream will cause profound mental changes, according to Dr. Broda Barnes.[4]

Also, when blood glucose drops, salt is lost in the urine. It is salt that keeps the plasma in the blood vessels. When this salt is lost, the plasma gets thin and enters tissues it should not. Mother describes these conditions: When the fluid goes into the brain, the condition is called migraine headache; when the fluid goes into the eyes, the condition is called glaucoma; when the fluid goes into the nose, you have a stuffy nose and the condition is called hayfever, sinus problems and post-nasal drip, or allergies; when the fluid goes into the middle ear, the condition is called Meniere's Syndrome, and you experience ringing and noises in the ear, loss of hearing, and dizziness. When fluid goes into the lungs, the condition is called asthma.

Such conditions as these may respond to a half-teaspoon each of *salt and soda* in an 8-ounce glass of warm water. You might want to add a teaspoon of honey. This mixture raises not only the sodium, but also the low blood sugar. It brings the adrenals out of shock and stimulates the thymus, which in turn will stimulate the tonsils, adenoids, and lymph glands to make antibodies. A child who suffers from asthma attacks in the early morning may find relief by taking the salt and soda drink before taking other measures. And giving the child an eggnog or some protein food right after this should help keep the blood sugar level up.

YOUR LOWEST EBB   If you have low blood sugar problems, your lowest ebb will probably be at three or four o'clock in the morning. Some people wake up then and cannot go back to sleep, the usual hypoglycemia symptoms often being compounded at night by irrational fears and nightmares. If this has been happening to you, then you might want to take a protein drink before you go to bed at night. Do the same if you wake up.

This early morning low ebb can actually be very serious. A tremendous number of what people think are heart attacks occur at this time. When the blood sugar, blood calcium, and blood oxygen levels drop, chest pains may result. This pain is usually what is known as angina, and if this condition progresses it may even cause a heart attack if fear sets in. Then more adrenaline floods into the body and the heart begins to pound harder still. A blood vessel can spring a leak as a result, causing a thrombosis.

This could be prevented by keeping the adrenal glands healthy, the pancreas functioning properly, the diet low in refined carbohydrates and sugars, and the diet and life-style free of unnecessary stimulants.

HYPOGLYCEMIA IN CHILDREN Children who overeat, or who do not want to eat at all, are likely hypoglycemics. They may have impaired memory, so when they state that they did not say or do something, they probably don't remember what they did. Low blood sugar children frequently have trouble learning, or they may fail in a particular subject. You will often find that the class in which the child is failing occurs around ten or eleven o'clock in the morning. Such a child may be mischievous and restless. However, children manifest different symptoms—another child might be considered lazy and show signs of mental fatigue, dullness, indifference, lack of initiative, and a severe inability to make decisions.[5]

It may come as a surprise that low blood sugar problems can be far more serious for children than for adults. One child we knew suffered from severe headaches that regularly awoke her at night. After being misdiagnosed as having a brain tumor, it was discovered that she suffered from low blood sugar. A change of diet (eliminating refined sugar and refined carbohydrates) and a protein drink before bed and another one around midnight relieved her of painful symptoms and allowed her to sleep peacefully.

Diabetes: The Refined-Carbohydrate Disease

A person whose pancreas simply cannot produce enough insulin to lower the blood sugar level is considered diabetic. Some diabetics take insulin injections to bring the blood sugar down to normal, but this is clearly not a cure.

Diabetes is one condition in which minerals are more important than vitamins. Scientific literature is showing increasingly the importance of minerals in preventing degenerative changes in the pancreas. Dr. Robert Atkins calls chromium, zinc, manganese, and magnesium the "Big Four." They are essential trace minerals that have key roles in metabolic pathways and are so frequently deficient in our overly refined Western diet.[6]

Nutritionally, we know that the cells of the pancreas that secrete insulin must have calcium in the intercellular fluid before they can respond to the stimulation from glucose. Manganese, chromium and zinc have each been shown to be vital in helping to remedy carbohydrate metabolism problems. Chromium works closely with insulin, and insulin's effectiveness is greatly decreased when there is chromium insufficiency. Zinc is a crucial trace mineral that speeds wound healing and is involved in the granulation and storage of insulin. Diabetics lose more zinc in the urine than do nondiabetics.[7]

In the 1950s, Dr. Walter Mertz, of the U.S. Department of Agriculture, isolated a substance secreted from the liver that allows body cells to process insulin. This substance he termed the *glucose tolerance factor* (GTF). Since the GTF is involved somehow in the entry of glucose into the cells from the blood, its absence can cause diabetes. According to Dr. Jeffrey Bland, "The glucose tolerance factor has been found to depend upon the essential trace mineral chromium, and this nutrient is often deficient in Western diets. Chromium is a mineral that is easily lost in the milling of grains and the processing of foods and may be commonly deficient in the 'average, well-nourished' American."[8]

A recent study has revealed an important correlation between low concentrations of magnesium in the serum (the liquid component of blood) and another vascular complication of diabetes, diabetic retinopathy (hemorrhaging in the back of the eye).[9] Although the reasons for low serum-magnesium in diabetic patients are still not clear,[10] the correlation is compelling. We do need all of the vitamins and minerals; they work together as a team.

Your diet can be supplemented by wheat germ, bran, desiccated liver powder, multi-mineral tablets (with all the minerals from natural sources), and brewer's yeast to assure an adequate supply of this and other vital minerals.

Irwin Stone, author of *The Healing Factor,* showed how tests on guinea pigs indicated that ascorbic acid (vitamin C) has a profound influence on the body's sugar utilization. Guinea pigs depleted of ascorbic acid showed a low glucose tolerance, but their tolerance was rapidly restored when they were fed ascorbic acid.[11] Since ascorbic acid assists the action of insulin, it is important that your body maintain optimum levels of this valuable vitamin at all times. Moreover, since ascorbic acid is a potent detoxifier that counteracts and neutralizes the harmful effects of many poisons in the body, and since it increases the therapeutic effect of different drugs and medicines by making them more effective, it may be that many diabetics could reduce their insulin requirements if they were supplied with sufficient amounts of vitamin C.

If you are one of the many people who suffer from diabetes, be sure to have five to six small feedings spaced evenly throughout the day. This schedule will give you a pickup each time your blood sugar starts to drop after not eating for three or four hours. Be sure to stay away from all sugar and refined carbohydrates, and be sure you get protein with every feeding. Since protein is metabolized slowly, it will help you maintain your blood glucose level.

The Importance of Breakfast

When you eat breakfast, you break an all-night fast. And what you eat then determines how you will feel all day. It is well worth considering the results of a study reported by the U.S. Department of Agriculture on blood sugar levels in relation to breakfast.[12]

When the 200 volunteers who participated in the study were given black coffee alone, blood sugar decreased and the volunteers experienced lassitude, irritability, fatigue, exhaustion, hunger, nervousness, and headaches. The symptoms became worse as the morning went on.

A breakfast of two donuts and coffee with cream and sugar caused a temporary rise in blood sugar, which fell to a low level after an hour. At that point, fatigue and inefficiency set in.

Then, a basic breakfast was selected: a glass of orange juice, two strips of bacon, toast with jam, and coffee with cream and sugar. The blood sugar rose rapidly at first, but then fell far below the pre-breakfast level within an hour and remained below normal until lunch time. When this same basic breakfast was served with oatmeal and sugar and milk, the blood sugar rose more rapidly, but also fell more quickly and to a lower level than after any other breakfast studied.

When the volunteers drank 8 ounces of whole milk fortified with 2.5 tablespoons of powdered skimmed milk, in addition to eating their basic breakfast of juice, bacon, toast, jam, and coffee, their blood sugar rose above normal and stayed around 120 milligrams throughout the morning. A feeling of unusual well-being was experienced.

When two eggs were served instead of the fortified milk, a high level of efficiency was maintained all morning.

All volunteers were given the same lunch, and blood samples continued to be taken at hourly intervals throughout the afternoon. In all cases the blood sugar increased soon after lunch. The subjects who had eaten eggs or fortified milk for breakfast showed high blood sugar all afternoon. They were able to work efficiently for the rest of the day. When the breakfast had allowed blood sugar to be low during the morning, the increase after lunch to a level of cheerfulness and efficiency lasted only a little while; then it fell to a low level which lasted throughout the afternoon.

The selection of a proper breakfast may prevent fatigue. *Going off to school or work without an adequate protein breakfast can affect your whole day.* The typical American breakfast of cereal, hotcakes, waffles, or coffee cake (all starches that turn to sugar rapidly) sets you up for a letdown. If you take time to understand the protein content of foods, you can prevent many of the health problems of today. Helpful suggestions for balanced meals can be found in Appendix A.

Breaking with Tradition

The warning has been sounded. Will you heed it?

My philosophy as a mother of four children was not denial but substitution. I made our own Easter candy. Each holiday or event was treated differently.

You, too, can learn to make great substitutes. You can learn how to make desserts or candies that actually build health because they are so loaded with natural foods. You can experiment in your kitchen. And don't be afraid to fail.

Buy a few good health-food cookbooks. One way to tell if it is a good book is to check the sugar content of the recipes. If they often say, "Add 2 cups of sugar," then don't buy that book. We should not bake desserts that need that much sweetening. But don't try to convert your old white flour, white sugar, and white fat recipes. Rather, start all over. You can find new recipe books on the market that avoid those products.

Finally, let your children have fun experimenting in the kitchen. Teach them how to avoid white sugar products, and inform them early in life of the impact on their health from different foods and drinks that are loaded with sugar.

**Guide to the Selection of Foods for the Maintenance of
Proper Blood Sugar Levels**

Complete Proteins (1)	*Percent of Carbohydrates (Approx.)*			
	5% (2)	10% (3)	15 – 20% (4)	50 – 100% (5)
Certified raw milk	Artichokes	Apples	Apricots	Alcohol
Fertile eggs	Asparagus	Beets	Bananas	Cakes
Fish	Avocados	Blackberries	Beans	Candied dried
Lean meat	Beans	Carrots (old)	lima	fruits
Plain yogurt	green	Cranberries	kidney	Candies
Poultry	soy	Currants	navy	Chocolate
Protein powder	sprouts	Gooseberries	Blueberries	Cigarettes
Serenity Cocktail	wax	Grapefruit	Cherries	Cocoa
Unprocessed cheeses	Beets	Limes	(sweet)	Coffee
	Broccoli	Onions	Corn	Cola beverages
	Brussel	Oranges	Figs	Cookies
	sprouts	Peaches	Grape juice	Corn syrup
	Cabbage	Rutabagas	Grapes	Donuts
	Carrots	Squash	Huckleberries	Drinks made with
	(young)	Tangerines	Loganberries	sugar, corn
	Cauliflower	Turnips	Mulberries	syrup, and
	Celery		Parsnips	glucose
	Chard		Pears	Fruits—canned
	Collards		Peas	and preserved
	Cucumbers		Pineapple	with added
	Eggplant		Plums	sugar
	Greens		Potatoes	Gelatin desserts
	Leeks		Prunes	made with
	Lemons		Raspberries	sugar
	Lettuce		Rice	Honey
	Melons		Yams	Ice cream
	honeydew			Jams
	muskmelon		**Other Foods**	Jellies
	watermelon			Macaroni
	Mushrooms		Almonds	Maple syrup
	Mustard greens		Brazil	Margarines
	Okra		nuts	(hardened
	Olives (ripe)		Cashews	fats)
	Peppers (green)		Chestnuts	Marmalades
	Pumpkin		Peanut butter	Pastries and pies
	Radishes		Peanuts	Pizza
	Rhubarb		Pecans	Popcorn
	Sauerkraut			Potato chips
	Spinach			Pretzels
	Strawberries			Puddings
	Tomatoes			Sherbet
	Watercress			Soft drinks
				Sugar
				Sweet rolls
				Syrups
				White flour and white sugar products

In order to guide you in the selection of foods that will help maintain proper blood sugar levels, the previous chart is provided. It lists foods in the following five categories:

(1) Complete proteins that should ideally be included in every meal.
(2) Foods of relatively low carbohydrate content. These may be eaten in liberal quantities *provided* an animal protein food is included in the same meal.
(3) Foods of moderate carbohydrate content. The quantities of these foods should be limited.
(4) Foods in the high carbohydrate range. Persons sensitive to sugars and starches should use these in very limited amounts.
(5) The very high carbohydrate foods, the use of which is to be avoided.

Columns 1, 2, 3, and 4 are all valuable to the diabetic or hypoglycemic who does not have a weight problem. If you have a weight problem, you should consume these foods in limited quantities and avoid column 4 altogether. Column 5 should be avoided by all.

NOTES

1. E. Cheraskin, M.D., and Dr. W. M. Ringsdorf, Jr., M.D., *Psychodietetics* (New York: Stein & Day, 1974), p. 157.
2. Carlton Fredericks, Ph.D., *Low Blood Sugar and You* (New York: Grossett & Dunlap, 1969), p. 20.
3. Paavo Airola, "What Is Hypoglycemia? Part Two, The Symptoms," *Let's LIVE,* April 1977, p. 84.
4. Broda O. Barnes and Charlotte W. Barnes, *Hope for Hypoglycemia* (Fort Collins, Col.: Robinson Press, 1978), p. 9.
5. J. L. Rodale, *Natural Health, Sugar and the Criminal Mind* (New York: Pyramid Books, 1968), p. 13.
6. Robert C. Atkins, M.D., *Dr. Atkins' Nutrition Breakthrough* (New York: Morrow, 1981), p. 195.
7. Ibid., pp. 195–196.
8. Jeffrey Bland, Ph.D., *Your Health Under Seige* (Brattleboro, Vermont: The Stephen Greene Press, 1980), p. 162.
9. "Hypomagnesaemia and Diabetic Retinopathy," *The Lancet,* April 7, 1979, p. 762.
10. Ibid.
11. Irwin Stone, *The Healing Factor* (New York: Grossett & Dunlap, 1972), p. 147.
12. E. Orent-Keiles and L. F. Hallman, "The Breakfast Meal in Relation to Blood Sugar Values," U.S. Department of Agriculture Circular no. 827 (1949).

✄ 6. The Protein Story

There is one certainty: You will never know optimal health
if your need for amino acids is not met in full.
—CARLTON FREDERICKS

People often say, "I'm bewildered by all I read and hear. Should I be on a high protein diet or on the high complex-carbohydrate diet I hear so much about. And should I eat vegetable or animal protein, or both?"

Anyone who has heard Gladys Lindberg speak knows that she believes protein to be the primary dietary requirement. When protein is eaten, your digestive processes break it down into amino acids, which pass into the blood and are carried throughout the body. Your cells can then select the amino acids they need for the construction of new body tissue, antibodies, hormones, enzymes, and blood cells. Thus an understanding of how much and what kind of protein you need requires some knowledge of the essential amino acids.

Getting the Amino Acids You Need

The amino acids are like the letters of the alphabet. The essential amino acids are like the vowels. Just as you cannot make words without vowels, so you cannot build proteins without essential amino acids.

It is generally accepted that there are twenty-two or twenty-three amino acids, some of which can be made by your body. For years, eight of these amino acids were considered *essential*—that is, you *must* get them from the food you eat because your body cannot manufacture them. Most authorities agree that the following eight are those that are *essential* to growth and repair: isoleucine, leucine, lysine, methionine, phenylalanine, threonine, tryptophane, and valine.

However, when missionary groups went into Africa to help feed the malnourished children in Biafra, studies revealed that these children needed at least two additional amino acids, histidine and arginine. Children usually cannot produce these in sufficient amounts quickly enough to provide for growth or emergency healing. The Biafran children could not gain weight until these two amino acids were added to their diet.

The term *nonessential,* applied to the other amino acids, simply means that you don't have to get them from food; they can be synthesized within the body itself.

The Three Protein Groups

GROUP I:

Animal Proteins. These are complete; they contain all the essential amino acids in adequate amounts.

Sources:

Eggs

Milk and milk products (unprocessed natural cheese)

Meat (liver and other glandular meats, beef, lamb, veal, pork)

Seafood (shellfish)

Fowl (chicken, turkey, etc.)

GROUP II:

Partially Complete Vegetable Proteins. These are partially complete; while they do contain all the essential amino acids, some are present in inadequate amounts.

Sources:

Brewer's yeast

Wheat germ

Soybeans

Nuts and seeds

(Although these foods may contain inadequate amounts of certain essential amino acids, they are rich sources of other amino acids. For that reason, they have an important place in the diet. They may be combined with complete animal proteins or the incomplete vegetable proteins to balance the amino acids.)

GROUP III:

Incomplete Vegetable Proteins. These are incomplete; they may be entirely lacking in certain essential amino acids or may contain them in such small quantities that their biological value is negligible.

Sources:

Beans

Peas

Lentils

Unrefined grains and cereals (corn, wheat, oats, rice)

(These are generally less expensive foods. Unfortunately, they alone will not support life, growth, or reproduction. They must be combined or ingested with the Group 1 or Group 2 proteins.)

Note: The foods listed in this chart are grouped according to their biological value from the standpoint of their protein content. *Biological value* refers to the *quality* and *quantity* of the amino acids as they occur in foods.

If one essential amino acid is low, all of the others are reduced to the same low proportion. For example, if you eat a food containing 100 percent of your lysine requirement but only 20 percent of your methionine requirement, only 20 percent of the protein in that food will be used as protein by the body. The rest will be used as fuel rather than for replenishing or building tissue. With a diet inadequate in amino acids, the body will eventually be forced to rob amino acids from its own tissues.

Your body reacts to the total lack of an essential amino acid as if *all* the amino acids were missing by going into what is called "negative nitrogen balance"; more nitrogen is excreted than is ingested.

Three Protein Classifications

Incomplete proteins are those lacking one or more of the essential amino acids; these are plant proteins. Complete proteins contain all of the essential amino acids; these are animal proteins. Bear in mind that the body should have all of the eight essential amino acids at the same meal to do its job of building and repair.

We have found it helpful to divide these two kinds of proteins into three groups: complete animal proteins, partially complete vegetable proteins, and incomplete vegetable proteins.

GROUP I: SOURCES OF ANIMAL PROTEIN *Eggs,* not meat, are considered the ideal protein food and are frequently used as the model for measuring amino acids. This should come as no surprise, since eggs contain everything needed to promote life. We recommend fertile eggs.

It is unfortunate that the cholesterol controversy has scared people away from eggs. Although it is true that eggs contain cholesterol, they also contain lecithin, which is also manufactured by the body and helps keep cholesterol emulsified.

Milk follows eggs in protein value. A quart of milk, or four glasses, provides 32 grams of protein. Drink plenty of certified raw milk and use other milk products (cottage cheese, cheese, yogurt, kefir, buttermilk) regularly. Powdered skim milk is an especially rich source of the amino acid methionine, a shortage of which may result in loss of energy, depression, and hair loss. Use natural products whenever possible—for example, cheese without fillers, colors, or extenders. Read labels.

Although *meat, seafood, and fowl* generally supply more protein by weight than eggs or milk, the value is not as high, because the amino acids are not in the optimal parallel quantity ranges. Seafood is slightly superior to meat in the value of protein, the ratios between the essential amino acids being better than in meats.

Highly marbled fat in steaks and roasts is not desirable, of course, nor is meat to which hormones and chemicals have been added. As a nation we need to start demanding sources of uncontaminated, untreated, quality range-fed beef. When enough people ask for this, it will become available.

When buying chicken, try to learn the supplier's source. It may be possible to find a supplier who can assure you that no chemicals have been used in the fattening of the fowl.

GROUP II: SOURCES OF PARTIALLY COMPLETE VEGETABLE PROTEINS   *Soybeans* have the highest protein value in this group. The only legume that is a complete protein, soybeans contain all of the essential amino acids. Their value is diminished slightly because of their short supply of the amino acids methionine and tryptophane. (Actually, tryptophane is not an easy amino acid to get; richest sources are dark leafy greens, eggs, milk, yogurt, soybeans, seeds, and nuts. It seems to be nature's weapon against depression and sleeplessness as it works in the brain and throughout the central nervous system. Much significant research has been done proving its merits as an antianxiety agent; in fact, people severe stress have benefited from taking L-Tryptophane in tablet form. Tryptophane is also involved in the production of niacin, a lack of which is associated with skin problems, digestive upsets, and nervous conditions.)

As meat becomes more expensive, it is important that we learn about the versatile soybean and its many uses, and begin to combine it with other foods to complement and increase their protein value.

Brewer's yeast and wheat germ are higher in protein value than most other vegetable or plant foods. It can be added to beverages or included in cooking. If a fortified protein drink such as the Serenity Cocktail, which includes brewer's yeast, is taken, you are assured of getting the right ratios of amino acids as well as other vital nutrients. Unfortunately, yeast and wheat germ are extremely high in phosphorus but low in calcium, so if you add brewer's yeast or wheat germ to your diet, be sure to add another source of calcium.

Many people consider *peanut butter* a complete protein, but we disagree. It is a vegetable protein low in methionine. If you add one-eighth cup peanut oil (no substitutes: if you use another kind of oil you lose the peanut butter taste) and non-instant powdered skim milk to one pound of nonhydrogenated peanut butter (no sugar added), you will have a complete protein equivalent to that found in meat. (Mix the peanut oil and the peanut butter well; then add powdered milk as needed to return the mixture to peanut butter consistency.)

GROUP III: INCOMPLETE VEGETABLE PROTEINS All *seeds, grains, and nuts* are incomplete proteins, although raw cashews and sunflower seeds are high in certain amino acids. The important point to remember is that these foods must be used in combination with other foods of high protein value.

Vegetables are on the bottom of the scale for protein value. To make up for their amino acid deficiencies, combine them with dairy products or nuts and seeds. For example, cauliflower and broccoli with sesame seeds and Brazil nuts, topped with a cheese or egg sauce, is a complementary combination.

Vegetarians must be especially careful to achieve the needed balance of amino acids by eating plenty of eggs, cheese, and milk. These foods are not part of a strict vegetarian diet, but we feel that you need to compromise to this extent if you want to stay healthy on a no animal product diet. See the following chart for suggestions on how best to combine foods to achieve complete proteins without meat, fish, or fowl.

Formula for Combining Amino Acids

Milk completes the amino acids when combined with:
  Grains (corn and soy; rice; wheat)
  Nuts and seeds
  Legumes (beans, etc.)
  Potatoes
Nuts and seeds complete the amino acids when combined with:
  Legumes
  Dairy products
  Grains
Legumes complete the amino acids when combined with:
  Rice
  Corn
  Wheat
  Nuts and seeds
  Dairy products

If you decide to be a total vegetarian, the advice of the Food and Drug Administration should be considered:

Select from a wide variety of plants to ensure that you are getting the amount and quality of protein you need. You also need to take vitamin B-12 as a dietary supplement, because plant foods contain only traces of this vitamin. The inclusion of even small amounts of milk, cheese and eggs makes it simpler to select a diet that is adequate in both quantity and quality of protein.[1]

Most cultural groups, primitive and modern, mix proteins, a wise practice that has been handed down from generation to generation. Mexicans, for example, eat corn tortillas and beans; the combination makes a complete protein. They also eat cheese, eggs, chicken, and some beef. The Orientals eat rice with soy, bean sprouts, and crisp vegetables, as well as fish and many products from the sea, chicken, and eggs.

Dr. Weston Price observed:

During these investigations of primitive races, I have been impressed with the superior quality of the human stock developed by Nature wherever a liberal source of sea foods existed . . . As yet I have not found a single group of primitive racial stock which was building and maintaining excellent bodies by living entirely on plant foods. I have found in many parts of the world most devout representatives of modern ethical systems advocating the restriction of foods to the vegetable products. In every instance where the groups involved had been long under this teaching, I found evidence of degeneration in the form of dental caries, and in the new generation in the form of abnormal dental arches to an extent very much higher than in the primitive groups who were not under this influence.[2]

In other words, primitives always seem to consume some form of animal protein (for example, insects, fish eggs, or sea foods).

Common Results of Protein Deficiency

What happens if you ignore your need for protein? Problems can range from the relatively simple—nail and hair problems, for example—to backaches, bursitis, and neuritis. A protein deficiency robs the basic component of your body—your cells—of the food they need to grow and thrive.

"Every human being begins life as a single cell, a fertilized egg; by the time he reaches adulthood, his body consists of 100 trillion cells. The cell is the fundamental component of all living things. As cells deteriorate, people age. As cells malfunction, people get sick. If cells were better understood, people might live longer and stay healthier."[3]

When you have unhealthy cells, cells that are missing the essential amino acids, the body will "cement" you together with scar tissue. That scar tissue appears in your eyes as *cataracts;* in your lungs as *emphysema;* in your liver as *cirrhosis;* in your kidneys as *nephrosis;* in your arteries as *arteriosclerosis;* in your nerves as *multiple sclerosis;* and in your brain as *senility* (when it obstructs the flow of oxygen to the brain). Usually vitamin and mineral deficiencies go hand in hand with protein deficiency, but this state is preventable, and often reversible, if we give our bodies *all* the nutrients it needs.

Protein is what every living cell in your body is made of. Furthermore, every cell must have a continuous supply of protein to maintain its life. Proteins are often referred to as the building blocks of the body, necessary for tissue repair and the construction of new tissue. Your muscles, hair, nails, skin, and eyes are made of protein; so are the cells that make up the liver, kidneys, heart, lungs, nerves, brain, and even your sex glands. The hormones secreted from the various glands—thyroxin from the thyroid, pancreatin from the pancreas, and a variety of hormones from the pituitary—as well as the soft tissues (such as the intestinal mucous membrane), hard-working major organs (like the liver, heart, and kidneys), and muscles are the most active protein users, and they have the richest stores of protein.

Next to water, protein is the most plentiful substance in your body. If all the water were squeezed out of you, about half your dry weight would be protein. About a third of this protein is in your muscles, a fifth in your bones and cartilage, a tenth in your skin, and the rest in your other tissues and body fluids.

FATIGUE Red blood cells must have protein to be replenished. Hemoglobin, the iron-containing material in red blood cells, is a protein (95%) molecule. Anemia results because of a lack of these red blood cells, which carry oxygen throughout the body.

Low blood pressure can also result when proteins are undersupplied. Your blood vessels are lined with little rings of muscles lying side by side. These tiny muscles can lose their tone and strength, and enlarge or stretch. When this condition exists, the blood vessel loses its "push" and the blood pressure drops.

Under normal conditions, if the diet is supplied with good-quality protein, the blood pressure remains normal. More red blood cells and energy-releasing enzymes are produced, and you feel vigorous.

Mother sees people every day who look and act very fatigued

and ill. When an adequate protein diet replaces their low-protein diet, these people start feeling wonderful. When their cells receive the nutrients they need, the result is increased energy.

SUSCEPTIBILITY TO INFECTIONS AND VIRUSES   A protein-deficient diet accounts for susceptibility to infections and viruses. All of our enzymes, the antibodies that are the white blood cells, the lymph cells, and everything our bodies use to fight infections are made out of protein. If you do not get enough protein, few bacteria-fighting cells can be produced. And remember, a vitamin C deficiency usually accompanies viral and infectious diseases, too.

Egg yolk, meat, milk, liver, and yeast have been shown to have the ability to build up your body's defenses. Changing from an inadequate protein diet to a good protein diet can greatly increase the amount of antibodies you produce.[4]

POOR HEALING   Wounds, cuts, burns, and bruises heal very slowly when protein intake is inadequate or poorly balanced. Sometimes a wound will pull apart and fill with scar tissue (an adhesion). If adhesions after an operation are severe, further surgery may be required to remove them.

POOR DIGESTION AND ELIMINATION   Sometimes people tell Mother they have trouble digesting protein. Protein is not normally assimilated if the stomach is not secreting hydrochloric acid. This is why Mother suggests almost everyone past the age of forty take hydrochloric acid tablets when they complain of indigestion. Because our digestive enzymes are largely protein, the body actually stops producing hydrochloric acid when a protein deficiency exists.

Daily Protein Requirements

Your Ideal Weight	Grams of Protein Needed
*Boys and girls through the age of twenty**	
29 lbs.	20 grams
44 lbs.	30 grams
59 lbs.	40 grams
74 lbs.	50 grams
88 lbs.	60 grams
103 lbs.	70 grams
118 lbs.	80 grams
132 lbs.	90 grams
147 lbs.	100 grams
162 lbs.	110 grams
176 lbs.	120 grams
191 lbs.	130 grams

* The usual recommendation for this age group is 1.3–1.5 grams of protein per kilogram (2.2 lbs.) of ideal body weight.[5] Our calculations are based on 1.5 grams.

Daily Protein Requirements

Your Ideal Weight	*Grams of Protein Needed*
Men and women over the age of 20*	
89 lbs.	40 grams
111 lbs.	50 grams
133 lbs.	60 grams
156 lbs.	70 grams
178 lbs.	80 grams
200 lbs.	90 grams
222 lbs.	100 grams
244 lbs.	110 grams

*Our calculations for this age group are based on the usual recommendation of 1 gram per kilogram (2.2 lbs.) of ideal body weight.[6] However, adding 10 grams of protein to the above recommendation as a safety margin will ensure your getting enough protein. Nursing mothers should add 40 grams of protein to the above recommendation.

LACK OF MUSCLE TONE   The walls of the stomach and the small and large intestines are made of circular muscles. Strength in these muscles is maintained when the diet supplies *all* the essential amino acids. When muscle contractions are weak, the food is not mixed well with digestive juices and enzymes; food is left undigested and the bowel becomes sluggish. This may lead to poor elimination. However, protein and B-vitamins in particular will strengthen those muscles.

There are other muscles that can suffer from a protein deficiency. Most of us, at one time, have been ill and experienced weight loss because we did not feel like eating. Usually that weight loss is a result of living for a while on our own muscle, which is protein. The body cannibalizes itself. Then when we feel our arms and legs, they may seem to be soft and flabby. If we are eating good-quality protein, if our bodies are digesting the protein properly, and if we are getting some exercise, our arms and legs should be firm. Parents should check the arms and legs of their children for muscle tone.

EXCESSIVE WATER RETENTION   Here is a protein deficiency that you should be able to observe in yourself. If you wake up in the morning and your eyes are puffy, or if you go to bed at night and find that your ankles feel swollen, you have an indication of water retention. This can be the result of a protein deficiency.

With your hand, squeeze your leg above the ankle. If the squeeze leaves an indentation, you may have edema (water retention). This is one of the ways a doctor checks pregnant women to see if they are getting enough protein. Although fluid retention is most common among pregnant women and elderly people, anyone who is careless about the choice of foods and fails to get complete proteins can have this problem. Learn to count your grams of protein daily.

If you have been retaining fluids due to an inadequacy of protein in your diet, you may actually lose weight on a high-protein diet, due to initial water loss.

POOR NAILS   Women frequently complain to Mother about their nails breaking, cracking, and peeling. Mother tells them that the body is a whole unit, and when something as visible as their nails exhibit problems, the source of the trouble is seldom where you can see it. Protein and calcium play an important role in nail health. The B-vitamins can also make a big difference in the quality and strength of your nails. Vitamins A and C, as well as minerals, including magnesium, have been shown to help nails. This nail condition may also indicate a thyroid deficiency.

Nail preparations and polishes formulated with protein are on the market, but any real change in the condition of the nails must come about as the result of a diet adequate in proteins.

LACKLUSTER HAIR   Everything we eat contributes to our internal cellular environment. Anything that doesn't help and benefit our bodies, day by day, is going to contribute to ill health. One of the first places you may notice deficiency symptoms is in the hair.

Hair products containing protein attract the buyer with problem hair. The hair does need protein for luster, growth, health, and beauty. But the benefits that hair products provide to the customer are temporary. Hair health comes from within. The secret of growing healthy hair lies in protein and the B-complex vitamins. Copper, zinc, and other elements also help promote hair health.

BONE FRACTURES   When we were born, our bones were mere gristle. As we grew older, minerals were laid down in our bones. If we have a severe protein deficiency, we lose the gristle and our bones become weakened. In that state they can fracture easily.

Another reason bones of the elderly break so readily is because these older people often do not have enough protein in their diets. They are also lacking in calcium. Many of them don't even drink milk, which provides both protein and calcium. Decalcified bones become porous, a condition known as osteoporosis. Such bones are so brittle that they can simply give way. Many elderly people who think they have broken a bone as the result of a fall have actually done just the opposite: a bone gave way, causing them to fall. Fractures in the elderly occur easily and they heal very slowly. A diet that is adequate in protein, calcium, phosphorus, and vitamin D is the best prevention and treatment for such brittle bones. Mother knew of one ninety-year-old woman with an unhealed broken hip. A new diet, rich in proteins, was tried, and she was soon on her feet. She stayed strong for five more years.

The need for first-class protein never diminishes; and it becomes doubly important as we get older. Ruth Weg, Ph.D., Associate Professor of Biology and Gerontology at the University of Southern California, came up with some significant findings. Older people require protein of higher quality, and they need the zinc that is found in animal protein. Their requirements for all nutrients are greater than when they were younger because, as Mother explains, their assimilation is poorer since they usually lack hydrochloric acid and digestive enzymes.

We found deficiencies and low levels of vitamins and minerals to be a serious problem for large numbers of the elderly. Inadequate intake, overprocessed foods, poorly balanced diets, drug-food interactions and/or digestive system disorders all contribute to the problem. Signs of malnutrition among the elderly manifest themselves as confusion, disorientation, insomnia, irritability, and loss of weight and appetite. The tissue changes that result culminate in illness, disease, and death.

The eating habits of many older people are quite alarming. Those who live alone rarely fix eggs or meat for themselves. They live on canned soups, canned fruits and vegetables, and bread. The average three and one-half ounce portion of soup contains, at the most, 3.5 grams of protein. Yet most elderly people don't even have milk to add to their can of soup. If you want to spare elderly parents or grandparents the agonies of broken bones and disease, one important thing you can do for them is keep them supplied with high-quality protein foods.

LIVER DAMAGE The liver has been called "the balance wheel of the body" because it performs so many important functions. It is the central clearinghouse for all unabsorbed nutrients, and it masterminds many of the body's metabolic processes. You do well to take good care of your liver; for if your liver fails to function, you are in serious trouble.

These are some of the functions of this vital organ: metabolizing carbohydrates, proteins, fats, and minerals; destroying harmful substances in the body; detoxifying drugs, poisons, chemicals, and toxins from bacterial infections; assisting with iron storage and the manufacture of the elements necessary for blood clotting; converting sugar into body starch (glycogen), storing it, and reconverting it to sugar when needed; and storing several trace minerals, vitamin A, and, to some extent, vitamins D, E, K and the B vitamins. To prevent liver damage must be a constant goal of good nutrition, since dietary sins harm the liver more than any other part of the body.

A low intake of proper protein can cause liver damage. Rats tested on a typical American diet—one high in refined carbohydrates and saturated fats, and deficient in magnesium—developed massive scar tissue in the liver. The damage was worse when the diet was also low in calcium, high in phosphorus, and when protein or the sulfur-containing amino acids, cystine and methionine, were undersupplied. When generous amounts of vitamin E were added, no scar tissue formed.[7] But when rats were kept on diets deficient in both protein and vitamin E, massive areas of cells died. Destruction of liver tissue, with resulting hemorrhage, allows the damaged areas to fill with scar tissue that is incapable of carrying on its cellular activity.[8]

"When diets are deficient in protein and choline, severe cirrhosis results quickly."[9] Excessive alcohol drinking causes the liver to swell and become fatty, resulting in cirrhosis. Choline aids in the decomposition of fat in the liver. Lecithin is a valuable source of choline, and eggs, which are a complete protein, are rich in lecithin.

The liver does have an amazing capacity to regenerate itself. If a rat is given an adequate diet and then two-thirds of its liver is cut away, the entire organ grows back within three weeks.[10]

Dr. Richard Kunin conducted a dietary survey among 132 of his patients. More than half of them were deficient in vitamin E, and a third of them were deficient in one or more of the B vitamins. Their deficiencies were considered serious. In addition, half of these patients were deficient in calcium, magnesium, and in the essential amino acid methionine. Ten percent were low in tryptophane and phenylaline, two other essential amino acids necessary for normal cell growth.[11] What is surprising about this is that these were patients who were nutrition-conscious, and they were in better shape than most people!

REPRODUCTIVE FAILURES The reproductive system is dependent on healthy tissues and normal glandular secretions and reactions. To function properly, male and female reproductive cells require certain amino acids. To say there is no life without protein is never more appropriate than when we consider the relationship of proteins to the reproductive system.

Many human studies strongly indicate that adequate protein (amino acid) nutrition, both prenatal and postnatal, is the prime factor in the birth of healthy, well-developed babies.[12] There is also evidence that one factor involved in reproductive failure is an inadequate nutritional environment furnished to the cells in the developing embryos.[13] While it is difficult to understand, it appears evident that a large segment of people in the United States live their lives on a scale of nutrition that could be rated no better than fair. Consequently, when they reproduce, there are many failures.[14]

MENTAL RETARDATION The effects of inadequate protein on the unborn child need to be emphasized. Mental retardation has been produced in rats by giving the pregnant mothers diets deficient in protein. Dietary deficiencies are more harmful in periods of greatest brain growth, and the earlier the deficiencies occur, the more damage takes place.[15] Later, when the brain is fully developed, it can withstand severe dietary deprivations, or even starvation, and will return to normal when the diet is improved.[16] Many other factors also play a role in retardation.

It is believed that deficiencies of high-quality protein cause the brain development of 70 percent of the world's children to remain subnormal. When infants are nursed, their brain development is generally more normal.[17] In developing countries, a child is taken off the breast when the mother has another child who needs to be nursed. The child who is no longer nursed then becomes underfed, particularly in all of the essential amino acids found in complete proteins, and becomes susceptible to many diseases. Mother urges pregnant women to be certain they are receiving 25 more grams of protein per day above what they would normally take. To nurse their babies, they will need still another 15 more grams per day—a total of 40 grams above their normal requirements. One reason many women cannot nurse their babies could be because they have not received enough protein.

Even if a baby is born bright, the brain can be damaged by an inadequate diet at any time during the child's first four years and especially during the first six months after birth. If a child's diet has been low only in calories, the brain will remain normal though small, but if the diet has been deficient in complete proteins, the brain cells will be decreased in number and show numerous abnormalities.[18]

The work of psychologist Dr. Ruth Harrell has recently been recognized. In the 1930s she began working with people who had allegedly suffered brain damage in surgery. In trying to teach them to speak and write, she found that their skills improved when she put them on adequate diets. Then, as a rehabilitation psychologist in neurosurgery at Johns Hopkins Hospital, she worked with patients who had the left hemisphere of their brain removed because of cancer. They no longer recognized friends and family members even though they survived their operations. Again she applied her "magic" of six meals a day (including a mid-morning, mid-afternoon, and before-bed meal) of chicken breasts, chopped sirloin, melon, fruit, eggs, wheat toast, and fresh orange juice. In one group of 15 patients, all regained the use of their minds and their memories after 5 weeks of saturation feeding and were able to return to homes and jobs. Her high-protein diet had helped regenerate their brain-controlled functions.[19]

In recent years, research has vastly improved our knowledge of the importance of protein in the functioning of the whole body. We all ought to be eating foods that are high in complete proteins—eggs, cheese, milk, fish, poultry, lamb, and beef. We need to "bring our brains to the school of nutrition," to borrow the words of Dr. Lendon Smith. He claims, "No teacher should be required to teach a child who did not bring his brains to school. . . . Every morning each pupil should report what his breakfast contained. If he had no protein and ate mainly carbohydrates, he should be sent home."[20]

Protein Individuality

These protein requirement charts are to be used only as guidelines for determining your optimal amount of protein intake. You may need more; or you might be able to get by with slightly less.

If you are trying to build muscles, you will probably need more protein. If you are undergoing any type of stress or if you are ill, you need more protein, since the antibodies needed to fight infection are made of protein. If you don't eat many carbohydrates or fats, for fear of gaining weight, then you need more protein. This is because your body needs fuel, and if it does not get it from carbohydrates or fat, then it will convert up to 58 percent of your daily protein intake to sugar for fuel. Less protein is then available for tissue repair. For this reason, Mother always recommends that complex carbohydrates be eaten with protein so your body doesn't have to steal protein to make energy. Any excess protein the body receives will be converted to sugar (glycogen) and stored in the liver and muscles. (See table, pp. 66–67.)

Count Your Grams of Protein

Now that you know how much protein you need, make sure you eat the right foods every day to get that amount. The following protein chart lists grams of protein in common foods. Calories and grams of carbohydrates are also given, so that you can choose complete-protein foods and count calories or grams of carbohydrates if you tend to put on weight easily.

Calorie, Carbohydrate, and Protein Guide

	Measure	*Calories*	*Carbohydrates (in grams)*	*Proteins (in grams)*
DAIRY AND EGGS				
Cheese				
American, pasteurized processed	1 oz.	107	.5	6.5
Cheddar	1 oz.	112	.36	7
Cottage cheese, 4% fat				
large curd	1 cup	235	6	28
small curd	1 cup	220	6	26
Cream cheese	1 oz.	100	1	2
Monterey Jack	1 oz.	106	.2	7
Swiss	1 oz.	107	1	8
Cream				
Half and half	1 cup	315	10	7
Sour cream	1 cup	495	10	7
	1 tbsp.	25	1	trace
Whipping cream, heavy unwhipped	1 cup	820	7	5
Eggs				
Egg (raw)	1	82	.5	6
Scrambled or in omelet	2 eggs	190	2	12
Milk				
Buttermilk	1 cup	99	11.7	8.1
Goat	1 cup	168	10.9	8.7
Human	1 oz.	21	2.1	.3
Low-fat	1 cup	121	11.7	8.1
Whole	1 cup	159	11.4	8.5
Nonfat instant dried	1 cup	244	35.5	24

Calorie, Carbohydrate, and Protein Guide

	Measure	Calories	Carbohydrates (in grams)	Proteins (in grams)
Nonfat dried	1 cup	435	62.4	43.4
Yogurt				
Whole milk, plain	8 oz.	139	10.6	7.9
Low-fat, plain	8 oz.	144	16	12
Low-fat, fruit	8 oz.	225	42.3	10
Butter				
one cube	½ cup	815	1	trace
about ⅛ cube	1 tbsp.	100	trace	trace
FISH AND SHELLFISH				
Bass	4 oz.	118	0	21
Crabmeat, steamed	4 oz.	105	0.6	20
Fish sticks,	4 oz. or 4			
breaded	sticks	200	8	20
Halibut	4 oz.	113	0	24
Lobster	4 oz.	103	0.6	19
Salmon				
fresh	4 oz.	246	0	25
canned, pink	½ cup	155	0	22
Shrimp, fresh	4 oz.	103	1.7	20
Tuna				
canned in oil,				
drained	½ cup	157	0	23
canned in water	½ cup	127	0	28
MEAT AND POULTRY				
Beef				
Chuck roast	4 oz.	226	0	20
Ground beef, lean	4 oz.	203	0	23
Heart, beef, lean and				
braised	3 oz.	160	1.	27
Liver, beef, fried in				
butter	3 oz.	195	5	22
Steak, lean sirloin,				
T-bone, porterhouse				
or rib, broiled	4 oz.	462	0	25
Lamb				
Lamb chop, rib,				
broiled	3.1 oz.	360	0	18
Lamb leg, roasted	3 oz.	235	0	22
Pork				
Ham, light cure, lean,				
roasted	3 oz.	245	0	18
Luncheon meat/				
boiled ham	1 oz.	65	0	5
	1 slice			
Pork chop	3 oz.	310	0	21
Poultry				
Chicken breast, fried	2.8 oz.	160	1	26
Chicken livers,				
simmered	4 oz.	187	3	30
Drumstick, fried	1.3 oz.	90	0	12

Calorie, Carbohydrate, and Protein Guide

	Measure	Calories	Carbohydrates (in grams)	Proteins (in grams)
Half broiler, broiled	6.2 oz.	240	0	42
Turkey				
roasted dark meat	4 pieces	175	0	26
roasted light meat	2 pieces	150	0	28
chopped or diced	1 cup	265	0	44
Veal				
Cutlet, broiled	4 oz.	265	0	30
Roast, rump	4 oz.	267	0	31

SOURCES: John D. Kirschmann, director, *Nutrition Almanac* (New York: McGraw-Hill, 1979); Catherine F. Adams and Martha Richardson, *Nutritive Value of Foods* (Washington, D.C.: U.S. Department of Agriculture, 1978).

NOTES

1. John D. Kirschmann, director, *Nutrition Almanac* (New York: McGraw-Hill, 1979), p. 1.
2. Weston A. Price, D.D.S., *Nutrition and Physical Degeneration* (Los Angeles: The American Academy of Applied Nutrition, 1939), pp. 263, 279.
3. "The Secret of the Human Cell," *Newsweek,* August 20, 1979, p. 48.
4. Adelle Davis, *Let's Get Well* (New York: Harcourt, Brace & World, 1965), p. 143.
5. *Nutrition and the M.D.,* vol. 7, no. 8, August 1981.
6. Richard A. Kunin, M.D., *Mega Nutrition* (New York: McGraw-Hill, 1980), p. 267; Hans J. Kugler, M.D., *Dr. Kugler's Seven Keys to a Longer Life* (New York: Stein and Day, 1978), p. 46.
7. Adelle Davis, *Let's Get Well,* pp. 209–210.
8. Ibid., p. 210.
9. Ibid., p. 211.
10. Ibid., p. 211.
11. Kunin, *Mega Nutrition,* p. 11.
12. Roger J. Williams, *Nutrition Against Disease* (New York: Pitman Publishing, 1971), p. 58.
13. Ibid., p. 52.
14. Ibid., p. 53.
15. Adelle Davis, *Let's Have Healthy Children* (New York: Harcourt, Brace & World, 1951), p. 38.
16. Ibid.
17. Ibid., p. 40.
18. Ibid., pp. 40–41.
19. Lendon Smith, M.D., *Feed Your Kids Right* (New York: McGraw-Hill, 1979), p. 227.
20. From personal conversation with Ruth Harrell and tape of appearance on TV talk show, C.B.N. 700 Club, interview with Pat Robertson, April 22, 1981.

✌ 7. Protecting the Heart

It is just impossible to assess the damage done by the anti-cholesterol theory.

—DR. WILFRID E. SHUTE

If you have been hanging onto outdated information—to a large extent erroneously reported—warning of the ill effects of cholesterol, we want to help set the record straight. Cholesterol isn't going to kill you—not the kind of cholesterol that comes from eating sensibly as a part of a total nutrition program.

With heart disease, the best protection is prevention. You may not get another chance. And we believe that it's what you put in your mouth that makes the difference. All evidence points to this inescapable conclusion: good nutrition prevents cholesterol deposits from forming; and the rate of synthesis of cholesterol in the body is influenced by the available supply of cholesterol from the outside. Elevated cholesterol levels are a symptom—correct the problem, get at the cause, and your cholesterol and triglyceride levels can be brought under control.

You can't get away from cholesterol, no matter how hard you try. Your body manufactures it! You probably don't know that by avoiding cholesterol foods—eggs in particular—you may be denying yourself the very help you need to prevent or reverse artery problems.

Some Facts You Ought to Know

Here are some facts about cholesterol that you may not know:

- The body must have cholesterol in order to function properly, and to manufacture vital hormones and chemicals. Production of adrenal hormones (cortisone) and sex hormones (estrogen—female hormones; testosterone—male hormones), of bile and vitamin D, depends on cholesterol.
- Cholesterol makes up a large part of the brain and cell membranes.
- Your skin excretes excessive cholesterol by the normal

sloughing off of cells daily. The ultraviolet rays of the sun on exposed skin converts this cholesterol to vitamin D-3. Cholesterol is the protective, insoluble skin molecule that resists water and prevents maceration (the softening and wearing away in water).

- The body makes 80 percent of its cholesterol within the liver and intestines. It does not come from dietary cholesterol, but rather from other elements such as fat, protein, and certain forms of carbohydrates.
- High-density lipoproteins (HDLs) and low-density lipoproteins (LDLs) are packages of cholesterol released into the blood. LDLs are considered harmful and HDLs are considered helpful.
- Cholesterol serves as a conductor for the transmission of nerve impulses throughout the body.

Many outstanding researchers and doctors have pointed out that if you believe you can ward off death from heart disease by altering the amount of cholesterol in your blood, whether by diet or by drugs, you are following a regime that has no basis in fact.[1] The cholesterol theory has always had serious flaws, and knowledgeable researchers and doctors have been saying for years that implicating cholesterol in heart disease is wrong.[2]

Dr. Richard Passwater has made the observation that, "Although people insist on examining all the diets of the world looking for one component, such as cholesterol, to blame as a cause of heart disease, they would be doing better to look for the *absence* of one component, such as vitamin E. Just as it is dangerous to worry only about cholesterol, it is dangerous to worry only about vitamin E. Total nutrition—supernutrition—is the main concern. Without it, we are predisposed to premature heart disease."[3]

The Much-Maligned Egg

It seems incredible that eggs, the most perfect food that God put upon this earth, have taken the brunt of the cholesterol scare! So widespread has been the fear of cholesterol that rarely (if ever before) has any diet campaign approached the success with which the American public has been indoctrinated against eating cholesterol-containing foods, especially eggs. That fear has touched all age levels.

Mother tells of a young woman who phoned to discuss the

health of her son who wasn't growing properly. When asked about the child's eating habits and if he received eggs for breakfast, the young woman responded with surprise, "Of course not! I'm not going to give him cholesterol!"

Mothers are actually giving their babies skim milk formulas. The magnitude of misinformation that has been picked up by the public is alarming. But what is so tragic is that millions of Americans have deprived themselves of essential factors in their diets and become convinced that by avoiding eggs, meat, butter, and dairy products, and by concentrating on eating cereals, grains, margarine, and other "cholesterol-free" foods, they are reducing their chances of becoming victims of coronary heart disease. We are in agreement with Dr. Linus Pauling, who says, "We must educate people away from the dangerous idea that you can control heart disease by not eating foods such as eggs, butter, and milk. This oversimplified idea is totally wrong."[4]

Have you been pouring your eggs from a carton instead of cracking them from a shell—thinking that, by doing so, you were avoiding cholesterol? In trying to improve upon God's design and eating what man has manufactured in artificial eggs, you are loading your body with such flavor "preservers" as trisodium and triethyl citrate, such emulsifers as diglycerides and propylene glycol monostearate, cellulose and xanthan gums, aluminum sulfate, and artificial colors. Even if we could pronounce all those names and really knew what they meant, common sense should tell us that human industry couldn't possibly improve upon the natural, fertile egg.

Dr. Fred Kummerow, a leading biochemist at the University of Illinois, reported his findings to a Federal Trade Commission and sent shock waves throughout the processed food industry. He had been conducting experiments with the polyunsaturated margarines and egg substitutes and found them to be significantly less nutritious than natural butter and eggs. In fact, he reported, they might be a major contributor to heart disease and strokes.

In his experiment, Kummerow found that test rats on a diet of egg substitutes showed all the signs of acute malnutrition, including early death. Three separate groups of nursing rats had their diet of mother's milk supplemented by unlimited amounts of egg substitutes, standard lab chow, or whole eggs. "After one week, the rats on egg substitutes developed diarrhea. At three weeks the egg substitute diet rats weighed only half as much as the other two groups. After two more weeks all the rats were weaned, and four weeks later, all of the rats on the egg-substitute diet were dead."[5]

THE OUTSET OF THE CHOLESTEROL CONTROVERSY What really happened at the outset of the cholesterol controversy was that the American Heart Association and other organizations started recommending that the public avoid eating egg yolks and that the food industry minimize the egg yolk content of commercially prepared food. The egg fell from the good graces of millions. And all the research proving the value of eggs hasn't put the egg back where it belongs in the thinking and eating habits of vulnerable Americans. Why eggs? An egg contains 275 milligrams of cholesterol, but there are actually only 5.7 grams of fat in a medium-sized egg. And your body manufactures many times that amount of cholesterol daily for normal functioning, even if your intake is zero.[6] Eggs also contain the cholesterol-manager lecithin—about 1,700 milligrams per egg.

Carlton Fredericks, in commenting about this, wrote: "Despite all the hue and cry, the case against eggs—which is the case against cholesterol—is in no way proved."[7] He also observed that eggs are rich in the very type of fat that prevents cholesterol from working the mischief it is supposed to create in the arteries. Eggs are also rich in choline, inositol, pyridoxine (B-6), lecithin, and cystine. These nutrients have been used successfully in the medical treatment of hardening of the arteries.[8]

THE RUSSIAN RABBIT EXPERIMENT In 1906, a Russian physiologist, N. Anitschkow, conducted research in which he fed mature rabbits egg yolks. Many years later, Mother attended a meeting where a doctor told how he had duplicated the Russian research and produced hardening of the arteries in the test rabbits. Mother listened in amazement as he stated, "We've now found the cause of hardening of the arteries—we know that cholesterol and excess fat are the killers. Don't eat egg yolks; don't drink whole milk; don't use cream and butter; avoid all cheeses, except low-fat cottage cheese. . . ." Her reaction to this announcement was the following:

When I first heard about the Russian experiment, I knew what any farm boy knows—rabbits don't eat eggs! I recognized immediately that this didn't prove that eating eggs would produce atherosclerosis in humans. To give rabbits eggs, you have to put a tube down into their stomachs and then pour the egg yolks into the tube because rabbits won't eat eggs. There is nothing in their metabolism to handle eggs. Rabbits are complete vegetarians. If a man were to eat the equivalent of what was given to those rabbits, he'd have to consume sixty eggs a day for one year to develop the same degree of atherosclerosis.[9] The probability of anyone eating that quantity of eggs ... is beyond all sense of reason.

I met the doctor after that meeting and reminded him that our ancestors have been eating eggs, meat, and these other good foods for thousands and thousands of years and that the first mention of heart attacks in scientific literature was in 1896, the second in 1912, and the third in 1919. Now we know that coronary heart disease is the most common cause of death in our country: hundreds of thousands of people die of heart attacks each year. I told him I felt that required an explanation— to blame it on something that's *always* been a part of our diets didn't make sense to me, that it had to be something of more recent origin like the refining of flour, and the introduction into the diet of high-carbohydrate foods, sugar, and hydrogenated fats.

The doctor called what I was talking about "a primitive diet." I responded, "Yes, I'm teaching people how to eat a primitive diet. People are coming to my home so ill they could drop dead in my living room. They've heard of someone who's been helped, so they are coming to me to learn."

He responded quickly, "Oh, Mrs. Lindberg, you must keep these people under medical supervision."

I was able to tell him that by the time they came to me they were almost bankrupt with doctor bills. That they'd been dismissed by their doctor, or told to go see a psychiatrist. But I also told him that I always did tell people to be sure and stay in touch with their doctor.

"A FANTASTIC HUMAN EXPERIMENT" The doctor recognized immediately that (in his words) this was "a fantastic human experiment." He urged, "Send them to me. I won't charge them. I will medically supervise them while you tell them what to eat." I was thrilled with his offer and so were the people. He was able to give them the medical supervision I was not able to provide, and I was relieved to have his medical help for these people. He did have a real researcher's heart and was genuinely anxious to see people's health improved.

The results were visible as one after another continued on my "primitive diet." I sent the more difficult cases to the doctor and, true to his word, he took their blood cholesterol readings, electrocardiograms, and did their total blood chemistry work. Then he would say, "Now eat exactly as Mrs. Lindberg tells you to eat." He related their blood chemistry back to me. One month later they would go back to him and each time he was astonished. He would call me and excitedly say, "What do you attribute this to, Mrs. Lindberg? Their blood cholesterol has dropped."

I told the doctor that I had people eat five times a day, taking the fortified Serenity Cocktail between meals, and adding all the vitamins and minerals including lecithin, kelp, yeast, liver tablets or powder. This raised their metabolism and their thyroid gland functioned better. This was helping to bring their cholesterol level down. I said, "People get in trouble because they eat the wrong foods. They are eating too many refined foods—foods that contain few, if any, vitamins or minerals. These are lifeless foods. People on my diet get fertile eggs, certified raw whole milk, raw butter, fresh fruits and vegetables, with meat, fish or fowl. I have them trim all the excess fat off their meat. These are the foods our ancestors ate. I also talk to them about controlling the stress factors in their lives, and I tell them to do more walking for exercise."

Many years have passed since that conversation and working with that fine doctor who is now retired. But many people and researchers alike are always looking for one thing—the magic bullet—to cure disease. It's not that simple; it isn't one thing. It's a combination of many things that brings people's cholesterol down and makes them feel energetic as they regain their health. I have said it before, it bears repeating: The body is always trying to heal itself, but we must give it the right materials with which to work.

What You Need to Know to Protect Your Heart

Linus Pauling has noted that during the last decade it has become increasingly evident that the great hope of 25 years ago that heart disease could be controlled by limiting the intake of saturated fat (as in meat and butter) and cholesterol (in meat and eggs) and increasing that of unsaturated fat, especially polyunsaturated fat (margarine, certain vegetable oils) had failed.[10]

The words *saturated, unsaturated,* and *polyunsaturated* are descriptive terms. A saturated fat is a completely closed chemical entity; that is, because it contains sufficient chemical parts to make it stable—thus the term saturated—it does not easily react with other chemicals. *Unsaturated,* on the other hand, describes a compound that has some "loose-ends," elements that will easily combine with other chemicals to form new compounds. When unsaturated fats bond with nutrients in the body, they carry them to their destination through the miles of blood vessels, and also help in building cell structure.[11] Those fats that have many "loose-end elements" which combine with other chemicals are called polyunsaturated fats; they are even more "willing" to form new compounds than unsaturated fats.[12]

These so-called unstable compounds, the polyunsaturates, readily combine with oxygen, which turns them rancid. All fats will eventually turn rancid, but natural fats, in their natural state, contain anti-oxidants that delay the process. In the preparation of today's cooking and table oils, however, these anti-oxidants are destroyed. Rancid fat in the diet harms more than the palate; it contributes to destruction of the fat soluble vitamins. We should be very careful with our unsaturated, natural oils (everything from cooking oil to cod-liver oil), keeping them refrigerated at all times. Since vitamin E is an anti-oxidant, and therefore helps keep oils fresh, we recommend squeezing vitamin E capsules directly into cooking and table oils.

Hydrogenated Fats

Vegetable fats are generally liquid at room temperature, but commercial products such as margarine and cooking fat are converted to solids by forcing hydrogen through the fat in order to "saturate" it. This process was developed around the turn of the century to prevent rancidity (by preventing oxidation) and to make fats more useful in cooking by raising their melting point.[13] Those goals were accomplished, but with unforeseen effects: with the fat molecules saturated with hydrogen, the fat can no longer fulfill its duties inside the body.

After hearing about the detrimental effects of hydrogenated fats, including margarine, one enthusiastic customer went home, got out her can of a well-known brand of white solid fat (popularly used by homemakers for pie crusts), scooped its contents into a hole in the back yard, and covered it with dirt, vowing never again to use hydrogenated fats. Planting a tree ten years later, the woman and her husband cut into the long-buried fat. They were amazed to discover the fat just as they had buried it; it hadn't deteriorated, and the bugs hadn't eaten it. Can you imagine what that kind of fat does to your arteries? Is it any wonder we've had a heart disease epidemic in this country?

Dr. Fred A. Kummerow and his colleagues at the University of Illinois at Urbana reported the results of their studies on hydrogenated fats at a meeting of nutritionists and related scientists of the 1974 Federation of American Societies for Experimental Biology. Kummerow's findings suggested that a fat found in margarine presents a greater health risk than many cholesterol-rich foods. Newspapers carried their story under such titles as "Margarine Found Health Hazard." Too bad the story didn't make the front page.

The researchers fed different diets to four groups of swine for eight months. (Swine were used because the weight of the aorta and heart of a pig is comparable to that of a human, and because pigs are similar to humans in their response to cholesterol.) Kummerow concluded from autopsies on the research subjects that hydrogenated fat is more atherogenic (capable of causing atherosclerosis) than nutrients such as butter, egg yolks, or egg whites. Identical results were achieved when the experiment was repeated. The greatest degree of atherosclerosis was detected in the pigs fed a hydrogenated fat with their diet. Second was the group whose feed was supplemented with sugar. Almost negligible damage was found in the pigs fed butter, and they found the very least disease in the group fed egg yolks or egg whites with their standard diet.[14]

The controversy over saturated versus unsaturated fats is complicated by the fact that we need both. Actually, natural oils and fats contain both, in varying proportions:

Safflower oil	84% unsaturated	7% saturated
Soybean oil	70% unsaturated	14% saturated
Egg yolk	53% unsaturated	30% saturated
Butter	37% unsaturated	56% saturated
Milk	33% unsaturated	62% saturated

(Percentages do not equal 100 percent)[15]

These unsaturated and polyunsaturated fats are needed for cellular membrane health and the production of prostaglandins (hormone-like chemicals that regulate vital metabolic processes throughout the body). They are important to growth, maintenance of skin and hair (eczema and other rashes have been associated with a shortage of fat in the blood and have been corrected when oils were ingested), regulation of cholesterol metabolism, maintenance of reproductive functions, and to keep blood platelets from getting sticky.[16] Fats are also essential for the production and movement of bile, an important digestive "juice" produced from cholesterol by the liver and stored in the gall bladder. Good sources of unsaturated and polyunsaturated fats are these oils: soybean, linseed, peanut, safflower, corn, and sunflower oils, as well as some fats in seafood and fish (for example, cod liver oil). Unsaturated and polyunsaturated fats are vitally important as sources of vitamins A, D, and E.

Fats that are predominantly saturated are lard, butter, and

fats from all meats. Certified raw butter is the best natural saturated fat. If this is unobtainable where you are, then we suggest sweet butter, which can be found in most supermarkets. Many people believe they are saving money when they buy margarine instead of butter, since the price per pound is less. Actually, that saving is far offset by the possible cost to their health.

Unit for unit, the vitamin A found in butter is three times as effective as the vitamin A in fish liver oils. And the natural vitamin D in one pound of butter is equal to that found in ten quarts of milk. Butter is the most digestible and easily tolerated of all fats because it has free-floating globules and is easily acted upon by the body enzymes. Butter also contains vitamin E in sufficient quantities to prevent oxidation. Butter is one of the important foods that provides the raw materials for normal sexual development.

A nutritious blend of butter and oil can be made that will stretch your dollar, give you the consistency of butter, and increase the unsaturated fatty acid content of the butter. Whip 1 pound of softened certified raw butter or sweet butter with 1 cup of soy or safflower oil (cold-pressed). Add 200 units of Vitamin E, and sea salt or vegetable salt to taste. Whip these ingredients together until the mixture is fluffy. Refrigerate in a covered container, freezing unused amount in another container. (If you use nice-looking containers, the butter can go straight from the refrigerator to the table.) One tablespoon of lecithin granules can be added to increase the butter's nutritive value.

WHAT ARE THE DANGERS?   One obvious result of an overconsumption of oxidized polyunsaturated fats is the appearance of ceroid bodies (also known as liver spots or "clinkers"), brown pigmentation on the hands and face. Ceroid pigment is actually dead body cells, or waste products, of the chemical reaction following the oxidation of polyunsaturated fats. Vitamin E protects polyunsaturates from oxidizing.

Heating oils to the smoking point increases their capacity for harm. When the polyunsaturated fat or oil is heated, a chemical reaction causes the polyunsaturate to bond with the oxygen in the air to form varnish. Studies have shown that animals can suffer total intestinal obstruction from these heated polyunsaturates.[17]

"The longer a polyunsaturated fat or oil is heated, the more dangerous it becomes," observe nutritionists Dr. Edward Pinckney and Cathey Pinckney. "Think of this the next time you visit a commercial establishment that deep-fries its foods. Almost all of these food suppliers re-use their cooking oil. They only add new oil to the vat to maintain the proper cooking level, as the old oil is withdrawn on the foods that have been cooked."[18]

Out of curiosity, I went to a local fast-food restaurant and learned from its owner that the oil in the fish and french fry cookers was changed once a week, and that it was very expensive to do so. I also learned that their franchise owners plan to introduce a chemical to the oil so it only has to be changed once a month! Why not ask your local fast-food establishment how often they change their oil. Remember: it's the highly heated or re-used fats that cause the trouble.

In an experiment designed to assess the extent of the problem, one group of animals was fed heated polyunsaturates and another, heated butter. The animals fed the heated corn oil had a markedly lower growth rate, they developed diarrhea, and their fur became rough; all of them developed tumors, and only one of the original 96 survived the forty-month experiment. However, all the animals fed butter survived without developing any tumors.[19]

"Dr. Roslyn Alfin-Slater, of the University of California at Los Angeles, showed that the feeding of heated polyunsaturates interfered with the reproductive performance of animals. And, Dr. A. L. Tappel of the University of California at Davis has demonstrated testicle damage in animals fed excessive polyunsaturates, due to the high concentrations of polyunsaturates absorbed by these organs. Surprisingly, the amount of heated polyunsaturates that caused the damage rarely was more than 10 percent of the diet. In one particular study, when the amount was raised to 15 percent of the diet, all of the animals died within three weeks."[20]

Additionally, claims J. I. Rodale, noted nutritionist writer, "Highly heated fat has been shown by some of our most prominent researchers to be a likely cause of cancer."[21]

Vitamin E

Drs. Wilfrid and Evan Shute are recognized worldwide for achieving outstanding results with cardiac patients by using vitamin E (alpha tocopherol). The effectiveness of vitamin E has been attributed to several major points, each of which has been established and confirmed by the Shutes' and others' tests and the laboratory reports:

1. Alpha tocopherol is an antithrombin: it helps dissolve fresh clots and prevents their formation in arteries and veins. *2.* Alpha tocopherol is an antioxidant: it decreases the need for oxygen in the tissues and organs of the body. Megavitamin levels of vitamin C and trace levels of selenium also share this function. It improves the transportation of oxygen by the red blood cells. *3.* Alpha tocopherol restores capillary permeability. *4.* Alpha tocopherol helps to dilate the capillaries and therefore acts to facilitate the circulation of blood throughout the body. *5.* Alpha tocopherol steps up collateral circulation (new blood pathways) by reducing the tendency toward abnormal spasm and by enlarging the size of the collateral channels. *6.* It can help increase the power and activity of muscles such as the heart.[22]

Vitamin C

Vitamin E is an oil-soluble antioxidant, and vitamin C is a water-soluble antioxidant; they complement each other. More and more research points to atherosclerosis (fatty degeneration of the inner surfaces of the arteries) as a long-term deficiency of vitamin C. "Vitamin E favorably affects the results of blood-vessel narrowing, as does vitamin C to some degree. Together, these two vitamins reverse the basic pathology," according to Dr. Shute and other researchers.[23]

This confirms Mother's beliefs about the way atherosclerosis develops and what she has been telling people to do. She explains:

Atherosclerosis develops slowly through several stages, usually over a period of many years. I believe that it begins with little hemorrhages of the inner lining of the arteries (the intima), when there has been a vitamin C deficiency. Then, because of a vitamin E deficiency, scar tissue fills in. This is repeated again and again through the years. The cholesterol in the blood should be able to pass through the artery wall, but because of this buildup of scar tissue, it cannot. Finally, these fatty globules and crystals begin to harden with calcium on the inside of the arteries forming plaques with fibrous scars. They bulge out into the arterial passage and interfere with the flow of blood through the coronary arteries and to the heart.

The blood that is trying to pass through the arteries is sticky and tends to clump. For years I've been telling people that bioflavonoids prevent blood from getting sticky. By eating two oranges daily (all the pulp with the white rind, not just juice alone, which also has vitamin C), we can help prevent clumping.

Dr. Emil Ginter, Director of the Biochemical Department of the Research Institute of Human Nutrition in Bratislava,

Czechoslovakia, is credited with doing the greatest research linking vitamin C deficiency to plaque formation leading to atherosclerosis.

In his experiments, Dr. Ginter used guinea pigs since, like humans, they do not make their own vitamin C. Ginter's controlled experiments showed conclusively that the amount of cholesterol in the arterial plaques averaged 30 percent higher in the vitamin C-deficient group.[24]

Ginter's studies have been going on for years and have produced strong evidence showing that if enough vitamin C is present in the blood, there is plenty of the beneficial high-density lipoproteins (HDLs) to counteract the buildup of fatty deposits in the arteries. Ginter found that 300 milligrams of vitamin C daily substantially reduced serum cholesterol levels in individuals with high initial readings but had no effect on those with normal readings.[25]

Dr. Constance R. Leslie, a hematologist at Pinderfields General Hospital in Wakefield, England, reports that vitamin C "has a controlling influence on all the factors that become abnormal in atherosclerosis." She believes that vitamin C is not only responsible for transport of cholesterol to the liver, but that it further acts to lower triglyceride levels.[26]

Impressive research literature shows that "vitamin C and E reduce blood platelet adhesion—a very important discovery, since blood clotting is one of the causes of many heart attacks. British and Swedish scientists have reported that vitamin C does this by reducing the stickiness of the blood."[27]

"Simply put, coronary thrombosis strikes when two conditions occur at the same time: the first condition is a narrowed artery, the second is sticky blood."[28]

The B-Vitamins

Many researchers have shown, through carefully controlled experiments, that the B-complex vitamins are critical in avoiding heart disease. Pyridoxine (vitamin B-6) has been found to be deficient in atherosclerosis patients. This nutrient is considered probably the single most important member of the B-complex family because it is a vital part of the coenzyme that helps form lecithin in our bodies. And pyridoxine is one of the vitamins that is not added back to "enriched" flour. Dr. Roger Williams notes that pyridoxine is lacking not only in enriched flour, but also in heat-sterilized milk, canned evaporated milk, and heat-processed milk powders. Tests with experimental rats show that they cannot thrive on milk treated in this way. Williams states: "All of these considerations lead us to conclude that in order to prevent atherosclerosis and heart disease, the avoidance of B-6 deficiency has a very high priority."[29]

Niacin or niacinamide, vitamin B-12, choline, PABA, and inositol are other key members of the B-complex family of vitamins important in the prevention of heart disease. It is wise to remember that pyridoxine (B-6), like other members of the B-complex family, is used in the formation of coenzymes that metabolize not only the fat, but also the sugar in our diets. And since sugar has been implicated with increased blood levels of triglycerides and heart disease, you will want to protect your heart by making certain you are getting all the B-vitamins.

Dr. Passwater in pointing these things out emphasizes the advantages of taking extra choline daily: "Heart disease is such a killer that sometimes it is advisable to forget scientific conservatism and go a little overboard just to be sure. One of the better sources of choline (which is used in making lecithin in your body) is lecithin itself.

LECITHIN   Lecithin is like a detergent, for it keeps cholesterol soluble in the blood. . . ."[30]

He shows that another important component of lecithin is linoleic acid, an essential polyunsaturated fatty acid. "The best sources of linoleic acid are wheat germ oil, whole milk, nuts, seeds, eggs, soybeans, and, of course, lecithin itself."[31] *Lecithin* comes from the Greek word *lekithos,* meaning "egg yolk," which, with soybeans, is one of its richest sources. But your body can only produce as much lecithin as you have available components and coenzymes to form whole lecithin molecules. According to Passwater, one of the problems with drinking skim milk is that the linoleic acid has been removed. Furthermore, skim milk does not contain the cholesterol needed by infants to make myelin sheaths for nerve fibers. Nature has always provided ample lecithin in the same foods that contain cholesterol, which may partly account for the reason that eating high-cholesterol foods has not been found to cause heart disease.[32] Lecithin also increases the capacity of bile salts to remove cholesterol.

More information on the value of lecithin reaches the nutrition magazines each month. Dr. Lester M. Morrison, M.D., D.Sc., a good friend of Mother's, published a classic study in 1958 on the value of lecithin. He was looking for a harmless natural alternative to the various drugs traditionally used to lower cholesterol levels, a natural food product that would be valuable both in treatment and prevention of excessive blood fats associated with atherosclerosis.

Dr. Morrison studied a group of patients with high cholesterol who had not responded to the usual methods of treatment. For at least a year, these patients had eaten fat-restricted diets, but did not take lecithin. Their cholesterol levels did not decrease despite these low-fat meals and cholesterol-lowering drugs. All his patients remained on the low-fat diet but added two tablespoons of lecithin three times each day to their diet. "After three months, twelve out of fifteen patients had experienced striking reductions in the levels of cholesterol in their blood. Even when the three patients who did not react to the lecithin were included in the results, the average fall in cholesterol was 30 percent."[33]

The commercial lecithin used in this study is a bland, water-soluble, granular powder made from refined soybeans. It is a natural phosphatide, an essential constituent of all living cells, and it appears to be vital to the normal functioning of body cells.

Dr. Morrison says, "The action of lecithin is noticeably different from that of other cholesterol lowering agents which owe their effect to 'blocking' the absorption of cholesterol and possibly essential fatty acids. Lecithin appears to enhance fat metabolism and lipid transport. As a phosphatide, lecithin is an important constituent of the blood lipoproteins. These phosphatides in the blood are the essential stabilizing agents of the fats."[34]

Since 1950, a number of researchers have reported that people with high blood levels of a *certain kind* of fat did *not* get heart attacks. In fact, this fat, a kind of cholesterol, is so good for you that it greatly diminishes your chances of having a heart attack. It is a fat-protein combination referred to as high-density lipoproteins (HDLs).

In contrast, research reveals that people with high levels of another fat-protein combination called low-density lipoproteins (LDLs) were almost certain to have heart attacks. It is postulated that HDLs help protect against heart attack in two ways. They appear to interfere with the cells' ability to take in unwanted LDLs, thus stopping the buildup of fatty deposits that can cause atherosclerosis and heart attacks. And the necessary HDLs aid the body in excreting excess cholesterol.[35]

You may ask, "Who has the good HDLs and who doesn't? And

if I don't have them, how can I get them?" Unfortunately, there are no precise answers for these questions. The best that doctors can currently do is to give a test that measures HDLs and LDLs. Dr. William P. Castelli, Director of Laboratories for the Framingham group, says that these tests, combined with good, early intervention, could help prevent or delay a heart attack in people shown to be at risk.[36] Women generally have higher levels of the beneficial HDLs than men, and this may account for the lower incidence of heart attacks among women.

There are a couple of factors that do seem to predispose one to the unwanted LDLs—smoking and lack of exercise. A healthy life-style balances work with play, exercise with rest. Excessive dietary sugar consumption is likely to bring about the wrong kind of lipoproteins in the blood—that is, less of the helpful HDLs and more of the harmful LDLs. This same expert mentioned exercise as being helpful and pointed to evidence showing that joggers and athletes who exercise vigorously every day have high levels of the good HDL.

H. Loomis, writing in *Science,* described the HDLs as a garbage collector that sweeps up arterial cholesterol and takes it to the liver where it can be cleared from the body in the form of bile, which is lost in the feces.[37]

About Triglycerides

Whenever cholesterol is discussed, knowledgeable people will also talk about triglycerides (neutral fatty substances found in the blood and fat cells). It is generally thought that triglycerides may be as important as cholesterol in the matter of heart disease.

Blood triglyceride levels increase when you eat refined carbohydrates. Read that statement again. Did it mention eggs, meat, or any of the other foods commonly associated with cholesterol? No, triglyceride levels increase when you eat refined carbohydrates, and this is a very interesting fact in any discussion of what *really* may cause heart disease and the buildup of plaque in your arteries.

We believe this helps explain why an overweight person who consumes a lot of refined carbohydrates runs the risk of heart disease. Not only does the added weight place a strain on his heart, but the triglycerides contribute to the plaque formation in the intima (the lining) of the arteries, a condition which can result in atherosclerosis. So, while cholesterol has received all the blame for this condition, several other substances are involved, including triglycerides.

Many authorities, including Dr. John Yudkin, author of *Sweet and Dangerous,* state that triglyceride levels are an important factor in predicting the likelihood of an individual developing heart attacks.[38] They also state that both triglyceride and cholesterol levels contribute to heart disease potential—however, you must bear in mind, whenever cholesterol *is* implicated in heart disease, it is cholesterol of a certain type of fat, namely LDLs.

Blood Cholesterol Levels

Lipid (fat) patterns vary from person to person, so you must find out from your doctor what your particular lipid profile pattern is. This profile reports the results of tests for cholesterol, triglyceride, HDLs, and LDLs. The person with high triglyceride levels (say, 250) would have a dramatic lowering of his readings on a low-carbohydrate diet. (A normal reading is 100.)

Blood-serum cholesterol levels vary, too. A "normal" level may vary between 150 and 300, 150 and 250, or 150 and 280 mg% (mg. of cholesterol per 100 mls. of blood), depending upon the textbook you check or the institution with which you confer. "People under stress have shown normal variances in their cholesterol of 10 to 20 percent. A normal, "average" male may have a serum cholesterol of 200 mg% one day and 240 mg% the next. The 40-point difference would not reflect a worsening condition; simply the average normal range for that individual during stress. One is just as likely to have heart disease without high serum cholesterol as with it."[39] Some researchers have shown that cholesterol levels may not be significant indicators of heart disease tendencies.

"Drs. Ray Rosenman and Meyer Friedman, of the Mount Zion Hospital in San Francisco, stated that 62 percent of their heart disease patients had serum cholesterol levels less than 260 mg%. . . . Only 20 percent of heart disease patients have serum cholesterol levels above 222 mg%. . . ."[40]

In considering the various risk factors related to coronary heart disease, and what can be considered a "normal" range of blood cholesterol, we must bear in mind that many variables affect cholesterol levels. We must also bear in mind that cholesterol readings by one's doctor can be unpredictable.

The Thyroid Gland

In his book *You Can Predict Your Heart Attack and Prevent It,*
Dr. Menard Gertler expressed the belief that low thyroid could
lead to an accumulation of cholesterol in the blood and other
tissues,[41] and that the addition of thyroid hormone could prevent
this.

Broda Barnes, M.D., is a recognized authority on thyroid
deficiencies. In his book *Hypothyroidism: The Unsuspected Illness,* he states, "By 1950, it was obvious that many cases of heart
attacks were accompanied by high blood cholesterol levels. To
most investigators, this suggested that the elevated cholesterol
levels were *causing* the attacks, but to me they signaled possible
thyroid deficiency."[42] This launched him into a study of 1,569
patients for a period of twenty years to determine the role of
thyroid deficiency to heart disease.

In reviewing the medical literature, Barnes found evidence
dating back to 1918 and 1925, which showed that thyroid therapy is an effective measure to prevent heart attacks. It's unfortunate that these early experiments clearly showing the
relationship between a thyroid deficiency and atherosclerosis
have been overlooked. "A rational approach to the prevention of
heart attacks calls for the recognition of thyroid deficiency—better late than never but preferably as early as possible—and its
proper treatment for the rest of life."[43]

EASY THYROID TEST   Barnes suggests an easy test that can
help you determine whether you have low thyroid. You will need
to take your basal temperature immediately upon awakening in
the morning. Shake your thermometer down well the night before, place it beside your bed, and as soon as you wake up, place
the thermometer snugly under your armpit for ten minutes.
(You are not to get out of bed until after this.) The normal range
is considered to be between 97.8 and 98.2 degrees Fahrenheit. A
basal temperature below 97.8 may indicate thyroid deficiency.
Conversely, the person who has an excess of thyroid hormone
will run a temperature above the normal range. (The temperature of a woman varies with the different phases of her menstrual cycle; on the second and third days of menstruation
comparable readings can be obtained.) Barnes states that infection, or even cancer, can elevate the basal body temperature. If
you find that your temperature is low, you should relate your
findings to your doctor who can further test you to make certain

if you have a thyroid deficiency. The thyroid gland can be stimulated naturally by taking kelp, a natural form of iodine. If the kelp doesn't help, your doctor can give further tests and prescribe thyroid accordingly.

Living in the Coronary Culture

Heart problems have become the plague of the twentieth century, as real, as much to be feared, and as devastating as any of the infectious diseases that ravaged the populace in former centuries.

Coronary heart disease is the most common cause of death in our country—more than 800,000 men and women die of heart attacks each year (1981 statistics). The annual death rate per 100,000 Americans for heart disease (most of which is coronary artery disease) is 331.3. This is almost double the death rate for cancer of all types. Men have heart-attack incidence three to four times as high as women; but the rates grow closer together as people age.

On the horizon in recent years appeared several medical procedures that seemed to offer hope. First, there were the heart transplant operations accompanied by worldwide fanfare. The desperation of people afflicted with heart ailments was appalling. People appealed to their doctors for transplants and even asked that their names be placed on waiting lists—so that when someone died, they could have the heart! The cost of $75,000 for a heart transplant didn't seem to stop anybody. Dr. Norman Shumway, of the Stanford Medical Center, and his surgical team did 161 transplants between December 3, 1967 and August 1970, and soon nearly all the patients were dead, according to Dr. Wilfrid Shute's *Vitamin E Book*.[44] Although his and others' results have improved in recent years, many now feel that transplants really aren't the answer; the quest goes on.

Coronary Bypass Surgery

After transplants came coronary bypass surgery, with its promise of reducing chest pain, prolonging life, and helping the coronary victim to withstand more physical activity. The technique was developed by surgeons in Cleveland and Milwaukee. In this surgery, the plugged-up parts of the three main coronary arteries that transport blood to the heart are "bypassed" by the insertion of grafts of veins taken from the legs. The grafted veins provide alternate routes for blood that would normally pass through the coronary arteries. Costs vary for this surgical procedure—for many reasons—but we have seen quotes of from $37,000 upwards to $60,000.

Dr. Henry Russek, Professor of Cardiology at New York Medical College in Manhattan, reported that "more lives are lost each year through bypass surgery on the heart than have been saved by it. . . . Fifty-five to 60 percent of these die during the operation or within a year of it. Or they suffer heart attacks which result in their becoming permanently disabled."[45]

BYPASSING THE BYPASS   Those on the forefront of nutrition research believe strongly—and they have the results and statistics to back up their beliefs—that there is another procedure that costs about one-tenth as much as bypass surgery, has a minimal risk factor, and causes very little, if any, pain. The treatment is called *chelation* and it appears to be a major breakthrough in the treatment of blocked arteries (arterio- or atherosclerosis).

Chelation therapy is aimed at stripping calcium deposits from the arteries and other parts of the body so that the material can be excreted through the kidneys. Physicians administer an amino acid solution called disodium ethylenediamine tetraacetic acid (EDTA) drop by drop into the bloodstream.

The word *chelate* comes from the Greek *chele,* which refers to the claw of a crab or lobster, implying a firm, pincerlike binding. The amino acid floats past a hardened area in the blood vessel, and its strong attraction for calcium literally picks up the offending chemical, like pincers, and pulls it right out of the area.

You may be wondering if chelation therapy can affect the calcium in your bones. Because the bone-forming cells (called osteoblasts) are not components of the blood vessel walls, the chelation leaves bone calcium where it belongs.

You may also be wondering whether chelation can remove the "good" minerals your body needs. The amino acid that is used has a strong attraction for calcium and lead in particular. In fact, the therapy originated in Detroit, Michigan, in 1948 when it was used to treat lead poisoning. After the treatment, doctors observed that the patient's arteriosclerosis also improved markedly. That observation prompted further experimentation. The treatment was used in medical centers on thousands of patients and not one fatality occurred as a result of the therapy.[46] However, losses of some of the other minerals in the body, such as zinc, manganese, and magnesium, can take place, so it is critical that the attending physician replace those essential minerals through nutrition and supplements.

Chelation has some risks, and like any other treatment procedure, the therapy sometimes fails. But member physicians of the American Academy of Medical Preventics (AAMP) have already administered more than two million treatments to over one hundred thousand patients, with a remarkable record of safety and effectiveness.[47] Hundreds of doctors testify that this therapy can eliminate the need for bypass surgery and that it has restored victims of severe angina to health, with complete freedom from pain and vastly improved tolerance for exercise. We have talked with families of formerly senile patients who regained their intellectual function when chelation therapy improved circulation to the brain.

Dr. Bruce Halstead, author of *Chelation Therapy,* says that "near miraculous results have been obtained in the treatment of atherosclerosis, sclerotic heart valves, coronary heart disease, intermittent claudication (leg pains due to lack of circulation), gangrene, angina pectoris, heart attacks, stroke, senility, scleroderma, arthritis, degenerative joint disease, and psoriasis. Studies have shown that the basis of most of these problems is poor circulation caused by hardening of the arteries or hypercalcinosis."[48]

We could relate the stories of a number of people we know to whom chelation therapy has proved beneficial. One case stands out, however.

A seventy-year-old woman whose arteries were clogged spent four weeks in the hospital following a triple bypass operation. For years she had been a semi-invalid, unable to travel even twenty miles to visit her children and grandchildren. After the operation, she still had many problems. She could walk slowly, painfully, with the aid of a cane on the carpet in her home, but she dared not venture outside. She was unable to climb stairs or do any of the things everyone had hoped she would be able to do after bypass surgery. Her son described her condition as "weak, tired—like senility, couldn't think, her remarks were out of focus."

One day she fell and injured her hip, back, and head. Her doctor confirmed what her family had suspected: her brain was not receiving enough blood. The prognosis was bad—another operation was needed to ream out the corroded arteries in her neck.

The elderly woman was readmitted to the hospital. However, as she was being prepared for the second surgery, a bruise on her head was discovered. It was a bruise that had not healed from the earlier fall. Surgery was postponed. In the meantime, the woman's son talked to her about chelation therapy and she agreed to try the treatment.

Her son describes what happened after the chelation started:

As I was driving her home, she started telling me things—bank account numbers, the amounts in those accounts, doing mental math to get percentages. She was very precise and concise. Sharp thinking, clear-headed.

A few days later she went outside, walked uphill to our mailbox, and then went out into the garden and started picking vegetables. It was like a miracle. Just two weeks before she could hardly walk on the carpet in her home without the use of her cane.

"That was three years ago. Since that time she has flown to Michigan during the winter, taken a thirty-day trip by bus, driven by car with us to Oregon, and is now wondering what trips she should take next. She wants to go to the Queen's Charlotte Islands in Canada. Her stamina is just amazing!" And she never went back to the hospital for surgery!

Not surprisingly, the American Medical Association has not endorsed chelation therapy completely, ruling it "not useful because the effects are not lasting." The pharmaceutical and health insurance industries also stand in opposition to the therapy.

Yet the Food and Drug Administration has approved EDTA for use in chelating lead and digitalis intoxication. Furthermore, the American Academy of Medical Preventics continues to accumulate extensive clinical data that clearly shows the health benefits that can be achieved from chelation, benefits that cannot be matched by other forms of therapy for arteriosclerosis and related disorders.

Carlton Fredericks best expresses the view we hold: "There are times when bypass surgery is lifesaving. On the other hand, I am aware that the statistics of survival after bypass surgery don't include some of the patients who survive the operation by a few years and then have a fatal attack. The omission in the procedure is an obvious one: if you repair clogged plumbing by inserting new pipes, but don't correct ... the initial problem, it must recur. That is why the chelating physician insists on necessary changes in life-style, cessation of smoking, intelligent choices of food, and proper use of vitamin, mineral, lecithin, and other supplements."[49] Lecithin, inositol, choline, chelated mineral supplements, alfalfa, vitamin C, vitamin E, garlic, rutin, kelp, some legumes, and sulfured amino acids have all been shown to act as chelating agents. These are things you can take as you take charge of your health.

NOTES

1. Edward R. Pinckney, M.D., and Cathey Pinckney, *The Cholesterol Controversy* (Los Angeles: Sherbourne Press, 1973), p. 3.
2. "A tremendous campaign has been waged to promote diets with low cholesterol, low saturated fat, and increased polyunsaturated fat. Despite this campaign, the death rate from cardiovascular disease has remained constant during the last 25 years, and it now seems to be almost certain that the assumption that heart disease is caused by a high intake of saturated fats and cholesterol is wrong." Linus Pauling, Ph.D., "Vitamin C and Heart Disease," *Executive Health,* January 1978.
3. Richard Passwater, *Supernutrition* (New York: Dial Press, 1975), p. 100.
4. Ibid., p. 81.
5. Richard Passwater, *Supernutrition for Healthy Hearts* (New York: Harcourt, Brace, Jovanovich, 1977), p. 80.
6. Pinckney and Pinckney, *The Cholesterol Controversy,* p. 22.
7. Carlton Fredericks, "Hotline to Health," *Prevention,* January 1975, pp. 44–47.
8. Ibid.
9. Menard M. Gertler, M.D., *You Can Predict Your Heart Attack and Prevent It* (New York: Random House, 1963), p. 124.
10. Linus Pauling, "Vitamin C and Heart Disease," *Executive Health,* January 1978.
11. "Fats and Cholesterol," *The Prevention Health Series,* no. 69, p. 10.
12. Pinckney and Pinckney, *The Cholesterol Controversy,* p. 40.
13. Ross Hume Hall, Ph.D., *Food for Nought* (New York: Harper & Row, 1974), p. 238.
14. Passwater, *Supernutrition for Healthy Hearts,* pp. 90–91.
15. Nutrition Search, Inc., *Nutrition Almanac* (New York: McGraw-Hill, 1973), pp. 206, 222.
16. Ibid., p. 80.
17. Pinckney and Pinckney, *The Cholesterol Controversy,* pp. 51, 130.
18. Ibid., p. 52.
19. Ibid., p. 51.
20. Ibid., p. 52.
21. J. I. Rodale and staff, *Cancer: Facts and Fallacies* (Emmaus, Penn.: Rodale Books, 1969), p. 55.
22. Wilfrid E. Shute, *Complete Updated Vitamin E Book* (New Canaan, Conn.: Keats Publishing, 1975), pp. 86–95; see also p. 213.
23. Shute, *Complete Updated Vitamin E Book,* p. 140.
24. Passwater, *Supernutrition,* p. 103.
25. Ibid., pp. 103, 104.
26. Constance Leslie, "Atherosclerosis and Vitamin C," *Lancet,* December 11, 1971, p. 1280.
27. Emil Ginter, "The Effects of Ascorbic Acid On Humans in a Long-Term Experiment," *International Journal of Vitamin Nutrition Research,* vol. 47, no. 2.
28. Passwater, *Supernutrition for Healthy Hearts,* p. 26.
29. Roger J. Williams, *Nutrition Against Disease* (New York: Pittman Publishing, 1971), p. 79.
30. Passwater, *Supernutrition,* p. 105.
31. Ibid., p. 106.
32. Williams, *Nutrition Against Disease,* pp. 73–74.

33. John Yates, "Lecithin Works Wonders," *Prevention*, February 1980, pp. 55–59.
34. Lester M. Morrison, "Serum Cholesterol Reduction with Lecithin," *Geriatrics*, January 1958, pp. 12–19.
35. Since this is a fairly recent discovery, there is little available literature. Significant information can be found in the following, however:
    Robert C. Atkins, M.D., *Dr. Atkins' Nutrition Breakthrough* (New York: Morrow, 1981), pp. 213–214;
    Passwater, *Supernutrition for Healthy Hearts,* pp. 37–38, 318–319;
    Jeffrey Bland, *Your Health Under Siege: Using Nutrition to Fight Back* (Brattleboro, Vt.: The Stephen Greene Press, 1981), pp. 62–63;
    Linus Pauling, "Vitamin C and Heart Disease," *Executive Health*, January 1978.
36. Passwater, *Supernutrition for Healthy Hearts*, pp. 37–38.
37. H. Lommis, "Preferential Utilization of Free Cholesterol from High-Density Lipoproteins for Biliary Cholesterol Secretion in Man," *Science*, April 7, 1978, pp. 62–64.
38. John Yudkin, M.D., *Sweet and Dangerous* (New York: Peter H. Wyden, 1972), p. 78.
39. Passwater, *Supernutrition*, p. 77.
40. Ibid.
41. Gertler, *You Can Predict Your Heart Attack and Prevent It*, p. 125.
42. Broda O. Barnes, M.D., and Lawrence Galton, *Hypothyroidism: The Unsuspected Illness* (New York: Thomas Y. Crowell, 1976), p. 176.
43. Ibid., pp. 186, 195, 196.
44. Shute, *Complete Updated Vitamin E Book*, pp. 16, 33, 34.
45. Passwater, *Supernutrition for Healthy Hearts*, p. 256.
46. Bruce W. Halstead, M.D., *Chelation Therapy* (California: Life and Health Medical Group, 1974).
47. Robert C. Atkins, M.D., *Dr. Atkins' Nutrition Breakthrough* (New York: William Morrow and Company, Inc., 1981), p. 247.
48. Halstead, *Chelation Therapy*.
49. Carlton Fredericks, Ph.D., *Eat Well, Get Well, Stay Well* (New York: Grosset & Dunlap, 1980), pp. 167, 168.

✃ 8. Digestion and Elimination

The solution to widespread digestive problems is not to find some foreign chemical that will stop "heartburn" and other digestive distress signals, but rather to find for the individual sufferer the right kinds of adequate food so that digestion and assimilation will take place easily and smoothly.
—DR. ROGER WILLIAMS

Proper digestion, good assimilation of food, and regular elimination are requirements for good health. These three functions are interdependent; one cannot proceed smoothly unless the others do.

Our mouths are the first step in the digestion process. Chewing food well breaks it down into particles that can be readily acted upon by the digestive enzymes, decreasing the likelihood of indigestion.

The salivary secretions begin the digestive process. Human saliva contains the enzyme pytalin, which is important in the digestion of sugar and starch. There are no sugar- and starch-digesting enzymes in the stomach, so not until sugar and starch reach the small intestine is an enzyme from the pancreas added to complete the digestive work on those nutrients. Proteins must be broken down into amino acids, large sugar molecules must be changed to simple sugars, and fats must be reduced to fatty acids before they can be absorbed into the blood or lymph vessels.

Food leaves the stomach in a semifluid state and passes on through the pyloric valve, which is the gateway to the first section of the small intestine, known as the duodenum. This valve opens and if there has been enough hydrochloric acid in the stomach, the pancreatic enzymes and bile from the liver are triggered to flow and start acting upon the food.

The pancreas is the best hidden of all the endocrine glands. Lying below and behind the stomach, this gland controls blood sugar and also takes part in the digestion of proteins, starches, and fats. "In the normal person, as much as two quarts of pancreatic juice enters the small intestine daily, largely after meals. It contains water, alkaline-forming materials which can neutralize the hydrochloric acid from the stomach, one fat-splitting, four carbohydrate-splitting, and eight protein-splitting enzymes."[1]

As food passes gradually into the small intestine, bile from the liver finishes up the digestion process. (If no food is being digested, the bile is stored in the gall bladder.)

Bile is especially important in the digestion and assimilation of such foods as cream, butter, oils, and other fats. If an insufficient amount of bile is available, the result will be gas and indigestion. Bile breaks up fat into tiny droplets that are then surrounded by the fat-splitting enzymes and quickly digested. Undigested fat makes it impossible for the protein- and carbohydrate-splitting enzymes in the intestine to do their job. Thus, a lack of bile interferes with the digestion of proteins and carbohydrates.

Thiamine (B-1) plays a significant role in the digestive process. When this vitamin is lacking, the stomach contracts less vigorously and food is not well mixed with digestive juices. Hydrochloric acid is secreted in small amounts or may be absent altogether. The mucous that protects the delicate walls of the stomach and intestines is produced in smaller amounts. And, finally, the flow of bile, along with pancreatic and intestinal juices, is decreased so that fewer digestive enzymes are produced. The result of all this is that food is incompletely digested in the small intestine and cannot be well absorbed into the blood.

Since the adrenal glands indirectly help stimulate the digestive juices, they need to be healthy, and you need plenty of protein for good digestion. Without adequate protein in the diet, food can not be completely digested. This is because the walls of the stomach, the small intestines, and the large intestines are made of circular muscles that can maintain their strength only if the diet supplies all the essential amino acids. If the diet is inadequate and the B-vitamin thiamine is lacking, the muscular contractions will be less vigorous.

A poorly functioning digestive system can show these symptoms: bloating, chronic indigestion, foul-smelling gas, heartburn, insomnia, irritability, fatigue, headache, pancreatitis, gastritis, underweight, or overweight.

The Small Intestine

Any food that is going to be absorbed by the body is absorbed in the small intestine, while unabsorbable material is pushed toward the large intestine or bowel, which is about six feet long.

Absorption or assimilation means the passing of foods from the intestines into the blood, which in turn carries this nourishment to every cell of the body.

Throughout the intestinal walls are folds and tiny fingerlike projections called *villi,* through which the food must be absorbed. The small intestine is about twenty-six feet long with a surface area of about four square feet. However, the villi increase the absorption area to thousands of square feet.

Each of the villi has tiny blood vessels (capillaries) and a small canal known as a lacteal, which is connected with the lymph circulation. Digested food passes from the intestines into the blood capillaries or lacteals.[2]

Experiments with deficiently fed pigeons resulted in atrophy and congestion in the intestines, with erosion of the mucous membranes and hemorrhages in the bowels. Similar experiments with monkeys produced ballooning in the intestines, distension in the stomach, thinning in the longitudinal bands of muscle, duodenum congestion, intense colitis, inflammation, and hemorrhages. Bacteria from the bowels was seen in the mucuous membranes, and there were small areas of carcinoma and cancerous growths.[3] Sir Robert McCarrison, who conducted these experiments, pointed out that an adequate provision of the vitamins and minerals found in fresh vegetable foods, and a diet wholly adequate in all nutrients, protects one against such gastro-intestinal lesions and related problems.

The intestinal wall in a healthy individual contracts almost continuously, with the result that vitamins and minerals from food, which are freed during the process of digestion, pass from the intestine into the blood and lymph, and then move into general circulation.

The Large Intestine

There are always millions of bacteria in the large intestine. The more food left undigested, the greater the number of bacteria that can grow on this undigested food and the fewer particles of digested food that are brought into contact with the absorbing surfaces of the intestinal walls. This condition may create an immunologic response in our bodies that may be an allergic reaction. Gas is formed in the bacterial breakdown of undigested food, and the result can be distention and pain.

Insufficient contractions and movement of the intestinal walls prevent wastes from being expelled. When waste bulk moves into the large intestine and stays there longer than it should, it is acted upon by bacteria. Some of these putrefying bacteria can produce certain products that are carcinogenic—cancer-causing —and may be related to colon cancer (cancer of the large bowel). And these carcinogens, if reabsorbed into our systemic circulation, may cause cancer in other parts of the body also.[4]

The large intestine is part of the digestive tract, but its primary purpose is the conservation of water. It is important that we drink enough water or fluids. Mother suggests one glass before each meal and one glass immediately after each meal. This glass of water taken at the end of the meal will not dilute the digestive juices in your stomach, since most of these juices will not have started flowing yet. Then, after that, do not drink any fluids for the next two and a half hours or you will slow down the digestive process by diluting the digestive juices in the stomach. Many people make the mistake of washing their food down with water. Instead, you should chew your food thoroughly so that it mixes well with saliva.

Waste material should remain in the large intestine no longer than 35 hours. This allows for the absorption of water to occur. Since the purpose of the large intestine is to conserve water, the longer the waste remains there, the harder and drier one's stool becomes, and this, of course, leads to constipation. Drinking enough water will help to keep the bowel movement soft.

Helping the Queasy Stomach

When digestive disturbances occur, food often gets blamed. People will complain of "heart burn," or a "sour" or "acid" stomach, and say that they have had "to put up with this for years." Some of them take antacid tablets and alkalizers to neutralize their stomach acidity. In 1980, the most popular of such products, Alka-Seltzer (a combination of aspirin, bicarbonate of soda, and citric acid), achieved sales of $90 million![5] There are, in fact, people so addicted to their favorite brand of antacid product that they treat it almost like candy. One patient developed calcium deposits in his eyes and kidneys after four years of continuous consumption of antacids.[6]

Antacids may adversely affect your bones—even when you take only the amount advised on the label, as Dr. Herta Spencer discovered. Her research showed that while antacids do not block absorption of calcium, they *do* remove some of the calcium that is already in the bones. Furthermore, what they leave behind may be even worse—aluminum. When you take an antacid that contains aluminum, the level of aluminum doubles in the blood. And that aluminum is known to deposit in your organs, including your brain—where it may snarl the chemical traffic that keeps your mind alert. Too much aluminum in the cells of the brain has even been suggested as a cause of senility.[7]

Other problems that may arise as a result of antacids are diarrhea and constipation—either one—since antacids can disturb a normal colon.[8] In a study of ulcer patients taking antacids, 66 percent had diarrhea.[9] Aluminum is also suspected as a cause of colon cancer.[10]

Prolonged use of antacids or large doses of calcium carbonate (found in many antacids) are hard on kidneys. Antacids reduce the flow of blood to those organs, clogging their delicate filters and tubes.[11] *The New England Journal of Medicine* commented on this: "In view of these hazards we cannot recommend the use of calcium carbonate for routine antacid therapy."[12]

Mother describes how she handles the problem: "If I did not have hydrochloric acid tablets and pancreatic enzymes, I would have a difficult time helping most people. Actually, taking the antacids is exactly the opposite of what they should be doing. Their problem is that they do not have *enough* hydrochloric acid, or if they have too much, they are not keeping the right kind of food in their stomach to take care of it."

Hydrochloric acid in the stomach also determines an individual's ability to tolerate bacteria-laden food. For example, the concentration of normal gastric juice in a human being is about 2 to 3 parts per 1000, while in a healthy dog, the concentration is almost twice as strong—about 5 parts per 1000. That is why a dog can eat tainted meat with no ill effects, while man, if he ate that same meat, could develop a severe reaction and even die. Increasing hydrochloric acid in the stomach helps prevent "turista"—an acute diarrhea that often afflicts visitors to foreign countries because of bacterial invasion from water or food. We recommend taking several hydrochloric acid tablets with each meal when traveling. And it is of course prudent to exercise caution in choosing food and drink. As Dr. Walter Guy writes, "Hydrochloric acid is . . . the protective agency against microbic life in food and water intake of the stomach."[13] Too much hydrochloric acid in an empty stomach can cause ulcers, however.

Hiatal Hernias

When the stomach lacks hydrochloric acid, another problem, common among older people, can result: the stomach balloons up through the diaphragm, forming what is called a hiatal hernia. The valve at the end of the stomach does not open when there is a lack of hydrochloric acid, so food remains in the stomach and ferments. It is the gas from this fermenting food that balloons the stomach.

Many people find that their problem is relieved within hours by taking hydrochloric acid tablets and digestive enzymes. How long they need to take these digestive aids depends on how well their adrenal glands recover. The addition of fiber-rich foods—alfalfa, bran, raw fruits, and raw vegetables—to the diet also helps the condition.

State of Mind

Of the many things that hinder the process of absorption and digestion, not all are related to the food you eat. Your emotions and your general state of mind have a great deal to do with the digestion process. Mealtime contention in homes is far too common. Anger, disgust, sadness, excitement—all these feelings may enter in and disturb your digestion. As Proverbs 15:17 puts it: "It is better to eat soup with someone you love than steak with someone you hate."[14]

Allergies

Hydrochloric acid serves to activate another secretion—the enzyme pepsin—which aids in the breakdown of proteins for their further digestion. If protein is not completely digested, the body cannot get all that it needs. But complete digestion of proteins requires a number of digestive enzymes—each of which works effectively on certain types of linkages within the proteins being digested. A lack of these protein-splitting enzymes helps explain why we have food intolerances, food likes and dislikes, and food allergies.

A USDA report on nutrition research states that over 22 million Americans can be classified as allergic. The most common allergens are airborne; the offenders include pollens, household dust, feathers, and animal dander. There is no 100 percent cure for such allergies, but significant success has been achieved by building up the mucous lining of the respiratory tract. This helps prevent airborne particles from penetrating the lining to cause sneezing, sniffling, itching, a runny, stuffy nose, and watery eyes. Vitamins A, E, and C are particularly important for a healthy lining.

Foods can also cause allergic reactions. People who are allergic to such foods as milk, eggs, or whole grains usually react with skin and respiratory problems. Yet food allergies are linked to digestion. As Mother says, "You are never allergic to the food you digest."

Let us examine how the allergic response takes place. First of all, a food you have eaten is not completely digested because your stomach lacks essential digestive enzymes (hydrochloric acid, pepsin, pancreatin, and bile salts). The large, undigested protein molecules and fermented carbohydrate molecules then travel to the bowel, where they are absorbed into the system and cause problems. The bowel reacts to these partially undigested food molecules by producing histamine or a histamine-like substance that causes various symptoms. These symptoms may be the typical skin and respiratory problems or such symptoms as diarrhea, fatigue, irritability, eczema, and vomiting.

If you are producing too much histamine, you will *not* solve your problem by taking antihistamines. For when you take antihistamines, all you do is treat the symptoms, not the root cause. If you had been able to digest your food properly in the first place, and if your mucous lining had been healthy, you would not have produced any of the offending histamine.

In healthy individuals, the liver quickly destroys histamine by means of the enzyme histaminase; a sluggish or damaged liver cannot produce this substance. Ironically, the antihistamine drugs routinely prescribed for allergies may sometimes harm the liver and lessen its capability to destroy histamine. This is one reason why some people become so dependent on antihistamine products.

Whenever we encounter people with food allergies, we recognize, first of all, that they are deficient in *digestive enzymes*. Fortunately, these digestive enzymes can be taken in tablet form so that allergic individuals can completely and properly digest all their food and not have undigested food molecules causing allergic responses.

The adrenal gland will usually have become exhausted when a person is allergic. Mother tells her clients, "You never get over allergies until you make your own *adrenal cortical hormones*."

An exhausted adrenal gland will cause you to secrete low amounts of the digestive enzymes that you need to protect you from food allergies. However, it is now possible to get raw, freeze-dried, whole beef adrenal gland in tablet form. These tablets will support and feed your own adrenal glands, helping you to bring them back into top shape.

An interesting paper, published back in 1935, described a talk given before the California Medical Association about some remarkable work done on the adrenal hormones.[15] Although the research was accomplished nearly fifty years ago, the means of treatment used is still not readily recognized today. The article said that whole beef adrenal glands (ground up raw and mixed with peanut butter) and sodium chloride were given to a group of patients—with amazing results. Of the nineteen children and nine adults in the experiment, *all* were relieved of asthma. The raw adrenal was hard to eat in those days, but the raw, freeze-dried, whole adrenal gland now available in tablet form is not at all hard to take, and it works on the same principle as taking whole natural thyroid, rather than a synthetic part of the thyroid hormone. The sodium chloride acts as an additional support to the adrenal gland, bringing to mind Mother's remedy of salt and soda in water to counteract an allergy or asthma attack. (See p. 52.)

One B-vitamin, *pantothenic acid,* is known to be deficient in persons suffering from allergies. Pantothenic acid works to protect the adrenal cortex from damage, and it stimulates the adrenal glands to increase their production of cortisone and other hormones necessary for proper health. Skin reactions to allergens have been reduced by as much as 20 to 50 percent with the administration of pantothenic acid.[16] A deficiency of this vitamin also causes an increase in a type of cell called eosinophils, which multiplies during all types of allergies. A blood test to check the eosinophils could be administered to monitor the recovery of allergies when pantothenic acid is given, as a helpful gauge for determining the amount of pantothenic needed. People who suffer from allergies may require from 100 to 500 milligrams of pantothenic acid daily to maintain good health.

Vitamin C is another important nutrient for allergy sufferers. Abnormally small amounts of vitamin C are found in the blood of both persons with allergies and animals in which allergies have been produced. Vitamin C decreases the permeability of the cell wall, making it harder for allergens to penetrate a cell and cause damage. Vitamin C also makes cortisone more effective, and it has an antihistamine action while detoxifying foreign substances that enter the body. Some people may find they need only 500 milligrams of vitamin C to treat their allergies, while others may need as much as 10,000 milligrams.

Vitamins A and E are also very important since they are responsible for maintaining the health of our skin, mucous membranes, and respiratory tract.

Constipation

Constipation is defined as a hard stool rather than an infrequent one. *Executive Health* reported that some five hundred brands of laxatives are now sold over U.S. drug counters and that sales of these laxatives totaled over $200 million in 1980.[17]

Unfortunately, if used regularly, laxatives are known to irritate and overstimulate the intestinal muscles to a state of exhaustion. As a result, the individual becomes so dependent on these preparations that normal bowel function ceases to take place. In other words, laxatives can cause the constipation they are supposed to combat.

Generally, constipation is quickly relieved when adequate amounts of raw fruits and vegetables are added to one's diet. These are natural sources of the B-vitamins, especially thiamine (B-1) and pantothenic acid (B-5). Yogurt or acidophilus milk or culture should also be added to the diet, along with increased dietary fiber. Alfalfa tablets, which provide bulk, are a good source of the fiber that helps in elimination.

Mother also emphasizes the importance of *good bowel habits* and making sure the bowels move daily. Going immediately to the bathroom after breakfast is an excellent routine, and there should be one or two bowel movements a day. Parents should also help their children to develop the habit of going to the bathroom right after breakfast. And children should visit the bathroom after they get into their pajamas and before they go to bed at night. Small children can be potty-trained this way.

People often become constipated on trips because they get off-schedule. Teenagers are notorious for getting up too late and rushing off without breakfast and without a bowel movement. Sometimes I tell people to eat breakfast first, then bathe or shower—by that time they should be ready to go to the bathroom. Actually, the peristalsis (muscle contractions) caused by a decent breakfast should initiate the bowel movement.

Eating a combination of *prunes and senna leaves* may also help with elimination problems. One pound of prunes and three table-spoonsful of senna leaves should be placed in one quart of water and heated to a boil. Then the mixture should be set aside to cool and steep overnight. In the morning, take the seeds out of the prunes and put the entire mixture in the blender—juice, pitted prunes, and senna leaves. The result is a wonderful prune whip. Refrigerate it in a large glass jar and use a tablespoonful a couple of times a day. It is excellent on yogurt or cottage cheese. Nursing homes that serve this mixture find that their residents have far fewer problems with constipation.

We have seen X rays of bowels in which the muscles have lost their tone: waste material has settled in "puddles" along the colon. After ingesting brewer's yeast and B-vitamins, people with this problem soon begin to have stronger muscle contractions in their bowels. When they also take hydrochloric acid and digestive enzymes and eat a diet adequately supplied with vitamin A, their condition further improves.

People who are severely constipated may have to take either a laxative or have an enema as an interim measure, until good nutrition restores their bowels to health. Herb laxatives are to be preferred, but even they should not be depended upon.

Enemas should not be used except when absolutely necessary, but it is better to have an enema than to wait all night for a laxative to work. For an ordinary enema, use one quart of warm water with two level teaspoons of sea salt. The water will then be as salty as the blood, and it will flush the bowel without permeating its lining and flooding into the blood stream, as tap water would do.

Bad Breath and Perspiration Odor

People buy millions of dollars worth of breath fresheners and mouthwashes each year. But neither gargling nor sucking breath candies will keep breath from being offensive. Although decayed teeth or food particles lodged in the teeth may be responsible for mouth odor, most often it is the result of the gas of putrefaction flooding from the bowels into the bloodstream, through which it enters the lungs, causing bad breath. Body odor results from the same problem when the food gases escape through the skin, one of the primary organs of elimination.

People who take acidophilus and alfalfa tablets for their bowels often find relief not only from constipation but from bad breath and perspiration odors. Alfalfa, with its dark green color, is a very rich source of chlorophyll, which has for years been used as a natural deodorizer. Many believe it is the magnesium found in the chlorophyll that gives it deodorizing properties.

Intestinal Gardening

The large intestine secretes *lactobacillus acidophilus* and many other acids that (because of their acidity) prevent the growth of harmful bacteria. These acids are originally established in the intestinal tract by mother's milk when an infant nurses. Dr. Ilya Metchnikoff studied Bulgarian people who were over a hundred years old. He found that they all had one thing in common—their bowels were acid like a nursed baby's bowels. They had been given no antibiotics, they ate only natural foods, and they had been nursed for two or three years. For the rest of their lives, they drank quarts of yogurt. Yogurt got the credit for these people's longevity and amazing good health, and everyone in Europe started eating yogurt. But later investigations proved that the yogurt was simply feeding the real hero, the friendly bacteria acidophilus, established in nursing.[18]

Research has shown that the feces of breast-fed babies are acid. In contrast, the feces of infants given the usual cow's milk formula are alkaline.[19] The bacteria we carry in our intestinal tract have a very important impact on our health. These microorganisms complete the digestion of some of our food, and they are particularly efficient producers of vitamins, synthesizing nine vitamins, including the B-complex vitamins and vitamin K. Vitamin K is essential to the normal process of blood coagulation. It should be emphasized, however, that antibiotics destroy not only the specific causes of an infection, but also the natural intestinal bacterial flora. The result can be serious vitamin deficiencies, as well as dangerous intestinal infections and other related problems. Breast-fed infants have increased resistance to infections because of the lactobacilli (lactic acid bacteria) found in mother's milk. Formula-fed infants do not have this protection. That is why Mother likes to see people take the cultured acidophilus that contains the strains of lactobacilli so essential to maintain vigorous, acid, intestinal flora.

This product, found in natural food stores, is a bottled, liquid acidophilus culture that will colonize the intestine with friendly bacteria. It is beneficial and soothing to the digestive tract, and it helps to regulate bowel bacteria. Acidophilus is also available in tablet and capsule form (especially convenient for travel). It is an easy and safe way to keep one's intestinal tract healthy.

Fiber Reviewed

In 1973, the medical world sat up and took notice when Dennis Burkitt, M.D., a British medical researcher and surgeon, introduced the results of his studies investigating bowel disease in relation to dietary habits, comparing native diets in Africa with the dietary habits of Western civilization. He concluded that the decrease in fiber consumption in the West had had a greater impact on our health than any other change.[20]

Burkitt stated that rural Africans—whose diets are high in fiber-containing foods—have a much lower incidence of appendicitis, hemorrhoids, diverticular disease, cardiovascular disease, and cancer of the colon than that of people in the United States and other developed countries whose diets lack fiber. The rural Africans eat their food in its raw state and benefit from its cellulose (fiber).

One way in which it can be determined if you are getting enough fiber in your diet has to do with intestinal transit time— that is, the number of hours that elapse between the time you eat a meal and the time you eliminate the waste from that meal. Burkitt learned that transit time averages 35 hours for the Bantu native, compared with 77 to 100 hours for the average Englishman.[21] When transit time is too lengthy, poisons are reabsorbed into the bloodstream and can lead to all sorts of health problems.

Because the average American eats so many processed, lifeless foods, his stools are slow-moving, dehydrated, and hard. In order for the large intestine to move hard stool, the muscles in the walls of the colon must exert tremendous pressure. For many people, it is only a matter of time before they develop a ballooning along the colon wall. These "pouches" in the lining of the colon trap fecal matter and create an environment in the lower intestine that supports harmful bacterial growth and infection. This is the condition known as diverticulitis.

Dr. A. J. M. Brodribb, following up on Burkitt's report, studied forty patients with diverticulitis. He compared his patients with other people of the same age and sex who did not have diverticulitis and discovered that the diverticulitis patients consumed half as much fiber. Furthermore, they suffered twice the frequency of hemorrhoids and varicose veins, four times the frequency of hiatal hernia and inguinal hernia, and gallstones. The frequency of appendectomy was also doubled.

The patients were treated with two tablespoonsful of *wheat bran* daily for six months. More than three out of four showed tremendous improvement. Bowel transit time became faster, and the bran had a normalizing effect on the stool consistency. The bulk weight of the stools increased by almost 50 percent.[22]

Bran has become very popular since Burkitt's findings were relased. Mother has always cautioned people not to go overboard on bran, however. Instead, she advises them to get their fiber from fruits, vegetables, nuts, and alfalfa tablets, as well as cereal products. From her childhood, she remembers mill horses grinding wheat into flour. Each horse had a sack over its mouth, so it couldn't eat the bran and wheat germ. Thinking the bran would be good for the animals, she asked the miller why he didn't let them eat it. He explained that it would make them swaybacked and bowlegged because the bran, high in phosphorus and low in calcium, would have pulled calcium out of the animals' bones.

While all sources of fiber promote increased bulk and soft, moist stools that pass through the intestinal tract more quickly, an excessive intake of bran fiber can lead to the loss of important nutrients. No more than two tablespoons a day taken at one meal, has been recommended. If you are getting two servings of vegetables and two servings of whole grains—wheat and rice, or seeds and nuts—each day, then you are probably getting enough fiber.

Fiber is so important to the process of elimination that it is worth reviewing all that it does. Fiber increases the size of the stools and speeds up elimination. It encourages the growth of healthy bacteria that produce extra amounts of several important vitamins, and it discourages the growth of potentially poisonous and irritating bacteria. Fruit and vegetable fiber, in particular, contains pectin and lignin, which remove harmful substances such as lead, and also facilitate the removal of fats and cholesterol. Finally, fiber also provides silicon, a mineral nutrient that is valuable to the heart and may help prevent arthritis and atherosclerosis.

The average person, when he or she learns about fiber, immediately thinks in terms of eating more bran or cereals. But dietary fiber is a natural part of plants and plant products, including fruits, vegetables, and nuts. It is not the bran we need so much as food in its raw state. The amount of fiber varies from food to food, but it is always composed of cellulose, which forms the cell walls. Many animals can digest this cellulose material; humans cannot. In humans, fiber works like a broom to sweep out the debris in the digestive tract.

Another way to make sure you are getting enough fiber in your diet is to use *alfalfa tablets*. These can be purchased at a health food store. Start with two or three of these tablets, taken a couple of times a day, and increase that amount gradually until you are taking as many as ten twice a day. Ask any farmer about the virtues of alfalfa. He'll tell you that when he puts his horse out in the alfalfa fields, it becomes sleek and strong. Because the alfalfa root system goes down up to forty feet, alfalfa is able to draw vital minerals from the soil, including calcium and phosphorus in the correct ratio.

Flax-seed meal, an old-fashioned remedy, is also effective. Mother tells people to grind one cupful of seed (dry) in the blender and take a tablespoonful in a glass of water twice a day. Three tablespoons of acidophilus can be added to each dose. This combination will help keep the bowels regular, active, and healthy. The ground-up seed should be kept in the freezer so that it does not become rancid.

Maintaining the Kidneys

Poisons from the bowels are also thrown off in the urine. This is the function of our kidneys, another of our organs of elimination. An adequate intake of fluid is necessary for healthy kidneys.

Many years ago, a very popular book, *Arthritis and Folk Medicine* by D. C. Jarvis, M.D., stated that the first yardstick of health is urine and that sickness appears when the urine becomes alkaline.[23] To determine whether your urine is alkaline or acid, you can conduct a simple test using pH test paper (Nitrazine paper available at drug stores). This pH test will give you the acid-alkaline relationship of your body's system. Your urine pH should be 6.40 and show slightly green in color on the pH test paper.

If the urine is alkaline (testing blue), the chance of infection is increased and kidney stones can develop in the urinary tract. Jarvis says that the home remedy of two teaspoons of apple cider vinegar in eight ounces of water can turn this blue reaction to acidic yellow. (Some people prefer taking cranberry juice, and it will do the same thing. However, read the label on the cranberry juice and avoid any brand that contains sugar. Vinegar will keep the urine acid and infections cannot grow in an acid medium. Also, vinegar acts as a diuretic, so that travelers who take vinegar are likely to avoid the swollen ankles that are common on long trips.

People who have kidney stones and/or other kidney and urinary tract infections have usually been on restricted diets—diets forbidding milk and milk products, eggs, whole grain bread and cereals. Yet such diets are inadequate in almost every respect.

Many people hesitate to take large doses of vitamin C because of reports that the nutrient can cause kidney stones. Dr. Frederick R. Klenner, well-known vitamin C authority, had this to say: "I can state very emphatically that you will not develop a kidney stone by taking 10 or more grams of ascorbic acid each day. It is physiologically impossible for such a condition to develop."[24]

Restoring the System to Health

One woman who had been diagnosed as having colitis (and diarrhea) for several years was brought to Mother by her landlord the day before she was to go into the hospital for a colostomy. In a colostomy, the large intestine is removed and the end of the small intestine is made to form an opening in the person's side. A sack is attached to this opening to collect wastes from digested food, and this sack must be carefully monitored and frequently emptied.

The landlord had pleaded with this woman to see Mother before she had the operation. Mother agreed to talk to her about her diet and suggested that she go back to her doctor and ask him if she could take time to build herself up for the operation. It was Mother's hope that, given the right foods and nutrients, this woman could be helped back to health.

The doctor agreed that the operation could wait a while, and Mother put the woman on a good basic diet containing the vitamins, minerals, and fiber necessary to restore her system. She gave her hydrochloric acid tablets and pancreatic enzyme tablets to be taken after each meal to help her digest the proteins and fats in her new diet. And she gave the woman the home remedy for diarrhea—two tablespoonsful of gelatin mixed in a glass of water, several times during the day.

Three months later, the woman returned to see Mother. Her doctor had just examined her and declared that her bowels were in good shape. He told her she should continue doing whatever she was doing. She stayed on the nutrition program and was able to live a normal, happy life.

When digestive and eliminative problems are ignored or inadequately treated, the consequences can be severe. Yet, even serious and long-standing health problems may sometimes be corrected with proper diet and treatment of one's system.

NOTES

1. Adelle Davis, *Vitality Through Planned Nutrition* (New York: The Macmillan Co., 1949), p. 20.
2. Ibid., p. 21.
3. Sir Robert McCarrison, M.D., *Studies in Deficiency Disease* (Milwaukee, Wis.: Lee Foundation for Nutritional Research, 1945) pp. 86–122.
4. Carl A. Hyland, "Nutritional Aids for Digestion—An Exclusive Interview with Kenneth A. Conklin, M.D., Ph.D.," in *Let's LIVE,* March 1981, p. 102.
5. Milton Moskowitz, Michael Katz, and Robert Levering, *Everybody's Business: An Almanac* (San Francisco: Harper & Row, 1980), p. 232.
6. Joe Graedon, *The People's Pharmacy* (New York: Avon Books, 1976), p. 87.
7. William Gottlieb, "Antacids Are Hard to Stomach," in *Prevention,* April 1981, p. 88.
8. Ibid.
9. Ibid., p. 88.
10. Ibid.
11. Ibid., p. 89.
12. Ibid.
13. Kurt W. Donsback, Ph.D., "Hydrochloric Acid," in *The Journal of the International Academy of Nutritional Consultants,* 1981.
14. Proverbs 15:17, The Living Bible.
15. Tom Blaine, *Goodbye Allergies* (New York: The Citadel Press, 1966), p. 147.
16. Charles Gerras, ed., *The Complete Book of Vitamins* (Emmaus, Penn.: Rodale Press, 1977), p. 639.
17. "About Laxatives and 'BMs,'" *Executive Health,* vol. 8, no. 11.
18. Albert von Haller, *The Vitamin Hunters* (New York: Chilton Company, 1962), pp. 197, 200, 201.
19. *Modern Problems in Pediatrics,* vol. 2 (Basel, Switzerland: S. Karger; Philadelphia: the School of Medicine, University of Pennsylvania, 1957).
20. D. P. Burkitt, "Some Diseases Characteristic of Modern Western Civilization," *British Medical Journal,* vol. 1, p. 274.
21. Ibid.
22. Richard A. Kunin, M.D., *Mega Nutrition* (New York: McGraw-Hill, 1980), pp. 188–189.
23. D. C. Jarvis, M.D., *Arthritis and Folk Medicine* (Greenwich, Conn.: Fawcett Publications, 1960), pp. 59–60, 68.
24. Frank Murray, *Program Your Heart for Health* (New York: Larchmont Books, 1977), p. 311.

✕ 9. The Immune System: Helping Your Body's Defense Mechanism

The main value of [Dr. Fred] Klenner's work is in showing that any active viral disease can be successfully brought under control with ascorbic acid if the proper large doses are used ... It might prove to be the "magic bullet" for the control of the viral diseases.

—IRWIN STONE

Your body is equipped with a wonderful healing system capable of handling almost any condition of infection or ill-health—provided it is given the nutritional support it needs. This health-restoring mechanism is known as the immune system.

It has been proven that malnutrition leads to a weakening or a suppression of the immune system. Perhaps when you think of malnutrition, you think of starving people overseas. Those are extreme examples of malnourishment; but, in fact, malnutrition is medically defined as "*any* disorder of nutrition." In our country it is usually a case of overconsumption of the wrong foods or even undernutrition because of dieting. Difficult as it may be to think of people in affluent America as malnourished, a tremendous amount of research and other evidence suggests that the rise in degenerative diseases nationwide can to some extent be traced to improper nutrition. All metabolic activities are influenced by the state of one's diet. You have heard it said, "You are what you eat," but that is only a partial truth. A more accurate assessment would be, "You are what your cells metabolize."

Living Can Be Hazardous

One essential fact must be understood if you are to maintain health: the state of your nutrition directly influences your biochemistry and your immunological system. Take care of your immune system and it will take care of you. If you can gain an understanding of the immune system, you will have taken a giant step toward understanding the chronic diseases that are so feared today.

What helps us ward off sickness? Why do some people stand up better under stress than others? How can one person avoid colds, sore throats, or the flu, while another is constantly battling these ailments? Why are so many Americans now dying of cancer? Health questions go on and on, and we want answers particularly when our own health or the health of a loved one is at stake.

We are living in difficult and changing times. Nearly every aspect of our lives is affected by our environment. Our bodies are continually assaulted by pollutants of all kinds—both outdoors and indoors—in the air we breathe, the water we drink, and the foods we eat. Add to this the physical and mental stress to which almost everyone is subjected—the byproduct of society's rapid growth and expanding technology—and you begin to understand why living can be hazardous to your health.

The Resistance Factor

In seeking an explanation for why some people catch every illness that comes along, while others never seem to have a sick day, you encounter the word *resistance*. You will hear people talk about someone having "low resistance" and someone else having "good resistance." Or they will talk about "building up resistance." This is a recognition that the body is fortified with a built-in biological defense that protects it from invading germs and disease. But what do you need to do to ensure continued protection for yourself? At what level of immunity are you now operating? How strong is your defense against disease? These are some of the questions you should be asking as you seek ways to take charge of your health.

There is an ever-present battle going on in our bodies. Sometimes we become aware of it—for example, when we sense a cold coming on. Then we take measures to ward off the illness—we drink more fluids, get more rest, and do whatever we have found works best.

Much of the time, however, we aren't even aware that our body is waging a war and constantly defeating many invaders that can cause problems. This may be a new thought to you, but it's an old theory to many scientists, and one that is being looked at with renewed interest—the idea that most of us have cancer cells in our bodies much of the time. These are cells that can become transformed into malignancies by viruses, chemical carcinogens (pollution), food factors, or radiation, but do not develop in the healthy body because the body's immunological defense agents destroy them.

The body has all sorts of weapons at its disposal to fight off invading germs. As Mark Bricklin explains, some of these "weapons" "go by exotic-sounding names like *macrophages* and *leukocytes,* cells to which the body's intelligence agency has given a license to kill. Others go by such mundane-sounding names as sneezes (which kick germs out the front door) and the runs (which kick them out the back door)." There are many factors affecting how well these various weapons function, including previous exposure to similar germs, heredity, stress, emotions and nutrition."[1]

Usually we have some indication that a cold is on its way. A scratchy throat, drippy nose, and sneezing are good indicators. My ancestors had an old-fashioned home remedy that worked wonders. They dissolved one-half teaspoon each of salt and soda in eight ounces of hot water and drank the mixture. If a sufferer was not feeling better in fifteen minutes, he repeated the treatment. Sometimes honey was added. Mother has given this mixture to people for years, and it works most of the time. But why?

The stuffy or drippy nose and the scratchy throat indicate that fluid is leaking out of the blood and going *into* the tissues. This fluid is full of germs. The salt and soda brings your adrenal glands out of shock. So by taking this mixture whenever you start to come down with cold symptoms, you will stimulate your adrenals to stimulate, in turn, your thymus, tonsils, adenoids, and lymph glands to make antibodies. The antibodies will go after the infection and the battle will resume.

Mother then tells people to whip an egg into a glass of milk with a little honey and vanilla. This eggnog will quickly supply your body with desperately needed protein. Remember, antibodies are made of complete protein. This cannot be emphasized enough. A lack of protein will prevent recovery from infections, regardless of the amounts of vitamins you take or whatever else you do. When your whole defense mechanism is low, it is a warning that proteins are undersupplied. On the other hand, if protein is abundantly supplied and the diet is otherwise adequate, we can expect high resistance to diseases and infections.

Gamma Globulin and Antibodies

Although there are many mechanisms that help to protect the body against infection, two are particularly dependent upon protein intake: antibodies and white cells. Under normal circumstances, the liver produces proteins known as gamma globulins, or antibodies, whose purpose it is to combine with, and render harmless, various bacteria, bacterial toxins, and presumably, viruses. Studies of persons suffering from almost every type of infection, including polio, show that the gamma globulins of their blood are undersupplied. These globulins might be thought of as a militia guarding your health. Changing from an inadequate protein diet to a good protein diet can greatly increase the amount of antibodies you produce.[2]

Research interest in immunity has focused for years on gamma globulin, which is found circulating in the blood. When a virus invades the body, a specific antibody is manufactured to attack it. That particular antibody is then continuously produced in small amounts, and its output is increased immediately if the same virus appears. An adult's gamma globulin contains antibodies from vaccinations and from childhood diseases.

Physicians will sometimes "give injections of gamma globulin ... to persons suffering from infections, but unless the patient is too ill to eat or has severe diarrhea, his own body can produce far more gamma globulin than could be given by injection—provided he obtains adequate protein."[3]

Mother has another favorite, old-fashioned home remedy that she passes on to anyone who complains about high susceptibility to infections and fever. She mixes a raw egg yolk with ripe banana. Plain or mixed with milk, this is a good combination to give to children, whether well or ill, and it is also an excellent first food for babies. Egg yolk contains the mysterious "x" that Al Coburn, pioneer researcher, discovered had an anti-rheumatic effect upon highly susceptible rheumatic children.[4]

Mother cautions about giving antibiotics to children who have recurring infections. Thousands of people take antibiotics without apparent physical harm and without side effects. But others have experienced adverse reactions. Uninformed mothers frequently demand antibiotics for every sniffle and fever that their children develop. We believe their pediatricians must use their own judgment; however, we also realize many drugs can produce vitamin B-6 and other deficiencies that can result in more serious problems than the illness originally treated. Furthermore, bacteria can build up such a resistance to antibiotics that the drugs become ineffective. For these reasons, antibiotics should be reserved for emergencies.

The Immune Response

Your immunity system is spread throughout your body, a virtual network of silent lifesavers. In trying to understand how the body develops immunity to disease, investigators have been finding more and more clues that point to a crucial role for the thymus gland. Since the thymus of an adult human being is an organ that is barely discernible in the chest, its role in immunity has come as something of a surprise.

For over two thousand years, the thymus was considered nature's mistake. It was an enigma to researchers. The gland is an insignificant-looking little blob of yellow-gray tissue nestled in the front of the chest just behind the top of the breastbone. The thymus is large in relation to the rest of the body in fetal life and in early childhood. Then it grows less quickly, and, by the time an individual reaches puberty, the thymus weighs six times its original weight. At that point, it begins to atrophy.

When something atrophies, we tend to think of it as ceasing to function. That is why for years many researchers called the thymus a "useless gland." But far from being useless, the thymus is responsible for the production of a special kind of white blood cells called T-lymphocytes. They in turn manufacture the protein molecules called antibodies. These white blood cells remove external particles, including viruses, bacteria, and cancer cells—materials that *constantly* invade our bodies. The thymus, therefore, is the chief component of the body's defense force.

OUR FIRST-LINE OF DEFENSE AND VITAMIN A The skin, lungs, intestinal linings, and other areas of the body that are constantly exposed to germs act as the main barriers to disease-causing organisms. They have been compared to soldiers because they fight all foreign invaders with generalized defenses.

Mother explains the importance of healthy mucous membranes:

If the lining all through the body is healthy, and if it is kept healthy with vitamin A, then germs cannot live and, in fact, many bacteria and fungi are killed on contact. If vitamin A is lacking, the cells in the lining die too quickly, and germs thrive on dead cells.

The skin has four layers of cells. The fourth or bottom layer is kept healthy by the blood stream. If vitamin A is there, then these cells are normal and the normal cells work their way to the top layer in about thirty days. Now the top layer sloughs off in bathing. When that fourth layer is deprived of vitamin A, the cells die and the body rushes in with white blood cells and brings the debris to the surface and we see an eruption—a pimple, a carbuncle, impetigo, open ulcers, or a sty.... When I see teen-agers with facial blemishes, I suspect that young person is undersupplied with vitamin A.

Infections that we normally associate with a vitamin A deficiency involve the skin, eyes, lungs, and those areas normally protected by mucous membranes. What vitamin A does is to increase your resistance to germs and encourage your body's natural immune system to get to work.

Carlton Fredericks tells of 200,000 units of vitamin A, in one dose, repeated for three to five days, to be effective in stopping the onset of a cold. He explains: "Two types of colds can be aborted or mitigated with simple vitamin therapy. Vitamin A is effective for one type; vitamin C for the other—and never the twain meet, meaning that the simultaneous use of the two vitamins in the requisite high dosage is not only ineffective, but may prolong the cold. This is to say that a vitamin A responder gains no benefit from vitamin C; and the sufferer with a vitamin C-responsive cold profits not by vitamin A. There is no way to discern which type of cold one commonly gets, but logic dictates that vitamin A be tried first, for if it is ineffective, failure is the only penalty. If vitamin C is not effective, it may move the cold from the head to the chest."[5] An impressive amount of evidence suggests that vitamin A may well be the anti-infection vitamin most people need.

Even in the early days of vitamin research, discoveries pointed to the amazing anti-infection properties of vitamin A. As far back as 1938, in Germany, a Dr. Lindquist showed that, "in some unknown way, vitamin A was mobilized within the body and directed to diseased areas to combat infections."[6] And in Cambridge, England, Dr. Thomas Moore, of Dunn Nutritional Laboratory, "found that vitamin A deficiency actually weakened outer layers of tissues, enabling disease-causing viruses and bacteria to gain a foothold in laboratory test animals."[7]

Worldwide evidence continues to reveal the benefits of vitamin

A, in spite of those who warn that it can be toxic. Dr. Atkins comes to the defense of vitamin A, stating that

large doses of vitamin A, in the range I have described [100,000 units daily for 5 days, 50,000 units daily for the next five days, 10,000 units daily thereafter] . . . have never been proven toxic and can, as borne out by my patients' results, be a real help in dealing with the common cold.

I am especially concerned that vitamin A has such a widespread reputation for toxicity, because I feel that it has become the scapegoat vitamin. Whenever an opponent of the nutrition movement wants to prove a point, he cites the potential toxicity of vitamins A and D to support his ultimate conclusion that we should get off those dangerous vitamins and take our medications.

Worse still, vitamin A's therapeutic qualities have been underrated or ignored in the exaggeration of its potential dangers.[8]

See Vitamin A in Appendix B for more information on toxicity.

THOSE SWOLLEN GLANDS AND TONSILS   Most of us have experienced how it feels to have swollen tonsils. Once it was thought that the tonsils and adenoids were infected, and it was common practice to remove them in a child who had frequent "tonsillitis." In fact, the tonsils were only screening out of the blood the poisons that came from infection sometimes caused by constipation.

Mother's explanation of what happens when we have swollen tonsils and glands has been very helpful to hundreds of concerned parents:

When our tonsils and glands swell up, we swallow the infection picked up from the blood. If we have hydrochloric acid working in our stomachs, the infection is destroyed. However, many people do not produce adequate amounts of hydrochloric acid, and no longer have the friendly bacteria living in their bowels.

As long as the bowel is acid, putrefaction and disease organisms cannot germinate; in other words, you cannot reinfect yourself. Over a hundred viruses have been isolated that cause the common cold, and they are all found in the bowel.

When the lymph glands become swollen on the neck, under the arms, and in the groin, it always means there are toxins in the body. The lymph glands are doing their job. Mother describes this:

Our lymph nodes serve, first of all, as filtering beds that remove foreign matter from the lymph before it enters the bloodstream. They also serve as storage centers for the white blood cells and other antibody-manufacturing cells produced in the thymus gland. I could always tell when my children were constipated because their lymph glands would swell.

It is only when the adrenals inadequately function that any lymph tissue such as tonsils, adenoids, or lymph glands under the chin and behind the ears can become enlarged. Infections and allergies are very typical of inadequately functioning adrenals and enlarged tonsils are often an index of overall malnutrition.

Swollen tonsils and/or adenoids decrease rapidly in size when vitamin A, pantothenic acid, and vitamins B-6 and C are given several times daily with an otherwise adequate diet. In experimental "volunteers lacking pantothenic acid and vitamin B-6 so few antibodies and white blood cells could be produced that they had continuous infections, particularly sore throats, or acute pharyngitis."[9] These vitamins should be included in your regular daily dose of vitamins and minerals.

It should be emphasized, however, that the diet must be adequate in protein. If one of the essential amino acids is undersupplied, antibody production may decrease or cease entirely. Infections are especially prevalent when too little animal protein from meat, fish, poultry, milk, eggs, and cheese is eaten. Consequently, when you or one of your children is sick, you shouldn't try to make it on juices alone as so many do.

Gland Therapy

Going to the doctor and getting injections of thymus extract or taking raw, dehydrated thymus tablets will help your body's defense mechanism, and they are now being used in some cancer treatments. Generally, such a glandular product is not meant for prophylactic use over a long period of time unless there is a recognized deficiency. Sometimes results will appear within a week or two, and sometimes a month of daily supplementation may be required. A nutritionally minded doctor, a nutritionist, or an informed health food store or nutrition center will be able to advise you about such products.

Traditionally, most primitive cultures have eaten all of the glands and organs of an animal that was killed. Not too long ago, even many American families ate gland and organ meat. Today most people either don't know how to cook these meats properly or have acquired a distaste for them. The French, however, use glands and organs for gourmet cuisine.

You can get thymus in the meat department of your supermarket by asking for sweetbreads. If your butcher doesn't carry them, ask him to order them for you. I fix them by immediately cleaning and then freezing them. After they are frozen, I take a very sharp knife and cut them up. I then return them to the freezer in an ice cube tray. After they have frozen again, I pop them out into baggies and put them back in the freezer. When we want a special "Immunity Drink," I place two cubes in the blender, add a cup of tomato juice, and blend the mixture until smooth.

This is one way to get glandulars such as thymus, or brain, liver, and heart into yourself and members of your family. You can vary the flavor by adding yogurt, raw apples, bananas; and you can try apple juice instead of tomato juice. Honey or fructose can be added to sweeten, and vitamin C crystals, or crushed vitamin C (1,000 mg.), in the mixture will prevent oxidation. After several days of taking glandulars in this way, you will sense a marvelous pick-up. Eating glandulars will support the glands, but not stimulate them.

Vitamin C

Dr. Linus Pauling, the Nobel Prize–winning chemist, has reported studies that show that, by ingesting 1,000 milligrams of vitamin C daily (instead of the 60 milligrams recommended by the National Research Council), a person would catch 45 percent fewer colds.[10] Other studies have shown a 15 percent decrease in incidence and a 30 percent decrease in severity of the common cold.[11]

Many fellow scientists disagreed with Pauling. One such skeptic was Dr. Terence W. Anderson of the University of Toronto in Canada. Intending to disprove Pauling's claims, Anderson and his researchers conducted carefully controlled tests. However, in the end, they had to admit that vitamin C could substantially reduce the effects of the common cold. In a study involving over 1,000 subjects, the group that received 1,000 milligrams daily (increased to 4,000 milligrams during illness) had 40 percent more people free of illness, and those of that group who did become ill spent 30 percent fewer days indoors.[12]

Pauling believes that millions of people today are suffering from "sub-clinical scurvy." That is, although they may be getting enough vitamin C to prevent scurvy in its grossest forms, they lack sufficient vitamin C to ward off colds and other diseases and infections. Vitamin C is also used to produce the collagen—"glue"—the body uses to rebuild tissue and heal wounds.

Vitamin C is a potent, broad-spectrum, nontoxic virus fighter when used in large doses. Dr. Fred Klenner, the world's foremost authority on the clinical use of vitamin C, gives vitamin C by injection to patients with meningitis, encephalitis, polio, viral pneumonia, and many other serious diseases. Many of these patients were not expected to live. Antibiotics had been given without success. Every two to four hours Klenner gave vitamin C injections of 4,500 to 17,500 milligrams (4.5 to 17.5 grams). The injection dosages were based on a 154 pound man and were continued around the clock when needed. Many recovered quickly and could be "discharged from the hospital in three or four days."[13]

More than 10,000 studies over the past four or five decades have shown vitamin C to be effective in battling a long list of human ailments. It would be impossible to cover even a fraction of these many studies in this book. However, we do want to point out the work of several dedicated researchers, including the highly respected Albert Szent-Gyorgyi, M.D., Ph.D., Nobel Laureate for Physiology and Medicine.

Szent-Gyorgyi, who won the Nobel Prize in 1937 for his discovery of vitamin C, emphasizes that ascorbic acid (vitamin C) transduces protein into the living state and enables it to perform in our bodies.

The more ascorbic acid is available, the better the protein will work.... The ascorbic acid ingested by man is excreted only partly with his urine. *Its greatest part simply disappears!* What happened to it was a mystery. My studies indicate that *it is incorporated into the living machinery!*

This brings out a point which is important in relation to medical application. To have a well-functioning cellular machinery the ascorbic acid must be available while the machine is built.

(If we build a wall, the mortar must be applied to every brick. One does not raise a wall putting bricks together and then pouring cement over them.) *So one should not wait for the application of this vitamin until one gets ill, trying to put the situation right by taking big doses. We should take it all the time.*

To have plenty of ascorbic acid is especially important in our young years *when we build our body. But ascorbic acid should be available at all ages. The older we become the less we are able to store and use it, thus the more we need of it.*[14]

This wise and honored scientist, who was eighty-four years old at the time he made these observations, underscored the body's need for this vitamin which increases the cohesive force that holds living structures together. He also said: "I strongly believe that a proper use of ascorbic acid can profoundly change our vital statistics, including those for cancer."[15]

Dr. Fred Klenner routinely prescribes ten grams (10,000 mg.) of ascorbic acid daily to his adult patients for the maintenance of good health. His daily dosage for children is one gram per each year of age up to ten years, and ten grams daily thereafter (a four-year-old child, for example, would receive 4 grams or 4,000 mg. daily). We feel these are high dosages but time and research may prove his prescription correct.

Arthritis

Millions of Americans suffer from some form of arthritis, becoming virtual prisoners in their own bodies. Arthritis, characterized by inflammation and pain in the joints, can be caused by many things—among them, years of stress, emotional or physical. Cigarettes, coffee, alcohol, drugs, crash dieting, a lack of vitamins or minerals—these are but a sampling of today's stress inducers.

Those with arthritis most often have exhausted adrenal glands, which no longer can produce cortisone and other vital hormones. When doctors prescribe cortisone to relieve the pain, it is generally effective, but only as a stop-gap measure; it treats only the symptoms of arthritis. The adrenal glands are still not producing cortical hormones on their own so the arthritis is relieved only as long as the patient is taking cortisone—which cannot be indefinitely because of side effects from the medication. Mother believes in using whole raw adrenal glandular tablets from the adrenal glands of cattle, rather than cortisone. The tablets help support the adrenals, allowing them to repair themselves so that they can again secrete their own cortisone and other vital hormones.

There is some evidence to suggest a correlation between arthritis and infection elsewhere in the body, although it is not known whether arthritis is the cause or the effect. Presumably, because the adrenal glands are exhausted, the body is simply ill-equipped to fight the inflammation. When Mother talks to arthritics with an infection—typically in the teeth or bowels—she suggests that they take acidophilus and all the vitamins and minerals so the infection will clear up.

The Battle Against Cancer

The statistics of cancer are frightening. It claimed the lives of more than 400,000 Americans in 1981. Cancer is a formidable foe, generally regarded as the most dreaded of all diseases. But what is cancer? Basically, it is a group of abnormal cells growing independently of the body's centralized control. These are anarchist cells—cells gone wild, cells with the perverse capacity to break ranks, to sap the body's energy, to take all the fuels they want, and to starve the body's still-healthy cells.

Recent research has shown that cancer cells display antigenic activity. Antigens are chemical structures foreign to our bodies —that is, they are invaders. When an antigenic attack is detected, our immunological system sends out its "soldier" cells, which swing into action in a seek-and-destroy mission. The central dispatching post is our bone marrow, where approximately 3 million soldier cells (or their precursors) are produced every second of our lives. These white blood cells are sent out into the bloodstream, as well as to various outposts within the body (such as the lymph nodes). Immunological warfare is waged throughout the body, and the soldiers are constantly being replenished from within our bone marrow.

This is a very simplified description of the very complicated process that goes on constantly as our immune system does battle for us. But what happens when cancer takes over? The explanation appears to be that there is a breakdown of our immunological surveillance mechanisms. Researchers have thus been saying that if this is the case, then the goal of the immunotherapist and those in the forefront of cancer research should be to understand this mechanism, its breakdown, and how it can be started up again. This treatment of cancer is usually called immunotherapy and is a natural way for the body to help itself. So the danger of serious side effects is accordingly small.

VITAMIN C THERAPY   It is at this point that the role of vitamin C in combatting cancer becomes significant. Despite the vast sums of money and efforts expended during the last twenty-five years to find a cure for cancer, there has been essentially no decrease in the incidence of cancer or in the length of time of survival after diagnosis. But there have been very significant studies which show that large doses of vitamin C have a life-extending effect for patients with advanced cancer.

In 1971, Drs. Linus Pauling and Ewan Cameron began a five-year study of 1,100 terminal cancer patients. Dr. Cameron, Chief Consultant Surgeon at Vale of Leven Hospital, Loch Lomonside, Scotland, had advanced the thesis that considerable control over cancer might be achieved if we could find some way of stimulating our natural protective mechanisms to greater effectiveness.... He had emphasized the possibility of strengthening the intercellular cement and thus making the normal tissues stronger and more resistant to infiltration by a malignant tumor.

At this point, Pauling pointed out that the intercellular cement is strengthened by the presence in it of fibrils of the protein collagen, which act like steel rods in reinforced concrete.[16]

He suggested that an increased intake of vitamin C should result in the synthesis of more collagen fibrils with the consequent strengthening of the normal tissues. And when Cameron asked how much vitamin C should be given to patients, Pauling recommended 10 grams. (Most animals manufacture about this amount, calculated to the body weight of a human being, and Pauling believed that animals would not make this amount if it weren't needed to keep them in good health.) Cameron cautiously began clinical trials.

A comparison is made of 100 patients with advanced cancer who received vitamin C in amount usually 10 grams per day, beginning on the day when it was decided that conventional treatment would have no further value for them, and 1,000 other patients, ten matched controls for each of the ascorbate-treated patients (same kind of cancer, same age, same sex). The 1,000 controls were given the same treatment as the ascorbate-treated patients except for not receiving ascorbate. They were patients in the same hospital and were treated by the same physicians and surgeons.

The result of this study was that the ascorbate-treated patients have lived on the average over *four times* as long as the matched controls. Sixteen of the 100 ascorbate-treated patients have lived more than one year, whereas only three of the 1,000 controls had lived that long. Moreover, although all of the 1,000 controls have died, 16 of the 100 ascorbate-treated patients are still alive, and a dozen of them seem to be free of disease. "The results obtained are so promising that nearly all the cancer patients who come to Vale of Leven Hospital now receive the vitamin, as do so many of the cancer patients of other doctors in the neighboring regions."[17]

Cancer patients have a much greater requirement for vitamin C than normal healthy individuals, apparently because all available vitamin C is mobilized by the body in a valiant effort to boost natural resistance and repel the invasive malignant growth.

INTERFERON   Dr. Roger J. Williams says that, because so many years of effort have already gone into the problem of understanding cancer, a prudent scientist will hesitate before attempting to make any new suggestions or contributions in this area. Of course, we agree with these words of wisdom. Yet, in more recent years, one substance has been making the news in regard to cancer research and holding out hope to cancer victims and their families. Even the American Cancer Society has jumped on the bandwagon, investing $6.8 million in efforts to learn if this substance, which is produced in the body, can indeed slow the growth of cancerous tumors in humans. The substance is called *interferon.*

A handful of interferon enthusiasts have gradually unlocked some of its secrets, concluding "that it is a protein produced by cells in response to some stimulation, usually by a virus." Three varieties have been found: "One kind is produced by leukocytes, or white blood cells. A second type is generated by fibroblasts, cells that form connective tissue in skin and other organs. The third, called immune interferon, is apparently made by T lymphocytes, soldier cells that attack invaders and are part of the body's immune system."[18]

Although interferon cannot yet be produced synthetically, scientists have begun research using interferon isolated from donated blood. Dr. Jordan Gutterman, of the M. D. Anderson Hospital and Tumor Institute in Houston, conducted preliminary tests "on 38 patients with advanced breast cancer, multiple myeloma or lymphoma. . . . The results [of interferon] were encouraging. Seven of 17 breast cancer patients had positive results, as did six of ten with myeloma and six of eleven with lymphoma."[19]

Benjamin Siegel, a researcher at the University of Oregon Health Sciences Center in Portland, regards interferon as the body's first line of defense. It can wipe out a disease, but the body must produce *enough* interferon. And that's the hitch. Interferon is a natural, hormonelike substance that appears to regulate cell function and is produced by the body in response to viral infections, cancer, and other diseases. However, unless the body produces enough interferon, we remain hindered in our ability to fight off invaders. *Research has revealed that vitamin C increases the cells' production of interferon at all dose levels.*[20]

We have seen how rapidly the body under stress is depleted of vitamin C. The latest studies by Dr. Hans Selye show a correlation between stress and interferon levels:

Stress plays a role in obstructing the production of endogenous interferon.* Most significantly, cortisol, a stress hormone secreted by the cortex of the adrenal glands can apparently prevent or inhibit interferon production. Consequently, at times of peak stress, when plasma cortisol levels are high, the person's interferon levels are low. Stress control techniques are indicated to raise plasma interferon levels to insure maximum resistance against disease.[21]

There are other studies that point to synthetic hormones, cortisone and prednisone, as also suppressing interferon production. Drs. Michael Rytel and Edwin Kilbourne explain that these drugs, which are used for their anti-inflammatory properties, do their work at the expense of our natural interferon production. Their studies parallel the interferon-suppressive effects of cortisol, which is produced naturally by the body in the adrenal cortex in response to stress. This may help explain why we are more susceptible to viral infections, such as the common cold, during periods of high stress.[22]

We know also that high cholesterol levels are a common response to stress and that stress depletes the body of vitamin C and the B-complex vitamins in particular, as well as various minerals, including calcium, zinc, selenium and potassium.

Special blood tests, conducted at only a few preventive medical clinics, are now being devised to determine natural interferon levels. Once these tests have been perfected and standardized, a real breakthrough will have been accomplished. In the meantime, we as individuals must find ways to reduce our stress levels so that the body will, of its own accord, raise its interferon levels. We can help this process along by making sure we keep optimum amounts of vitamins and minerals in the body to help insure maximum resistance against disease.

Mother sees many people who are under chemotherapy or radiation treatment. These people are under the severest kind of stress. One woman who followed her complete approach to nutrition told Mother that she felt great while her doctor's other patients were nauseated and couldn't eat. Mother tells people, "Feed your defense mechanism so it doesn't get exhausted. Do everything you can to keep your body detoxified. The person who already has cancer needs to take acidophilus for his intestinal tract and needs mega-vitamins and minerals. Cancer cells thrive on glucose, so sugar must be kept out of the diet."

---

* Endogenous means grown from within the cell walls.

NONTOXIC THERAPY   Nontoxic cancer therapy is based on the use of enzymes, mega-vitamins and minerals, diet, nutrition, detoxification, and in some instances, the use of vaccines—all of which are designed to build up and maintain the body's own defense against disease.

A great many approaches have been tried, some of them with great success, others not as valuable or effective. Many important substances are being used. And we strongly believe that the best way to fight cancer is through preventive measures. Someday we hope proper nutritional therapy will be accepted and take its place alongside more conventional treatments.

OTHER NUTRIENTS ESSENTIAL TO THE IMMUNE SYSTEM
Zinc is a nutrient that has been much in the news in recent years. Individuals with low zinc levels have been found to have poor immunity and lowered resistance.

Selenium is another mineral that is necessary for the maintenance of good health and may play a role in preventing cancer. Statistical evidence for selenium's anticancer powers is impressive. Many studies confirm the correlation between high selenium concentrations and low cancer rates, although correlation alone is not proof of cause and effect. However, "Direct experimental evidence confirms that selenium can help prevent cancer."[23]

Gerhard N. Schrauzer, Ph.D., of the University of California at San Diego, who has been in the forefront of selenium research, speaks of selenium supplementation as a "method of cancer prophylaxis applicable at the individual or community level."[24] He suggests that the best way to get selenium is through "the combination of a selenium supplement and a high-selenium diet. I recommend anywhere from 150 to 250 mcg. of supplemental selenium a day."[25] And he recommends more seafood, more cereal and bread products, and a decrease in sugar consumption.

Dr. Richard Passwater speaks of the protective action of vitamin E and selenium in terms of their anti-oxidant and free-radical scavenging activity. He says that "without vitamin E or selenium, your body cannot defend itself against carcinogens or wild cells; with extra vitamin E and selenium, your body cannot be damaged by many invaders or wild cells."[26]

Sugar is highly suspect as a substance that distracts the body in its vigil against infection. Sugar also weakens the immune system by replacing in the diet natural foods that would supply the body with the vitamins, minerals and protein it needs.

Schrauzer issues strong warnings about sugar and its relationship to breast cancer. "High-sugar diets should be avoided. It has been shown that breast cancer patients very often have carbohydrate dysfunction. And breast cancer mortality correlates directly with sugar consumption in different countries. It is, in fact, the food item with which breast cancer mortality statistics correlate most strongly. Where cancer predisposition is suspected, this change of diet should be made as early in life as possible."[27]

All this confirms what Carlton Fredericks wrote in his book, *Winning the Fight Against Breast Cancer,* a book that every woman should read. He says,

The factors in nutrition that raise resistance to cancer are all anti-oxidants, and these are also the factors which delay aging . . . Vitamin E and selenium, for example. Add to the list vitamin C, and finish it with the high-quality proteins that supply sulfur-containing amino acids, which I cited before as a virtual description of eggs. Add the vitamin B complex to aid liver function in control of estrogen. . . .[28]

THE HEALTH OF YOUR LIVER   The functioning of a healthy liver is vital to the body's defense and well-being. Located under the diaphragm just above the stomach, the liver is the largest organ in the body. Thousands of chemical reactions take place in the liver every second during life. Only one of the functions of a healthy liver is its ability to destroy harmful substances, to detoxify drugs, poisons, chemicals, and toxins from bacterial infections. A healthy liver, then, is a master key to our body's protection from chemicals and toxins.

Adelle Davis' book, *Let's Get Well,* reported a study in which sixty-eight people seriously ill with cirrhosis of the liver were given a high-protein diet supplemented with multi-vitamins and two tablespoons of yeast at each meal. This diet induced "rapid recoveries" in all, even the most advanced cases. "In another group of patients with cirrhosis, the severest scarring was replaced by normal tissue within a few months after the diet was made adequate; and as long as such a diet was adhered to, there was no return of liver damage."[29]

To hasten liver regeneration, a diet high in complete proteins, vitamin C, the B-complex, lecithin, and especially vitamin E is necessary. Desiccated liver, which is 100 percent liver, dried at a low heat for vitamin protection, and powdered or compressed into tablet form, is a good way to rebuild the liver.

To avoid cancers and other diseases, we should eliminate the smoking habit, improve our diet, and avoid strong chemicals and radiation. We should also learn how to handle stress. Beyond that, we should do everything possible to stimulate and revive the body's immune system to preserve, restore, and regain health, and to protect against future disease.

NOTES

1. Mark Bricklin, "Increasing Your Resistance," *Prevention,* May 1981, p. 42.
2. Adelle Davis, *Let's Get Well* (New York: Harcourt, Brace & World, 1965), p. 143.
3. Ibid., p. 144.
4. We were awakened to the importance of eggs many years ago, when we read the account of Dr. Al Coburn and his unrelenting efforts to solve the rheumatic fever that was killing forty thousand Americans a year in the early forties. See Paul de Kruif, *Life Among the Doctors* (New York: Harcourt, Brace & Co., 1949).
   Coburn's research began in 1939 and continued through 1941. The diet of dangerously rheumatic children, rich and poor alike, was reinforced with two boiled eggs and two frozen egg yolks daily. Despite the fact that there were incidences of streptococcus sore throat among the children, all rheumatically susceptible, not one of them contracted the disease.
   In subsequent experiments, diets supercharged with eggs were given to more highly susceptible, heart-endangered rheumatics and, amazingly, the children escaped rheumatic fever.
   There seemed to be an "x" quality in eggs, some substance that could correct the allergic defect of children born rheumatically susceptible. Mother feels that the "x" quality is gamma globulin, which builds our immunity.
   When Coburn was called into the Navy at the start of World War II, Dr. Lucille Moore saw his historic experiments through to conclusion.
   Since the advent of antibiotics, we no longer hear much about rheumatic fever.
5. Carlton Fredericks and Herbert Bailey, *Food Facts and Fallacies* (New York: Arco Publishing Co., 1972), p. 235.
6. Roland Evin Horvath, in *Pathways to Living,* vol. 14, no. 1, p. 2.
7. Ibid.
8. Robert C. Atkins, M.D., *Dr. Atkins' Nutrition Breakthrough* (New York: Morrow, 1981), p. 146.
9. Davis, *Let's Get Well,* p. 140.
10. Linus Pauling, Ph.D., *Vitamin C and the Common Cold* (New York: Bantam Books, 1970), p. 86.
11. Ibid., p. 69.
12. Charles Gerras, ed., *The Complete Book of Vitamins* (Emmaus, Penn.: Rodale Press, 1977), p. 295.
13. Irwin Stone, *The Healing Factor* (New York: Grosset & Dunlap, 1972), pp. 72, 73.
14. Albert Szent-Gyorgyi, M.D., Ph.D., "How New Understandings About the Biological Function of Ascorbic Acid May Profoundly Affect Our Lives!" *Executive Health,* May 1978.
15. Ibid.
16. Linus Pauling, "Vitamin C and Cancer," *The Linus Pauling Institute of Science and Medicine Newsletter Reprint,* vol. 1, no. 2.
17. Szent-Gyorgyi, "New Understandings."
18. "The Big If in Cancer," *Time,* March 31, 1980, pp. 60–66.
19. Ibid., p. 66.
20. Dominick Bosco, "How Vitamin C Boosts Immunity," *Prevention,* May 1971, p. 88.

21. Richard Kaplan, D.O., "We Can Raise Our Own Interferon Levels Through Stress and Nutrition," *Let's LIVE*, May 1981, p. 158.
22. Ibid.
23. Jonathan Uhlaner, "Selenium: A Mineral Made to Fight Cancer," *Prevention*, February 1980, p. 129.
24. Ibid., p. 132.
25. Ibid.
26. Richard Passwater, Ph.D., *Supernutrition* (New York: Dial Press, 1975), p. 126.
27. Uhlaner, "Selenium," p. 132.
28. Carlton Fredericks, Ph.D., *Winning the Fight Against Breast Cancer: The Nutritional Approach* (New York: Grosset & Dunlap, 1977), p. 83.
29. Davis, *Let's Get Well*, p. 212.

✄ 10. Lively Longevity: Aging Without Growing Old

We don't really know exactly what causes aging but there are enough research results available that show that an average life expectancy of at least 110 years, while staying physically fit and mentally alert, is definitely possible.
—DR. HANS J. KUGLER

Mother has a simple test for establishing how old you are: pinch the skin on the back of your hand—if the skin snaps back, you are young (regardless of your chronological years); if it crawls back, you are old. Elastic skin is a sign of ample collagen, the strong, cement-like material that binds the cells of your body.

No one wants to get old as we generally think of it—the muscles having become soft, the bones brittle, the personality cantankerous, and the mind senile. While others have searched for the legendary "fountain of youth," Mother has been searching for something else—a way to help people stay healthy, energetic, and attractive. Her search led to nutrition.

What is aging? The question is not an easy one to answer. But it is easy to say what aging is *not*—it is not senility and poor health. Those are conditions generally brought on by chronic malnutrition and inattention to what the body needs to maintain its vigor at *any* age.

Though senility is not the same as aging, the two, unfortunately, are often equated. Everybody ages, of course, but only some become senile; senility is not the inevitable result of aging. Memory loss, inability to store new information, and certain personality quirks, these distinguishing signs of senility are senseless and preventable.

Mother's "Secrets"

People are generally amazed when they learn Mother's age. They want to know her "secrets." But Mother has none; everything she has learned, she shares. She has spent years finding

out what the body needs, how it responds, and what things contribute to optimum health. Book after book has appeared on the
market to claim that megadoses of certain nutrients, and substances believed to be nutrients, are of no known value to the
elderly or anyone else. Yet Mother is walking evidence that they
are of value. Furthermore, there are many other people like her
—among them, the ageless Gayelord Hauser, Carlton Fredericks, Bob Hope, and Lois and Art Linkletter.

One eighty-three-year-old gentleman with a jaunty air about
him picks up his vitamins, minerals, and brewer's yeast and ex-
claims, "Scotch and water and a tablespoonful of brewer's yeast.
What a lift!" One suspects he'll be around a long time. And
there's the eighty-two-year-old woman who regularly comes into
one of our stores, a constant source of amazement. She's been on
the Lindberg program for thirty-two years. She rides her bicycle
every day and gets upset when no one will ride with her. She
attributes her good health to proper nutrition, exercise, and
faithfulness to Gladys Lindberg's help and advice.

Another "older" gentleman (in his mid-eighties), who regularly replenishes his supply of vitamins and minerals, says, "Especially vitamin E, ladies, especially vitamin E. You wouldn't
believe how many womenfriends I have. . . ." This intelligent,
dignified older man has maintained remarkable health. His vig-
or, wit, and charm are a match for any man forty years his junior.

Such people as these have aged without growing old. Nutrition
has played a major role in preventing their physical and mental
deterioration. Many of the senior citizens we see have maintained a zest for living, loving, working, and growing. They are
still striving to be the very best they can be.

Mother has always maintained that you can improve with age,
that you can retain an attractive appearance and vitality while
enjoying optimum health. But health is not something that just
happens; it is an ongoing investment that involves your total
life-style.

Your Cells

We must look at what happens to our cells if we hope to answer the question, "What is aging?" Cell function is the basis of
all life. As each of us grows older, our trillions of body cells
gradually change. The best way to maintain health and vitality
is to keep these cells performing in harmony.

Every cell has a limited life, after which it reproduces itself through a process called "mitosis," or doubling. Then the cell dies. At any given time, thousands of your cells may be dying, while thousands more are being reborn, some faster than others. Fat cells, for instance, reproduce slowly, while skin cells reproduce approximately every ten hours.

This constant process of cell replacement is an advantage; but one type of cell is an exception to the process. When you were born, you were given your lifetime supply of brain cells, and when these cells become worn out, they are never replaced. Scientists tell us that, by the age of thirty-five, a person is losing 100,000 brain cells a day. Fortunately, the initial surplus is so great that this loss is scarcely noticeable.[1]

Is There a Biological Time Clock?

In 1968, Dr. Leonard Hayflick published an interesting paper which demonstrated that human cells have a definite number of cell divisions. This suggested that there was a limit to the human life span.[2]

However, in February of 1974, S. Gelfant, at the Miami Symposium on Theoretical Aspects of Aging, reported that in cell cultures a certain number of cells stop dividing, while others continue to divide, and that cells that have stopped dividing can be stimulated to divide again.[3]

"Human studies have shown that in a partial vitamin E deficiency, red blood cells are destroyed about eight to ten percent faster than in an adequate vitamin E state."[4]

Scientists have speculated that some biological time clock exists within the cell and controls the rate of aging. If this is true, then immortality for mankind may be achieved, they say, when some major breakthrough enables them to intervene in the cell's mechanism and "stop the clock" of aging.

Jeffrey Bland, Ph.D., of the University of Puget Sound, Tacoma, Washington, has described the cell as a kind of tiny biochemical factory that, at any one time, is involved in thousands of different chemical reactions, each of them vital to health and life. The cell membranes are largely responsible for the success of these functions. According to Bland,

That's because it's the membranes which actively transport all the vitamins, minerals, trace metals, nutrients, hormones, and other chemical messenger substances on which the cell depends for its very existence.

These vital substances don't merely "ooze" through the membrane to reach the places within the cell where they're needed. We now feel there is a kind of "push-pull" mechanism in which the membrane actively selects what it is going to take in and what it is going to expel. There also seem to be particular "ports" on the cell membrane which are programmed to recognize various substances—kind of like molecular doormen.

In other words, without the active cooperation of the cell membrane, the cell is not going to get what it needs to go on leading a useful life.[5]

Bland points to the many diseases, from cancer to diabetes, that are associated with altered or abnormal cell membrane structure. "In the case of diabetes, it appears that for some reason the cell membranes will not take up glucose or blood sugar. In the case of cancer, it seems that something happens to the cell membrane which prevents such abnormal cells from being attacked and destroyed by the phagocytes of the immune system."[6]

Life-Sustaining Nutrients

VITAMIN E   When you think in terms of cell protection, think vitamin E. The function of vitamin E is being made clear through the work of many fine researchers—among them, Dr. A. L. Tappel, of the Department of Food Science at the University of California at Davis. Tappel's findings suggest that anti-oxidants reduce the rate of "peroxidation," or oxidative damage, caused by chemicals such as the ozone in smog.[7] Vitamin E is the fat-soluble anti-oxidant, and vitamin C is the water-soluble anti-oxidant that works with vitamin E.

A cell cannot function fully when part of it has been degraded by oxidation, so the presence of an anti-oxidant—a substance that hinders oxidation—is of the utmost importance. Damaged organs can't perform their functions, can't dispose of their waste metabolites, and can't renew themselves. The need for vitamin E, therefore, would be greater as we get older; but the value of this vitamin, in retarding aging or in preventing the loss of healthy functions in many parts of the body, is such that the body needs to be adequately supplied at any age. The optimum time to begin using vitamin E is when it will do the most good, before aging has a chance to gain a foothold—in the twenties and thirties. However, the need for vitamin E, as for other vitamins, of course begins in infancy.

Ozone is so damaging that those who live where ozone levels

are high should heed Tappel's hypothesis regarding peroxidation:

When radiant energy, which can penetrate throughout the body entering every cell, strikes a polyunsaturated lipid that is present as a nutrient, one of two things happen. If enough vitamin E is present, the radiation will have little effect. If, however, there is an intracellular deficiency of vitamin E, the energetic rays will strike a lipid molecule and knock loose a hydrogen atom. This would typically initiate the peroxidation of polyunsaturated lipid . . . (forming free radicals). The free radical flies about within the cell under terrific force and without any pattern to its movement until it strikes another molecule and causes all sorts of damage. Lipid peroxidation is, therefore, widely regarded as the mainspring in the aging process.[8]

Tappel reports that the survival of rats exposed to three to fifteen parts per million of ozone is decreased if the animals' supply of vitamin E is inadequate.[9]

Dr. D. Warshauer and his associates at the Section of Infections and Immunologic Diseases, School of Medicine, University of California at Davis, found that a deficiency in vitamin E increases susceptibility to ozone-induced lung damage. The deficiency reduces pulmonary defense to infection and makes the organism more susceptible to invasion by bacteria. The membranes of cells are weakened, and since the membrane is the cell's first defense barrier, its integrity is essential for warding off potential threats to the cell's biochemical machinery.[10]

Denham Harman, M.D., of the University of Nebraska, has been working with anti-oxidants for over twenty years, and he has discovered that a number of them, including vitamin E, can prolong the lives of mice. In fact, he reports that sick old mice seemed to get younger when given massive doses of vitamin E. Although Harmon has shown that resistance to disease decreases with age, these older mice developed fewer infections and their immune systems dramatically improved.[11]

Other researchers are giving attention to the links between anti-oxidants, immunity, and aging. Ronald R. Watson, Ph.D., of Purdue University, writes: "The immune systems in young children and in older people are less effective than in mature adults. The longer you live, the more severely infections hit you. That's why when flu vaccines come around, complications to the vaccine usually develop in young people and older people." He has been testing the effects of diet on the immune systems of people in nursing homes and conducting animal studies with vitamin E; these latter have produced the results similar to Harmon's. According to Watson, "Vitamin E boosted one aspect of the immune response, important in the body's anticancer defenses, within a week of giving it to mice."[12] Other nutrients found to act as anti-oxidants are vitamins C and A, selenium, zinc, manganese, and the enzyme superoxide dismutase (SOD).

An impressive number of researchers agree that vitamin E stabilizes and even slows the aging process.

Carlton Fredericks explains that an individual who receives less than the ideal amount of vitamin E may, as the only *visible* consequence, age more rapidly. Though the aging process has generally been considered normal, accumulating evidence now indicates that it is a sickness, in part due to improper diet. Sterility from vitamin E deficiency is rare, but premature or accelerated aging from want of this vitamin may be common.[13]

So it seems that a person who receives an optimal level of vitamin E should be able to avoid unnecessarily rapid cellular aging. But this question arises: How much should I take? Dr. Evan V. Shute, after thirty years of clinical work with vitamin E, states, "We think that the average normal female should have 400 units a day and the average normal male about 600 units a day." Recommended dosages are frequently increased for individuals with heart, circulatory, and other conditions. Shute offers other doctors this advice: "Dosage is the most important factor in successful vitamin E therapy." In other words, "if you use vitamin E, use enough."[14] See Vitamin E in Appendix B for further information on diabetes and heart conditions.

Dosage recommendations by other specialists in nutrition vary. Certainly 400 units daily is adequate. But Mother has been taking 1,200 to 1,600 units for several years. Before that, she took 400 to 800 units.

VITAMIN C   Dr. Irwin Stone, author of *The Healing Factor,* says that aging is a chronic, 100 percent fatal disease from which everyone suffers and which is present at birth and gains momentum as we go through life. His recommendation—one we fully endorse—is that treatment of this "chronic disease" should not be directed against acute symptoms that may develop in later years, but at preventive measures starting at birth and continuing throughout life.[15]

Statistics on the human life span are startling. The drop in infant mortality and in deaths from childhood diseases has changed life-expectancy charts for the early hazardous years, but life expectancy for persons past the age of sixty has remained nearly constant since 1789.

Stone believes that the proper use of ascorbic acid (vitamin C) *throughout life* may provide the long-awaited breakthrough in geriatrics. Most importantly, use of ascorbic acid should also prolong the period of vigorous and healthy maturity, not merely the life span.[16]

PANTOTHENIC ACID   Pantothenic acid is also believed to have anti-aging properties. Roger Williams, who discovered this important vitamin, found that when he gave mice a nutritious diet and treated them with pantothenic acid, they lived 653 days, 103 days longer than his control mice. In human beings, this would be equivalent to an increase in life span from 75 to 89 years.[17] Pantothenic acid has also been found to benefit arthritis, a common complaint among the elderly.

LECITHIN   Lecithin is being hailed as a nutrient that can activate and energize sluggish body processes so that aging can be controlled and perhaps someday even halted. The intake of two tablespoons of soy lecithin daily is said to help control cholesterol, improve the health of the heart, and offer hope for a longer and more youthful life.[18]

MINERALS   One thing we can do to make certain that we age with dignity is add minerals to our diet. Up to 80 percent of Americans suffer from often-dangerous nutritional deficiencies, and mineral deficiencies are especially common. Minerals in our foodstuffs are depleted at every step, from harvest to consumption. Lack of minerals can cause fatigue, sleeplessness, poor skin and muscle tone, vision problems, stiff joints, inability to think clearly, and susceptibility to infection. Furthermore, mineral deficiencies can cause premature aging.

DeWayne Ashmead, Ph.D., sets forth the theory that as a person becomes older, increasing accumulations of aluminum in the body (taken from the environment, largely) cause calcium to be removed from the blood and deposited where it does not belong. When this occurs, the body's balance of calcium and zinc is disturbed and excessive amounts of zinc leave the body. The result is senility. Supplementing the diet with extra zinc brings about a more natural balance between the calcium and zinc in the blood and tissues, which reduces the chances of atherosclerosis and possibly senility. According to Ashmead, the right balance of chelated minerals with vitamins is important because vitamins are responsible for picking up minerals and placing them in enzymes so that the minerals can activate the enzymes.[19]

Menopause

Someone may be wondering if nutrition can help menopause, and, of course, the answer is yes. What you eat can help you deal with some of the unpleasant side effects of menopause. As a woman's chemical balance shifts during this time, her nutritional needs change as well. Actually, nutrition for menopause should start twenty or more years before and include what is recommended on Mother's complete program.

Menopause is also a form of stress. If you are like the majority of women and have a difficult time with this phase of your life, this could indicate adrenal exhaustion.

Stringent weight-reducing diets may induce "loss of bone as well as soft tissue; calcium losses during pregnancies not compensated for adequately by prescribed prenatal supplements (especially in women with prepregnancy calcium deficiencies); failure to continue calcium supplements in mothers who breastfeed their babies; and calcium and bone losses associated with hormonal changes in menopause."[20]

Many interesting studies have been done in which calcium supplements were given to one control group, while no calcium was given to others in the same study. The results of these studies indicate beyond a reasonable doubt that a daily minimum intake of one gram of calcium, and perhaps more, is needed to maintain normal bone density.[21]

Not to forget the men, one study revealed "... how the continual physical activity of vigorous old men of 100 *or more* keeps the balance between bone formation and destruction such that their bones remain mineralized, dense and strong. So, along with calcium, don't forget to walk an hour or so a day."[22] That's good advice for both men and women.

One of the things that women especially worry about is getting a "dowager's hump"—that hump that develops at the back of the neck. Here again, the problem may be one of calcium being stripped out of the bones, causing height loss and a hump. "Recent studies indicate that at least 26 percent of all women over 60 have osteoporosis severe enough to cause deformity, height loss, and pain."[23]

Minerals for the blues of menopause include magnesium. A calcium tablet with magnesium is often suggested. An antistress program with daily supplementation of these minerals, in addition to all the other vitamins and minerals, is the most reasonable and comfortable way to get through menopause. This should be a delightful time of life—the concern over pregnancy is gone, the children are grown, and it should be a time when husbands and wives enjoy each other and do some of the things they've had to put off doing for years. Take charge of your health so you can be healthy enough to enjoy these years.

While we are on this subject, we need to say something about estrogen as well. Estrogen was the fifth most-prescribed drug in the country in 1980 for menopause relief. Instead of taking estrogen Mother recommends you take vitamin E for the symptoms of menopause. The hot flashes and night sweats often disappear when upwards to 800 units of vitamin E are taken daily. Mother went through menopause when she was in her fifties and never took estrogen. She took vitamin E and never had any complaints. She recommends that all women taking estrogen after menopause read Carlton Frederick's book *Winning the Fight Against Breast Cancer: The Nutritional Approach.*

Fredericks reports recent findings of the National Cancer Institute: "Estrogen, given in large doses over a prolonged period, has induced tumors of the breast, cervix, endometrium, pituitary, testicles, and bone marrow in mice, rats, rabbits, hamsters, and dogs. And he said, without reservations, that these animal studies are definitely applicable to women."[24]

Other studies have shown that "the administration of estrogen for both menopausal and postmenopausal women strikingly increases the risk of breast and uterine cancer—by a factor from 5 to as much as 14."[25]

We feel that's too high a price to pay for stopping hot flashes. Mother tells women that hormones should be taken as a last resort. Taking either the pill or estrogen therapy is, we believe, a calculated risk.

Let me just emphasize that women are under a tremendous amount of stress during their child-bearing and menopausal years. If stress is piled upon stress, if the diet is inadequate, and if the woman is not receiving supplements, the ravages of menopause, in particular, superimposed upon already existing deficiencies, can really play havoc with a woman's health.

Women need to be aware that good nutrition will help protect them against heart trouble after menopause. They should be taking, among other things, lecithin. Mother always tells women that they should be eating eggs, nature's source of that all-important lecithin. She also tells them to take alfalfa tablets because these contain potassium, which is so essential for the heart. "When your heart beats, that's potassium," she says. "And when it relaxes, that's calcium."

The Senility Syndrome

The deficiency of *any* essential nutrient, if continued for a long time, will hasten the onset of senility, but a deficiency of niacin (vitamin B-3) is implicated in rapid development of the senility syndrome. If the initial flush produced by niacin is too irritating or uncomfortable, start at a low dosage and work up slowly, over a few weeks. Interestingly, people with niacin deficiencies generally have more side effects than others when they begin to use this vitamin.

Ascorbic acid (vitamin C) is also considered an antisenility vitamin and is therefore especially needed by senility-prone elderly people.

Anti-Aging Therapies

CELL THERAPY   Many types of "rejuvenation" procedures have come and gone, but in recent years cell therapy has been used with growing acceptance throughout the world. Actually, therapy with cells or cell units is old indeed. Skin transplants from animals to humans were mentioned by Hippocrates, and physicians have long held the opinion that incorporating human or animal organs from a young and vital body may have a therapeutic effect. Dr. J. Stein points out that both Aristotle and one of the oldest known medical documents, the Papyrus of Ebers, mention a number of preparations made from animal or human organs. And in the sixteenth century, Paracelsus offered this prescription: "Heart heals heart, kidney heals kidney."[26]

Dr. Paul Niehans, a Swiss surgeon, is credited with having developed cell therapy as we know it today after saving a dying woman with an injection of a suspension of animal parathyroid glands.[27] As his research progressed, he discovered that the cells from animal embryos, injected into the muscles of an older or exhausted person, had a rejuvenating effect. It was also observed that injections of cells from specific embryo organs could improve the same organ in an individual. Thus, heart diseases were treated with heart cells, liver problems with liver cells, and so forth—just as Paracelsus had suggested—and the adult body did not reject the embryonic cells.

Niehans had administered more than 50,000 cell injections in his laboratory in Switzerland between 1931 and 1971, when he died at the age of eighty-nine. His technique consisted of injecting fetal cells or the cells of newborn animals into his patients. It has been reported that many famous people, including Winston Churchill, Charles de Gaulle, King George VI, Pope Pius XII, the Duke of Windsor, and Charlie Chaplin, have received these treatments.

Several years ago we had the pleasure of meeting Dr. Joachim Stein of Heidelberg, Germany, who had worked with Niehans for years. In connection with the University of Heidelberg, Stein developed the Cybila Laboratory, where freeze-dried cells from healthy, grass-fed animals are processed and sent around the world. We learned that both smoking and the use of alcohol destroy newly implanted cells.

Unfortunately, cell therapy is not available in the United States.

GLANDULAR THERAPY   Glandular therapy, hailed as "the ultimate in nutritional research," is causing a lot of excitement among health-conscious people. The raw glandular supplements used are specialized nutrients intended to improve the nutritional environment of the body's own glands and organs. The rationale for using such raw glandulars and organ concentrates is the same as the rationale underlying cell therapy—that is, cells help like cells. For example, adrenal concentrate is used to support adrenal gland function.

The sources of these enzyme- and hormone-active, whole food, tissue concentrates are animal, mostly beef. And the materials are left "raw," meaning that at no time during the processing or tableting are they exposed to temperatures higher than 37° centigrade (98.6°F), thus preserving their intracellular components. The targeting effect a specific glandular concentrate has on a depleted or malfunctioning gland or organ is nothing short of amazing. However, not everyone needs glandular therapy, and its use should be directed toward correcting a dietary or metabolic deficiency.

GEROVITAL (GH3) THERAPY   Not to be confused with the over-the-counter vitamin preparation, Gerovital is a treatment that was developed in Rumania by Dr. Ana Aslan. Aslan has achieved worldwide prominence from her use of Gerovital H3, which is a buffered form of the procaine (novocaine) used by your friendly dentist. The effectiveness of GH3 as an anti-aging drug is being hailed everywhere, and even in this country, the FDA has finally given it investigational status.

At the Geriatric Institute in Bucharest, where she originally studied the effects of Gerovital on three groups of inpatients and over 2,500 outpatients for over five years, Aslan reported that the drug accomplished the following: it eliminated depression, produced muscle vigor, reduced high blood pressure, and relieved symptoms of both arthritis and cardiac chest pain.[28]

Since this initial five-year study, many other studies and reports have come out under Aslan's supervision in cooperation with as many as 400 doctors throughout Rumania. We have had several friends who have gone to Bucharest for weeks of GH3 treatment, and they brought home sufficient injections for a year. However, we have not seen the fantastic results claimed for GH3.

Changes in Life-Style

The future will determine whether raw glandulars, cell therapy, nucleic acid supplements and injections, or some other "miracle drug" will be the key to the prevention of aging. Open-minded doctors who recognize the wisdom of continuing such research will be leading the way in exciting new developments. In the meantime, our most effective weapon against aging is our own willingness to change self-destructive behavior such as smoking, drinking alcohol, being overweight, inadequate nutrition, lack of exercise, excessive stress, and lack of satisfying work, rest, and leisure activity.

Smoking is one of the worst habits a person can maintain. Not only is tobacco use considered the greatest accelerator of aging in human beings, but it is the primary cause of many diseases and it creates maximum risk for heart problems and lung cancer. Smokers are particularly prone to severe respiratory diseases, especially emphysema, which is extremely disabling. High blood pressure is aggravated by the use of tobacco; and a decrease in the supply of blood to the brain can interfere with cerebral function and cause a stroke.

Drinking alcoholic beverages can cause mental and emotional problems and wreak havoc with the nervous system. Increasingly, evidence points to the deleterious effects alcohol has on the pancreas, esophagus, stomach, heart, liver, and almost every other organ in the body. Furthermore, drinking leads to multiple vitamin deficiencies.

The alcoholics Mother has worked with usually have a long history of low blood sugar, which complicates their addiction. She has discovered that for some people, meeting nutritional needs ends their craving for alcohol.

According to the AMA, one in every five Americans is *overweight*,[29] a condition directly related to ill health, loss of vitality, and mortality. The mortality rate among people who are 20 percent overweight is 30 percent greater than that of those who maintain their proper weight, while the mortality rate for those who are 40 percent overweight is increased by 70 percent.

However, dieting can be either a health-building or a health-destroying process. Dieting extremes often lead to serious nutrient deficiencies and health problems. When people decide to lose weight, they rarely give themselves sufficient time, becoming discouraged when results fail to appear immediately. Mother advises patience and following sound nutrition principles, and taking vitamin and mineral supplements to make certain the body receives all the essential nutrients. Some people are afraid that if they take vitamins and minerals, they will gain weight. Mother encounters that fear frequently, but it has no basis in fact.

Exercise improves the quality of life, enhances blood circulation, and permits greater food intake, thus increasing each cell's nourishment while helping to prevent obesity. Exercise enables your body to maintain a vital reserve, which has a protective effect during stress. At a three-day conference on aging and the role of exercise in prevention of physical decline, researchers from across the United States, Canada, and Western Europe offered incontrovertible evidence that physical activity can retard factors that have always been considered the inevitable consequences of the aging process. They emphasized that the body is the one machine that breaks down when it is *not* used; in fact, it works better the more it is used.[30]

Excessive stress can add years to the way you look and contribute to many disorders, most notably heart attacks. For this reason, you should do whatever you can to minimize stress in your life.

Undernutrition can be a problem for people who just don't en-joy their food or even the thought of eating. There are others who become undernourished or malnourished because they are afraid of gaining weight. Because such people show many signs of defi-ciency symptoms, they often look older than their age.

Protein deficiency is a special problem for those without an appetite, so Mother encourages them to drink small amounts of a delicious fortified protein drink several times a day. She also has them take digestive enzymes and hydrochloric acid, since their problem is often compounded by an inability to digest food well.

A less tangible factor in the aging process is our *involvement with life,* our refusal to live an aimless existence. Staying busy, learning new things, developing fresh interests, and maintain-ing some type of enjoyable leisure activity keep many older people both young in spirit and physically mobile. In other words we believe that our positive outlook on a long and healthy life is an important part of our physical well being. Our mind, spirit, and body must all be nurtured if we want to experience total health.

A NEW BEGINNING   It is never too late to start over. A new beginning is possible at any age. Preventive medicine places most of the care of your body into your own hands.

We cannot hold our doctors responsible for our health—or for our lack of it. Their responsibility is to help us when we are sick. They are involved in what is called "crisis medicine." That is what they are trained for, and we should be thankful that we can call upon them in times of need.

Nor can we expect the government to look after our health. The government does what it can to control communicable dis-eases and to reduce pollutants in our water and air, but it is our personal responsibility to learn what contributes to illness and break whatever bad habits we may have acquired. If we hope to prevent disease and untimely aging, what we really need is more respect for the human body. This can lead to a longer life cycle— certainly one more active and happy.

NOTES

1. Abram Hoffer, M.D., Ph.D., and Morton Walker, D.P.M., *Nutrients to Age Without Senility* (New Canaan, Conn.: Keats, 1980), p. 28.
2. Leonard Hayflick, M.D., *Scientific American,* vol. 218 (1968).
3. S. Gelfant, paper read at the Miami Symposium on Theoretical Aspects of Aging, February 7, 1974.

4. Dominick Bosco, *The People's Guide to Vitamins and Minerals* (Contemporary Books, 1980), Chicago, Ill.: p. 165.
5. Jeffrey Bland, Ph.D., "How Vitamin E Can Slow Cellular Aging: A New Discovery," *Prevention,* June 1976.
6. Ibid.
7. A. L. Tappel, "Will Antioxidant Nutrients Slow Aging Processes?" *Geriatrics,* October 1968, pp. 97–105.
8. A. L. Tappel, "Where Old Age Begins," *Nutrition Today,* December 1967, pp. 2–7.
9. Ibid.
10. Bland, "How Vitamin E Can Slow Cellular Aging."
11. Roland Evin Horvath, *Pathways to Living,* vol. 12, no. 5.
12. John Yates, "A New Pathway to a Longer Life," *Prevention,* December 1980, pp. 97–98.
13. Carlton Fredericks, *Look Younger, Feel Healthier* (New York: Grosset & Dunlap, 1972), p. 136.
14. Dr. Wilfrid E. Shute, *Vitamin E Book* (New Canaan, Conn.: Keats, 1975), p. 186.
15. Irwin Stone, *The Healing Factor* (New York: Grosset & Dunlap, 1972), p. 115.
16. Ibid., pp. 113, 115.
17. Dr. Roger J. Williams, *Nutrition Against Disease* (New York: Bantam Books, 1973), pp. 146–147.
18. Carlson Wade, "Lecithin—A Food to Reverse Aging," *Natural Food and Farming,* July 1979, p. 5.
19. DeWayne Ashmead, Ph.D., "The Role of Minerals in Preventing Senility and Aging," *Bestways,* January 1981, pp. 34–39.
20. "New Reports on the Dangers of Too Little Calcium in Your Diet," *Executive Health,* November 1977.
21. Ibid.
22. Ibid.
23. Ibid.
24. Carlton Fredericks, *Breast Cancer: A Nutritional Approach* (New York: Grosset & Dunlap, 1977), p. 11.
25. Ibid., p. 13.
26. Dr. K. Schmid and Dr. J. Stein, eds., *Cell Research and Cell Therapy* (Thoune, Switzerland: Ott Publishers, 1967), p. 19.
27. Ibid.
28. Gary L. Couture, Ph.D., and Lee Gladden, Ph.D., *How to Win the Aging Game* (Newport Beach: Harbour House, 1979), pp. 198–208.
29. Ivan Popov, M.D., *Stay Young* (New York: Grosset & Dunlap, 1975), p. 51.
30. "On Walking," *Executive Health,* July 1978, pp. 1–2.

11. Take Charge of Your Health: A Comprehensive Program

> For forty years I have been trying to help people stay in good health, teaching them the principles of good nutrition. It is our responsibility to take charge of our own health.
>
> —GLADYS LINDBERG

Mother doesn't believe in taking vitamin and mineral supplements and continuing to eat a poor diet. She encourages people to adopt a *comprehensive* nutritional program: to learn how to eat right, count grams of protein, keep their blood sugar up, and manage their weight.

This chapter tells you how to start Gladys Lindberg's nutritional program and stay with it for the rest of your life. Her balanced nutritional program has had fantastic results for the past 40 years, truly standing the test of time.

Take Charge Reference Chart

To help you learn how to take charge of your health, we've simplified Gladys Lindberg's nutritional program into easy-to-understand chart form. The first page of the chart offers various desired eating patterns: the "war on weight plan," the "stay healthy plan," and the "strength and energy plan." Each plan tells you when to take your vitamins and minerals, when to take fortified drinks, and when to eat your meals. You'll notice that an "all possible combinations" category allows you freedom to vary from your normal program.

The key is to take the fortified drink a couple of times a day, incorporating it into your five feedings a day needed to keep your blood sugar at an optimum level. The snacks or fortified drinks recommended during mid-morning and mid-afternoon crowd out the coffee breaks, cigarettes, donuts, and candy bars that might have tempted you in the past.

Take Charge Reference Chart

	War on Weight Plan (Dieter)	Stay Healthy Plan (Average Person)	Strength & Energy Plan (Athlete or Active Person)	Choose Your Plan (All Combined)
Morning	fortified drink *plus* balanced vitamin-mineral formula	breakfast *plus* balanced vitamin-mineral formula	breakfast *plus* balanced vitamin-mineral formula	fortified drink *or* breakfast *plus* balanced vitamin-mineral formula
Mid-Morning	fortified drink (about 3 hours after breakfast)	fortified drink *or* snack	fortified drink	fortified drink *or* snack
Noon	skip regular lunch	skip regular lunch	lunch (if hungry)	lunch *or* skip
Mid-Afternoon	fortified drink (in early afternoon)	fortified drink (if snack used earlier) *or* snack (if fortified drink used earlier)	fortified drink	fortified drink *or* snack
Evening	light dinner	dinner	dinner	fortified drink *or* dinner
If Early Dinner and Retiring Late	skip	small fortified drink *or* snack	fortified drink *or* snack	fortified drink *or* snack

EXTRA° SUPPLEMENTS You may want to add additional supplements* to your diet in addition to the vitamin-mineral program outlined in Appendix B. These are suggestions that have helped many people that fall into one of the following categories.

SERIOUS ATHLETE
>   Morning and evening
>   3 to 5 wheat germ oil capsules
>   15 raw liver tablets
>   Bee pollen (optional) in tablet or granulated form

PERSON UNDER EXTRA STRESS
>   Morning
>   15 raw liver tablets

*See pp. 161–66 for a description of supplements.

Noon
 Extra vitamin C (1,000 mg. or more)
Evening
 Extra vitamin C (1,000 mg. or more)
 Vitamin B–complex tablet

TO INCREASE IMMUNITY
Morning
 15 raw liver tablets
 Raw glandular tablets (thymus) (see dosage recommendation on bottle)
Noon
 Extra vitamin C (1,000 mg. or more)
Evening
 Extra vitamin C (1,000 mg. or more)
 Vitamin B–complex tablet
 Raw glandular tablets (thymus) (see dosage recommendation on bottle)

IMPROPER ELIMINATION
Morning and evening
 Acidophilus liquid (3 or more tbls.) or tablets (see label)
 5 to 10 alfalfa tablets

IMPROPER DIGESTION
After meals or fortified protein drinks
 3 to 4 tablets betaine hydrochloride with pepsin (commonly called "hydrochloric acid")
 3 to 4 tablets pancreatic enzymes with bile

Fortified Protein Drinks

Notice on the Take Charge Reference Chart (p. 150) that fortified protein drinks may be taken with a meal, instead of a meal, or instead of a snack. Try to take these drinks up to three times a day. They provide complete protein, many of the vitamins and minerals in their natural state, and additional factors or nutrients that are still unidentified. The following pages tell you how to make seven fortified drinks, from Mother's Serenity Cocktail, which contains a host of ingredients, to a very simple fortified milk drink.

You may want to take betaine hydrochloride with pepsin and pancreatic enzymes with bile, available in tablet form, to aid in the digestion and assimilation of these drinks.

The Serenity Cocktail, Gladys Lindberg's ultimate formula,

has evolved over the years. It started out when she first became familiar with the properties found in yeast and mixed it into our milk and food. Then she began to add raw liver powder. She knew, however, that brewer's yeast and liver are high in the mineral phosphorus but low in calcium, so she began to add other ingredients, including calcium and bone meal, to balance the formula. She named her drink the Serenity Cocktail after the inner calmness it gives your body.

Listed below is the formula for the Serenity Cocktail. The various ingredients can be purchased at your health food or nutrition store.

SERENITY COCKTAIL MIXTURE

        1 lb. protein powder (unsweetened)
        1 lb. brewer's yeast (not torula yeast)
        1 lb. soya lecithin (granulated or powdered)
        1 lb. powdered skim milk (noninstant)
        1 lb. whey (if unavailable, add an extra pound of skim milk)
        8 oz. raw liver powder
        8 oz. bone meal powder
        4 oz. calcium gluconate powder
        1 oz. magnesium oxide powder (or dolomite powder)
        2 oz. (approx. 14 tsp. or 60,000 mg.) vitamin C crystals
    4–8 oz. fructose (more if desired)

Mix ingredients thoroughly in a large paper bag. Turn the bag upside down repeatedly, shaking well. When thoroughly combined, store in a tightly sealed container. (Makes approx. six pounds.)

SERENITY COCKTAIL DRINK

Add to your blender:
        ½ pint (8 oz.) certified raw milk
        1 fertile egg (optional)
        ½ frozen banana or ½ peeled apple
        1 to 2 rounded tbsp. Serenity Cocktail Mixture

Until you become accustomed to the Serenity Cocktail, blend in only a tablespoon of the dry mix. Over a period of days you can increase the amount of mix used from one to two tablespoons, or even more. To make the drink more flavorful, add a spoonful of concentrated frozen orange or apple juice, or sweeten it with honey, sorghum, blackstrap molasses, or even more fructose. It doesn't taste like a chocolate malt, but as you develop a taste for it, you'll reap the rewards in your feeling of well-being. When we mix it for our friends, they are often surprised that it can taste so good.

One glass of the Serenity Cocktail gives you about 19 grams of first class, complete protein: 5 grams from 2 tablespoons of the Serenity Cocktail mix and 14 grams from the egg and milk.

The next two fortified drinks provide you with almost all the B vitamins in natural form, and include all the essential amino acids as well. These drinks do not contain vitamin C, so if you do not drink them right away, be sure to add vitamin C crystals or crushed tablets to prevent oxidation of the fruit. Brewer's yeast and raw liver have a difficult taste to mask, so you may want to experiment with adding different fruits or sweeteners, or even substituting fruit juice for the milk. These two drinks are definitely a meal in themselves. The health rewards you'll get from them are well worth depriving your taste buds of a little pleasure.

SUPER ANTISTRESS YEAST-LIVER DRINK

6 oz. certified raw milk
1 tbsp. brewer's yeast
1 tbsp. powdered skim milk (non-instant)
1 tsp. powdered raw liver
1 tbsp. blackstrap molasses or honey

    Blend with a banana or an apple.

ANTISTRESS YEAST DRINK

6 oz. certified raw milk
1 tbsp. brewer's yeast
1 tbsp. powdered skim milk (non-instant)
1 tbsp. blackstrap molasses or sorghum

    Blend with a banana or an apple.

The following two fortified drinks are for those who want only the essential amino acids. They contain protein powder but do not contain yeast, liver, and other ingredients. (As a result, they do taste better!) The added protein is vital to the diet and will help keep the blood sugar elevated. These drinks can be used for weight loss or weight gain, depending on whether you take them in the place of or with a meal. Again, the milk can be replaced with fruit juices or water (but the protein content of the drink will suffer).

POWER-PACKED PROTEIN DRINK

6 oz. certified raw milk (use lowfat milk if reducing)
1 raw fertile egg
2 rounded tbs. of protein powder (unsweetened)
1 tsp. vanilla to taste
1 tsp. honey or fructose if desired
ice cubes, if desired

Blend and enjoy.

SUPER-ENERGY PROTEIN DRINK

6 oz. certified raw milk
1 raw fertile egg
1 tsp. cold-pressed soy oil or linseed oil*
1 tbsp. soya lecithin
2 heaping tbsp. powdered skim milk or protein powder
½ apple, peeled and cored
1 tsp. vanilla to taste
1 tsp. honey or fructose if desired
ice cubes if desired

Blend and enjoy.

Variations (one or two of the following, omit if reducing): 2 heaping tsp. frozen orange juice; fresh or unsweetened frozen strawberries, boysenberries, or any other fruit; ½ ripe banana;** ½ apple; 2 tsp. peanut butter, or yogurt.

The last two fortified drinks are for people just starting out on a nutritional program, or those who want a quick, inexpensive drink to replace a snack. They are not intended to replace meals, but to supplement them. Blend them to taste; they are delicious.

---

*Calories from oil provide 2½ times the energy of carbohydrate calories and are essential for healthy skin and hair. These oils contain valuable linolenic and linoleic acid. These are essential unsaturated fatty acids.
**If you enjoy bananas in your fortified drinks, you may want to peel a quantity of them and store them, in sandwich bags, in the freezer for convenience.

FORTIFIED MILK DRINK OR TOPPING

1 pt. certified raw milk

½ c. powdered skim milk (non-instant)

>Blend together and refrigerate for cereal
>toppings, cooking, or just drinking.

EGGNOG DRINK

2 c. certified raw milk

2 raw fertile eggs

1 tsp. vanilla

1 tsp. honey, or ½ banana

>Blend and top with grated nutmeg. Serves two.

Proper Eating Patterns

Mother has tried to keep her program simple. Basically, she puts everyone on the same program while adjusting the quantity of the drinks and the other foods included at mealtime. After all, you may have a family that includes an eight-year-old and a sixteen-year-old, while you are forty and your father, who is living with you, is seventy. You all eat from the same table, but the portions can be adjusted.

The following pages discuss the various plans within Gladys Lindberg's nutritional program (outlined in the Take Charge Reference Chart on p. 150). If you are willing to follow through and stay with the program, you can experience dramatic results.

WAR ON WEIGHT PLAN   If you wish to lose weight, take a pint of the Serenity Cocktail (to which two eggs have been added) and divide it into three equal portions. For breakfast, have a teacup (approximately 5.5 ounces) of the Serenity; one-fourth of a cantaloupe, or a whole orange with all the white pulp, or one-half of a grapefruit with pulp, or an apple.

Three hours later, have another 5.5 ounces of Serenity, and three hours after that, drink the remaining Serenity.

For dinner, have a small portion of fish, chicken, beef, or lamb and a large salad with lots of raw vegetables. Use a dressing of 1 tablespoon cold-pressed oil and vinegar with seasonings. Remove the fat on the meat and take the skin off the chicken. If you find yourself having hunger pangs, snack on raw vegetables.

The vitamin-mineral supplements in Appendix B (p. 182) are very important for reducing. For example, stored fat has difficulty converting to energy with a vitamin B-6 deficiency. Fat is also burned more rapidly with sufficient amounts of protein. Oils, such as soy or linseed oil, are needed to provide the diet with linoleic and linolenic acid. Diets lacking linoleic acid may damage the adrenal glands and decrease energy production. The oil also delays hunger pangs since it keeps food in your stomach longer.[1] And the importance of vigorous exercise cannot be overemphasized.

Drink plenty of water and take the digestants after drinking the Serenity Cocktail, if you experience discomfort or indigestion. Be sure to take alfalfa for the bulk and potassium they supply. Weigh yourself each morning without your clothes. If you watch the clock and do not go too long before sipping the Serenity, you will not be hungry. You will be thrilled as your weight falls off.

STAY HEALTHY PLAN   Eat your normal breakfast in the morning.

Take 5.5 ounces of the Serenity Cocktail around ten or eleven o'clock in the morning. Around two or three o'clock in the afternoon take another 5.5 ounces. These two servings should take the place of lunch. Have a regular nourishing dinner around 6:00 P.M. By nine or ten o'clock at night, your food should be digested and your stomach empty, so take a small drink again (about 5 ounces) before bed. This will keep your blood sugar level up. This gives you one pint of Serenity for the day, with up to 38 grams of protein (using 4 tbsp. of the Serenity Mix with milk and two eggs). Many people tell Mother that they sleep better, they do not have cramps in their legs or that "restless" feeling, and they wake up in the morning feeling refreshed and well-rested.

STRENGTH AND ENERGY PLAN   Eat a good breakfast. Take the Serenity Cocktail to work with you. Drink 8 ounces mid-morning and another 8 ounces mid-afternoon. If you are hungry, have lunch. Have a nourishing dinner. Before bed, drink another 8 ounces of the Serenity. If you follow this program, by day's end the Serenity Cocktail with milk will have contributed 39 to 54 grams of complete protein toward your daily protein requirement.

The eating patterns we have outlined are guidelines, not rigid rules. You must be flexible, so that your meals do not become monotonous. You can substitute nutritious snacks for the fortified drinks and vary the type of fortified drinks you take.

Although you may be flexible in what you eat, you do need consistently to have at least four or five feedings a day, never going longer than three (and at the most, four) hours between feedings. And do try to take a fortified protein drink three times a day, although once or twice a day can still be of great benefit.

Nutritional Meals Are a Must

BREAKFAST   Breakfast is the most important meal of the day. How you "break the fast" from the night before actually determines the way you will feel during the day. You can become fatigued and inefficient from eating food inadequate in quantity or quality. (See pp. 55–56, and sample breakfast on p. 170.)

In our family, no one ever leaves for work or school, no matter how big the rush, without breakfast. Those family members who don't like a traditional "big" breakfast can have a complete meal mixed in the blender. It may consist of certified raw milk, fertile eggs, protein powder, fresh fruit, and toast. Remember that eggs can be fixed a variety of different ways. Whenever possible, eat fresh fruit, not the juice from the fruit. Many people think all they need in the morning is juice. What juice does is flood the bloodstream with sugar. Although it does give an immediate pickup, a letdown will come within a few hours. Juice passes through the starch-digesting enzymes in your saliva too quickly. Fresh fruit, however, mixes well with your saliva since it requires chewing, and will not provide that immediate pickup. Remember that the white part of citrus fruits provides valuable bioflavonoids.

Cereal alone is usually inadequate for breakfast. You need the kind of protein found in eggs. If you do eat cereal, make a granola type to which you add seeds and nuts. Milk or fortified milk, bananas, and berries add to the completeness of the meal. My own children sometimes enjoy cereal as an after-school treat, but they are not allowed to have it alone for breakfast. It must be in addition to their regular breakfast, with eggs or a fortified drink.

Processed cereals are out of the question. Next time you shop, look at a box of refined and sugared breakfast cereals. Read the ingredients and compare the cost per pound. You will be amazed at how little nourishment your cereal dollar buys. Eggs are still the best nutrition dollar buy in town.

LUNCH   What you should have for lunch depends on what you had for breakfast, whether you are taking the Serenity

Cocktail or fortified protein drinks (either with or between meals), and how many calories you can consume. In any case, a well-balanced lunch includes carbohydrates, proteins, vegetables, and fruits. After these requirements have been met, "extras" may be added as appetite permits.

Let's consider the sandwich, a staple of the American lunch. In your selection of bread you will want to be sure no dough conditioners, preservatives, bleaching agents, or colorings have been added. The best quality bread has included in its list of ingredients powdered skim milk and wheat germ. Bread with these two foods added need not be "enriched." Use only whole grains, not white bread. For variety, try these various types of bread: 100 percent whole wheat, soya (made from soy beans), stone ground whole grains (7-grain bread), oatmeal bread (no white flour added), pumpernickel, and rye. It is strongly recommended that no other highly refined carbohydrates be permitted in the lunch.

Sandwiches should contain more filling (at least 3 ounces) than bread. (If you are concerned about calories, most sandwich fillings can be eaten plain, without bread.) Meat, fish, eggs, and cheese are top quality protein foods and should be used as the base of the lunch. (See page 66 for daily protein requirements.) One-third of the protein requirement should be met at lunch time. Whenever possible, use lettuce, alfalfa sprouts and/or other sprouts, or watercress on sandwiches. These items will contribute to the vegetable category. The following are suggestions for sandwich fillings. Note that the gram figures in parentheses indicate the number of grams of protein in a three-ounce serving (as listed in "Composition of Foods," USDA handbook no. 8).

(1) Natural cheese. Unprocessed cheeses made with certified raw milk are the most valuable because of the unheated protein. Various cheeses are: Cheddar (21 gm.), Swiss (23 gm.), Brick (22 gm.), Camembert (17 gm.), and Jack (21 gm.).

(2) Chopped liver. Add a little onion, and mayonnaise, and season with sea salt and pepper (22 gm.).

(3) Canned tuna or salmon. Mix with mayonnaise, chopped celery and onions, lemon juice, and seasoned salt. Drained solid tuna (25 gm.); Red Sockeye salmon (17 gm.).

(4) Fertile egg (at least one per sandwich). Scramble or hard-boil and mix with soy bacon bits or chopped celery, mayonnaise, and seasonings (one egg = 6 gm.).

(5) Leftover meat. Pot roast (22 gm.), sliced roast (20 gm.), crumbled hamburger (21 gm.). Can be mixed with mayonnaise, mustard, relish, or other seasonings, depending on the type of meat used. Be sure to use greens with this kind of sandwich.

(6) Turkey or chicken. Either sliced, or chopped and mixed with relish. Cranberry sauce is especially good spread on sliced turkey. Turkey or chicken salad can be made using chopped celery, hard-boiled eggs, mayonnaise, and seasonings. Roasted turkey flesh (27 gm.), roasted flesh and skin (23 gm.), fried drumstick (28 gm.).

(7) Meat loaf. A favorite for sandwiches. Use for a really high-powered lunch. Be sure to fortify meat loaf with soy flour and powdered skim milk instead of bread crumbs, to increase its protein content. Add catsup or mayonnaise. "Composition of Foods" lists meat loaf at 13 grams. A Fortified Meat Loaf would measure much higher.

(8) Peanut butter or other nut butters. Use only nonhydrogenated, pure (no salt or sugar added) nut butters. Almond and cashew butters are especially tasty. Nut butters are not a complete protein, as some of the essential amino acids are very low. Fortify with peanut oil, powdered skim milk (non-instant), and a little honey. This makes it a complete protein. No jams or jellies, please! Peanut butter (24 gm.).

(9) Avocado. An excellent source of saturated fatty acids. Add mayonnaise or yogurt seasoned with salt and pepper. Add lettuce, sprouts, or watercress. California variety (2 gm.). Another source of protein should also be included in the lunch, since the protein count is so low.

Do not use bologna or other processed luncheon meats because of the presence of sodium nitrate and sodium nitrite (evidence is mounting against these two preservatives as being contributory to cancer).

Use real butter, not margarine. Raw butter is better yet. If you have to skimp on your food budget, this is *not* the place to do it. To gain extra unsaturated fatty acids, "extend" the butter by adding soy or safflower oil. (Blend 1 pound of pure creamery butter with ¾ cup soy or safflower oil.)

Use mayonnaise made from cold-pressed oils, whole eggs, and seasonings. This type of mayonnaise is superior to most supermarket salad dressings and mayonnaise. Better still, make your own.

Use dark green lettuce leaves whenever possible—the darker the leaves, the more valuable the vegetable. Watercress and sprouts, as already mentioned, are excellent instead of lettuce and provide variety. Learn to do your own sprouting; this is unbelievably economical and will help your food budget immeasurably.

Include raw vegetables in plastic containers or sandwich bags in every lunch. Prepare in advance, keep covered, and refrigerate until needed.

Always include fresh, seasonal fruit as well. Because of the dangers associated with pesticides, thoroughly wash all fruits. There are some fruits you can peel completely; to avoid contact with air (and the browning that results), wrap peeled fruit tightly in a sandwich bag. Important: fruits are partially digested with the saliva in one's mouth, so remind your children to chew well. If you have to use canned fruits, get them water-packed rather than in syrup. Dried fruit can be used occasionally, but it should not take the place of fresh fruit.

After protein, vegetable, and fruit requirements have been met, extras such as the following may be added as appetite permits: trail mixes with nuts and seeds, cottage cheese with pineapple chunks, tuna or chicken salad, yogurt with honey or fresh fruit, soup or grated carrot and raisin salad.

Sweets or refined desserts should not be eaten. This is especially true for children, whose small appetites are easily satisfied. To allow refined foods in their diet means crowding out more valuable foods. Stomach space should not be wasted on useless carbohydrates. Mothers who allow devitalized foods to be eaten are asking for trouble.

Potato chips and other highly advertised luncheon "treats," even when claims are made that they are "enriched," are also not a part of a nourishing meal.

Be sure to avoid all synthetic "juices" and drink mixes. Purchase only pure fruit juices with no added sugar, colorings, or chemicals. They may cost a bit more, but pure fruit juices are far superior to synthetic types. *Never* drink canned or bottled soft drinks. Milk is actually preferable to fruit juices with lunch, because of its protein. We recommend certified raw milk, if available.

DINNER   At the end of a long day, we should enjoy a leisurely dinner, served in a pleasant atmosphere. No problems should be discussed at dinner time. Anger, stress, and anxiety can restrict the flow of the gastric juices that digest our food.

Get in the habit of making meat-stock soup or chicken soup. Soups are nourishing and easy to prepare. Have an entree of rare beef or lamb, a steak or chop, poultry, or fresh (or frozen) fish. Add a slightly cooked vegetable (green or yellow) and a green salad. Fresh fruit and cheese for dessert, a wonderful European custom, top off a delicious, well-balanced meal. Adjust the quantity of food according to your size, activity, and weight.

If you eat an early dinner, around 5 P.M., and don't go to bed until ten or eleven o'clock, your stomach will be empty by bedtime. If you eat breakfast the next morning at seven o'clock, you will have fasted for almost 14 hours—much too long. You need to put something in your stomach before going to bed, to help keep your blood sugar level up. Young children and older people, especially, need this small extra feeding to help them sleep through the night. Either a small snack or a fortified protein drink will do the trick.

SNACKS Most people snack on candy bars, soft drinks, french fries, or donuts for a between-meal lift. Adults add stimulants such as coffee and cigarettes. Nutritious snacks and fortified protein drinks give you that same lift while providing you with valuable nutrients rather than empty calories. Nutritious snacks include cheese and crackers, various trail mixes (made with all sorts of nuts and seeds), fruits and vegetables, and even small sandwiches.

If you have children, make sure to have an area of your refrigerator where they know they may go at any time for permissible snack foods.

Nutritional Supplements

All of the nutritional supplements we have mentioned—from the ingredients of fortified protein drinks to aids to digestion—can be purchased from your local health and nutrition store. If for some reason they do not carry an item, they would probably be willing to order it for you. The following pages discuss the supplements in greater detail.

ACIDOPHILUS If you have ever taken antibiotics, which destroy some of the friendly bacteria in your intestines, you need acidophilus. It contains millions of live friendly bacteria of the lactobacillus acidophilus and bulgaricus strains that naturally colonize in the intestine.

Mix one or two tablespoons of the liquid with juice, or take one or two of the freeze-dried acidophilus capsules. If you have not been taking acidophilus, take either form both morning and night for six weeks. Thereafter, take it just once a day, unless fighting a cold or infection.

Most liquid acidophilus bottles have code dates on them, notifying you of the time when the friendly bacteria will start to die. Read the label: don't buy acidophilus and let it sit on your kitchen shelf too long.

ALFALFA   Alfalfa, the "father of all foods," is a plant that sends its roots deep into the soil to extract minerals usually inaccessible to plants. It contains protein and vitamins and is a good source of minerals, chlorophyll, and fiber. It also contains eight enzymes that help in the proper assimilation of food. Alfalfa is used as a diuretic, for aiding gas pains, stomach ailments, ulcerous conditions, dropsy, and arthritis, and even in lowering cholesterol.[2]

Start with two or three alfalfa tablets, taken morning and night. Increase that amount gradually until you are taking as many as ten, twice a day. They have a mild laxative effect if too many are taken. You will have to determine your limits for yourself; you may appreciate the laxative effect.

BEE POLLEN   Bee pollen is plant pollen that bees have gathered and stored in their hives. One of nature's richest foods, it contains all the nutrients essential for the human body. It is expensive, however, and should be taken only in small quantities, so one cannot rely on it as a source of all nutrients. Many people find it effective in relieving allergy symptoms, and it is a good supplement for athletes.

Take one teaspoon of the granulated bee pollen a day, or one or two tablets or capsules. We prefer the high desert variety, gathered away from "civilization."

BLACKSTRAP MOLASSES   Like alfalfa, sugar cane is a deep-rooted plant that draws many valuable vitamins and minerals from the soil. It is refined into table sugar and different grades of molasses, blackstrap having the strongest flavor and the most nutrients. It contains about half the sugar of the original cane sugar. It is a potent source of calcium—more so even than milk—contains more potassium than any known food, and provides 3.2 mg. of iron per tablespoon.

Many people mix a tablespoon of molasses into fortified protein drinks to sweeten the taste and increase the nutrient content. Taking too much molasses may have a laxative effect.

BONE MEAL   Bone meal is exactly what it sounds like—actual ground bones from cattle. It contains twice as much calcium as phosphorus, which is the proper ratio of those minerals in your body. It is available in powder form, for mixing into drinks, and in tablet form.

BREWER'S YEAST   Brewer's yeast, originally a by-product of beer, contains generous quantities of all the major B vitamins (except B-12), sixteen amino acids (making it a complete protein), and eighteen or more minerals, including selenium and chromium, which are not found in many other foods.

One of the best-known properties of brewer's yeast is its ability to increase energy. It also increases the nutritional value of all foods to which you add it.

Manufacturers are learning to make brewer's yeast that doesn't taste too bad, but flavor will never be its greatest virtue. It should be used in conjunction with high-calcium supplements such as calcium gluconate to offset its phosphorus-calcium imbalance. It is available in powder form, for mixing into drinks; in flakes, for sprinkling on other foods; and in tablets, for those who travel or don't particularly like the taste of brewer's yeast.

VITAMIN C CRYSTALS   Vitamin C crystals or powder, aside from their nutritive value, prevent oxidation of the ingredients, especially added fruits. When you add vitamin C to fortified drinks, you can mix the drink in the morning and refrigerate some of it for later consumption in the evening.

FRUCTOSE   Fructose can be used as a sweetener in fortified drinks, helping to mask strong-tasting ingredients such as brewer's yeast and liver. It is a simple sugar found in most fruits, many vegetables, and honey. It is sweeter than table sugar (so you need not use as much), and it can enter some of the body cell without aid of insulin from the pancreas. Therefore, it does not cause the wide fluctuations in blood sugar levels that regular sugar does. It also provides calories for energy, so the body doesn't have to convert valuable protein into energy. It is available in powder form, like regular sugar.

CALCIUM GLUCONATE   Calcium gluconate helps to balance those food supplements that are higher in phosphorus than calcium, such as brewer's yeast, lecithin, and liver. Available in powder form, it is preferable to calcium lactate because it is virtually tasteless. It mixes easily into milk.

GLANDULARS (RAW)   Raw glandulars are produced from the glands of grazed livestock and are usually freeze-dried into tablet form to preserve their enzymes, hormones, and essential fatty acids. The more popular glandulars are adrenal, thymus, liver, pancreas, spleen, thyroid, and pituitary.

The adrenal glandulars are used to help support and boost your own adrenal glands, giving them a chance to repair and build themselves up after being exhausted by stress.

The thymus glandular is taken to build up immunity. Thymosin, obtained from whole thymus tissue, can increase T-cell number and function, which is crucial to normal immune response and most antibody response.

Whole pancreas glandulars or extracts have been shown to lower blood sugar levels in diabetics; in fact, they are what diabetics took before insulin was isolated.

Many people believe that when glandulars are taken, the stomach breaks them down into separate amino acids, rendering them useless. Some of the glandular proteins retain their original characteristics, however, entering the bloodstream and the tissues.

When taking glandular tablets, refer to the dosage on the label (usually a couple tablets, morning and night). Glandulars are not meant for long-term consumption unless there is a recognized deficiency. Taking them for three or four weeks should give you the desired results.[3]

LECITHIN (SOYA)   The word *lecithin* comes from the Greek word for "egg yolk," one of its main sources. It is also found in soybeans (from which the supplement form is derived) and corn.

Lecithin is known to have an emulsifying action on fats, which helps keep the arteries free of cholesterol deposits. It is also a constituent of our brain and nervous system.

Lecithin is available in an almost tasteless granulated form, of which one tablespoon provides about 250 mg. of choline and inositol, both B-complex factors. It is also available in capsule form.

LIVER (RAW)   Liver is packed with vitamins (especially B vitamins and vitamin A), minerals, protein, and certain factors yet to be isolated. It is high in phosphorus and low in calcium, so be sure to balance it with calcium-rich foods.

Many studies indicate that liver may help protect us against stress. One study showed that of three groups of laboratory rats placed in 68° F water, the regular-diet-fed group and the extra-B-vitamin-supplemented group swam for 13 minutes before surrendering to fatigue, while almost all the rats on the liver diet swam for two hours.[4]

Liver is available in powder or tablet form. If you take the Serenity Cocktail, you don't need to take extra liver tablets. If you take a protein drink, however, you should take ten or more liver tablets, morning and night, especially if you are a serious athlete. Ten tablets provide you with the equivalent of ¾ ounce of fresh, defatted raw liver (over ½ pound of liver in a week).

MAGNESIUM OXIDE Your body needs about half the amount of magnesium as it does calcium. Besides its many other functions, magnesium helps promote absorption and metabolism of other minerals. Adding magnesium oxide to fortified drinks helps to bring the calcium-magnesium ratio up to par.

Magnesium oxide is available in powder form, for mixing into drinks, but it is more commonly taken in mineral tablet supplements.

PROTEIN POWDER The best protein powders, which provide all the essential amino acids, are those whose main ingredient is milk protein or caseinate. Soy protein is used as the base in many formulas, because it is less expensive. It is low in methionine, however, so make sure a soy-based powder also includes this essential amino acid. Never buy a protein powder with fructose listed as the first ingredient. (This of course means that the product contains more fructose than any other ingredient.)

Protein powder is usually available in one-pound cans. Because it does not usually contain brewer's yeast or liver powder, it does not alter the flavor of a fortified drink. Two tablespoons of protein powder usually provide 10 to 16 grams of protein. When protein powder is mixed with eight ounces of milk, the protein content increases to about 18 to 24 grams.

SKIM MILK (POWDERED) Powdered skim milk (non-instant) contains all the amino acids and is therefore a good complement to brewer's yeast, which contains all the essential amino acids but is low in a few. It is also a good source of calcium and trace minerals.

It has an almost sweet taste, due to the milk sugar (lactose) it contains. It can be added to any food or drink to bolster its nutritional value.

WHEAT GERM OIL Dr. Thomas K. Cureton, of the Physical Fitness Institute of the University of Illinois, has spent twenty years researching the effects of wheat germ oil on humans in exercise. He discovered that wheat germ oil had statistically significant effects on several types of endurance performance: total body reaction times, basal metabolism rates, and oxygen intake debt.

To maximize the influence of wheat germ oil, Dr. Cureton recommends taking ten capsules (6 minims each) of wheat germ oil a day for five weeks.[5] (One teaspoon of wheat germ oil equals 9 minims.)

WHEY   In making cheese or cottage cheese, milk is curdled and separated into two parts: the curd, or milk solid (from which cheese is made), and the whey, or milk liquid. Whey contains many of the vitamins of milk and is also an excellent source of milk minerals. (Milk's protein remains in the cheese itself.) It is a source of milk sugar (lactose), which gives it a sweet taste and aids in the growth of acidophilus organisms and the control of putrefactive colon bacteria. It is available in powder form.

AIDS TO DIGESTION   Many people, especially those past the age of 40, have problems digesting their food. They are troubled by indigestion, heartburn, burping for hours after a meal, bloating, foul smelling gas, insomnia, irritability, fatigue, headaches, pancreatitis, gastritis, underweight, overweight, or even allergies.

To help you digest your meals, take two or three tablets of betaine hydrochloride with pepsin (commonly referred to as hydrochloric acid). It is a protein digestant. Each tablet provides about 5 drops of hydrochloric acid. It takes about three cups of dilute hydrochloric acid to digest a meal, so don't be afraid to take more than one or two tablets if you are not getting results.

Pancreatic enzymes with bile should also be taken, since they complete the digestion of protein and help you digest carbohydrates and fats, including the fat soluble vitamins. One or two tablets are usually sufficient, but many people need to take more.

Fortified drinks are highly concentrated foods, and you may need help in digesting them even if you have no trouble digesting regular meals. Remember to start out with small quantities of fortified drinks, increasing your consumption slowly so that your body has a chance to begin producing more of the enzymes they require for proper digestion.

Health Rules to Live By

Now that you've learned how to eat properly—and more importantly, why—all that's left to do is try the program. You'll be amazed at the changes that take place. One co-worker, after starting out on the vitamin-mineral program, with fortified protein drinks, told me that this was the first time she had ever been able to grow strong fingernails and thick, healthy hair.

Your increased sense of well-being, your boundless energy, and the knowledge that you're practicing prevention are worth all the money in the world, a handsome reward for following a good nutritional program. The following eleven rules are Gladys Lindberg's "Health Rules to Live By." Understanding and following them will enable you to *take charge of your health!*

1. Avoid all white bread and white flour products; instead, use whole-grain or multigrain breads without preservatives. Become a label reader; make certain you are actually getting what you are seeking. (This applies to all the food products you buy, not just to breads.) You will also want to replace the white flour in your kitchen with whole wheat pastry flour, a light, soft-wheat flour that can be used in all your baking. Regular whole wheat flour, with its coarser texture, is good for bread or rolls. You can also use soy flour to increase the protein content of any recipe. Try adding three tablespoons of powdered skim milk (non-instant) to one cup of the flour of your choice.

2. Always keep powdered, non-instant skim milk on hand to increase the protein content of all recipes and blender drinks. This is an excellent and inexpensive way to fortify the diet. Soy flour and powdered skim milk added to your favorite meatloaf recipe really increase the protein content.

3. Use unrefined brown rice and grains. Use only whole grain or freshly ground cereals. Granola cereals, which you can fortify with nuts, and seeds, are also acceptable.

4. Substitute cold-pressed oils that have not been hydrogenated for all your hardened fats. Store these oils in the refrigerator after they have been opened. Keep them fresh by squeezing a few capsules of vitamin E into the bottle. (Vitamin E is an anti-oxidant and will help prevent the natural oil from becoming rancid.)

5. If you salt your food, be sure to use sea salt (evaporated sea water), which contains all the trace minerals. (Sea water is reported to have the same mineral content as our blood.) Kelp granules may also be used. An excellent natural

source of iodine, it looks like pepper but tastes like salt. Potassium chloride (salt substitute) can be mixed with sea salt to give equal amounts of sodium and potassium.

6. Eliminate all white sugar from your pantry shelves. To sweeten your foods until your tastes change, use small amounts of raw, natural honey, concentrated juices like frozen orange or apple, molasses (rich in minerals), or fructose, which does not force the pancreas to secrete insulin rapidly and is actually 60 percent sweeter than sugar. Health food stores carry concentrated berry syrups that are natural, delicious, and sweet. Barley malt and rice syrup, also natural sweeteners, do not create fluctuations in blood sugar levels, and they are absorbed more slowly and evenly than sucrose sugars. Although sorghum is sucrose, it is still better than white sugar. All these products should be used only temporarily, until you get over the idea that everything must be sweet.

7. Mother encourages everyone to count the grams of protein consumed during the day. Start by getting some idea of how much you are eating now, and then fortify your diet with the Serenity Cocktail or a fortified protein drink. With these drinks, you can easily get five feedings a day, instead of three large meals, and you will not experience the mid-morning or mid-afternoon letdown that comes from a drop in blood sugar level.

8. Many families are discovering the pleasures of raising their own uncontaminated foods while helping to ease the strain on their budgets. If you cannot raise your own fruits and vegetables, be sure to thoroughly wash or peel those you purchase. Washing fruits and vegetables in water to which a few tablespoons of vinegar have been added helps to eliminate any pesticide residue. The Environmental Protection Agency has issued warnings on the effect of pesticides: it is known that certain pesticides can lead to genetic mutations, birth defects, and even cancer. Become informed and take precautions.

9. Eat as many foods as possible in their natural raw state to ensure receiving the "magic" enzymes that regulate your life processes and profoundly affect your health. Too many families today are living on heat-treated, enzyme-deficient foods. By eating unprocessed foods, you stand a better chance of providing your body with the raw materials it needs.

10. When food must be cooked, avoid overcooking it. Use a minimum of water; steam slowly and briefly if possible. The remaining liquid can be added to soups, sauces, or gravies. Do not throw vitamins and minerals down the drain. The less water and heat used, the more food value saved.

11. Take your vitamins and minerals every day (see Appendix B). We cannot adequately stress their importance to our health. They make up for deficiencies in our diet and help protect us from the stresses of life; they are a great health insurance policy.

NOTES

1. Adelle Davis, *Let's Get Well* (New York: Harcourt, Brace & World, 1965), pp. 78, 81, 82.
2. Dr. F. M. Pottenger, Jr., *News Letter of the Academy of Applied Nutrition,* September 1948; Nutrition Search, Inc., *Nutrition Almanac* (New York: McGraw-Hill, 1979), p. 176.
3. Jonathan Rothschild, "Glandulars in Human Nutrition," *Let's LIVE,* May 1981, pp. 99, 100, 102.
4. Bill Gottlieb, "Liver: The Food That Protects Against Stress," *Prevention,* September 1977, p. 148.
5. Thomas Kirk Cureton, Ph.D., *The Physiological Effects of Wheat Germ Oil on Humans in Exercise* (Springfield, Ill.: Charles C. Thomas, 1972), pp. 290, 442.

✂ Appendix A:
Meal Suggestions

Breakfast #1 (28 g. protein)

Protein		Calories
12 g.	2 eggs (fertile if possible), poached, sunny-side up, in omelet, or scrambled—cooked at a low temperature When eggs are broken to scramble or to make an omelet, add	150
	1 tbsp. soy or sesame seed oil	125
8 g.	1 oz. natural cheese	
	(light-colored cheeses are best)	130
	Fresh fruit in season	60
	1 orange or ½ grapefruit	
	(eat all the white pulp)	
	or	
	½ melon (any type)	
	or	
	1 cup fresh berries	
	As calories and weight permit, add toast—100 percent whole multigrain—or potatoes, rice, or cornbread	60
	or	
4 – 8 g.	Whole-grain cereal, cooked or granola type, topped with fortified milk* (4 to 8 ounces)	75 – 150

*Certified raw milk (if available) fortified with one cup powdered skim milk. This increases the milk's protein from 34 grams per quart to 53 grams (one cup powdered skim milk = 19 grams).

Breakfast #2 (24 g. protein)

Protein		Calories
*16 g.	High Protein Hotcakes (recipe below) served with choice of toppings (see suggestions on p. 171)	400 – 600
	Fresh fruit in season (compatible with topping used on hotcakes)	60
8 g.	Herb tea, 1 cup certified raw milk, or decaffeinated coffee	159

*Protein based on 4 hotcakes 5 inches in diameter.

HIGH PROTEIN PANCAKES

Sift together:

⅔ cup soy flour	3 eggs separated (beat whites)
½ cup wheat pastry flour	3 tbsp soy oil or melted butter
⅓ cup powdered skim milk	1 cup milk
1 tsp baking powder	½ cup plain yogurt
¼ tsp sea salt	2 tbsp honey

Mix dry ingredients. In another bowl add egg yolks, oil, milk, yogurt and honey. Mix until smooth and add dry ingredients. Batter should be of medium thickness. Fold in egg whites. Rub medium hot griddle with oil; then wipe with paper towel. Cook until golden brown, light and fluffy.

Top pancakes with one of the suggestions below, rather than syrup.

PANCAKE TOPPINGS

Blend raw apples with plain yogurt, adding vitamin C crystals to prevent oxidation (which turns apples brown); a few fresh or frozen strawberries make the sauce pink.

Blend fresh or frozen blueberries or strawberries into plain yogurt; sweeten slightly with real maple syrup as necessary.

Blend 1 or 2 tsp. frozen orange juice into plain yogurt.

Blend fresh seasonal fruit into kefir.

Simmer unsulfured apricots until soft; blend until smooth; add drained, unsweetened crushed pineapple.

Heat peanut butter and a small amount of honey; blend until smooth.

Lunch Suggestions

Protein		Calories
25 g.	½ can tuna or 4 oz. salmon, with lettuce and fresh vegetables as a large salad	150
	Fresh fruit in season	60 – 100
	Whole wheat bread (if your weight permits)	50 – 100
	If you take the Serenity Cocktail or a protein drink, reduce the quantity of the lunch	

Dinner Suggestions

Protein	Calories
20 – 25 g. 6 oz. chicken or fish, or ¼ lb. lean, rare meat of any kind (liver and glandular meats are excellent if you like them and know the source)	100 – 200
Vegetables, slightly cooked	60
Raw salad with oil and vinegar dressing (1 tsp. oil per person)	150
If weight permits, add complex carbohydrates such as a baked potato, yam, brown rice, corn bread, bran muffin, or whole-grain roll.	150
Fresh fruit	
Herb tea or decaffeinated coffee	60 – 100

HIGH-POWERED MEAT LOAF

2 chopped onions   ½ cup wheat germ
1 green pepper   ½ cup soy flour (no substitute)
2 lbs ground round   ½ cup powdered skim milk
1 lb ground heart   3 tablespoons catsup
3 eggs   1½ tablespoon sea salt
Pinch of thyme and basil   ¾ cup fresh milk

Saute onions and pepper lightly in a little oil. Add the rest of the ingredients and mix well. Mold into a loaf in a shallow pan and bake at 350° for 50 minutes.

This High-Powered Meat Loaf recipe, created by Gladys Lindberg, has been very popular for many years and has the added distinction of having been published in books and newspapers throughout the United States.

Snack Suggestions

PEANUT BUTTER CANDY

Ingredients

2 lbs. crunchy peanut butter (non-hydrogenated, no sugars, salt, or stabilizers)

1 cup powdered skim milk (non-instant)

1 pound seed mixture (a packaged blend, such as a backpacker's mix, or your own selection of raisins or currants, sunflower seeds, chopped walnuts and peanuts, raw cashews, and toasted sesame seeds)

¼ cup unfiltered honey or sorghum

Procedure

Mix peanut butter and powdered milk until smooth. Add honey and seed mixture. Knead and roll like refrigerator cookie dough. Wrap in foil. Chill and slice.

Alternatives

Add blackstrap molasses instead of honey; add toasted wheat germ with sunflower seeds and raisins instead of seed mixture; add granola cereal instead of seed mixture.

WHEAT GERM CANDY

Ingredients

    1½ lbs. fresh roasted peanut butter, non-hydrogenated
        (crunchy or plain)
    1 cup molasses
    ½ cup honey
    1 tablespoon vanilla
    ¼ tsp. salt
    ½ cup calcium gluconate (this balances the high phosphorus
        content of wheat germ)
    ½ cup currants or raisins, washed
    2 cups fresh wheat germ (vacuum-packed if possible)

Procedure

Place raw wheat germ in flat pan and place under the broiler for a few minutes. Stir until it takes on a "golden" or "toasted" appearance. *Caution:* Do not leave the wheat germ to do something else—it can *burn* very quickly! Toasting gives a delicious nutty taste, but toast very lightly as heat will destroy some of the B vitamins.

Mix peanut butter, molasses and honey, vanilla, salt, calcium gluconate in a large bowl. Add currants or raisins and mix well. Now, add wheat germ, ½ cup at a time until it is all kneaded in together. You may even use more wheat germ to make a firmer candy.

Roll as refrigerator cookie dough and wrap in wax paper— refrigerate until chilled. Slice to desired thickness.

Alternatives

Roll in walnut size balls—press with a fork, place on a cookie sheet and chill. Will look like peanut butter cookies.

OR: Roll into walnut size balls—roll in wheat germ or chopped nuts. Chill.

Appendix B: Vitamins and Minerals

PREFACE

To understand the important role vitamins and minerals play in the rebuilding process of the body, think about what happens in just sixty seconds of life. Researchers have learned that every minute in the human body three billion cells die and three billion cells are created! To properly replenish these cells, your blood needs to contain forty different chemicals, including oxygen, hormones, enzymes, and vitamins and minerals. When any of these are lacking, the body cannot make the necessary repairs properly, and if deficiencies are not corrected, disease will result.

To really take charge of your health, there are some basic facts about vitamins and minerals that you need to understand. To begin with, vitamins are classified as water-soluble and fat-soluble.

The Fat-soluble Vitamins

The fat-soluble vitamins are A, D, E, and K. They are called "fat-soluble" because they dissolve in fat and in substances that dissolve fat. These vitamins are stored in the fatty part of the liver and other tissues.[1] Vitamins A, D, and E are available in oil capsule form, while vitamin K must be prescribed by your doctor. Some people complain that they can't take fat-soluble vitamins because they burp the taste of the oil. Such people may switch to synthetic or dry forms of these vitamins. However, if you can't assimilate these fat-soluble vitamins, then how can you expect to assimilate all the unsaturated fatty acids that your body also needs? The root cause of the difficulty may be a lack of hydrochloric acid in the stomach, which leads to a lack of the pancreatic enzymes and bile that actually digest the fats. And the reason not enough hydrochloric acid is made has to do with exhausted adrenals or other vitamin deficiencies. It's easy to see how important it is to be in good health for your vitamins to be assimilated properly.

The Water-soluble Vitamins

The water-soluble vitamins dissolve in water and are not stored by the body to any great extent. These vitamins include:

Vitamin C
Citrus Bioflavonoids (sometimes called vitamin P)*
B-complex vitamins
    B-1 Thiamine
    B-2 Riboflavin
    B-3 Niacin
    B-6 Pyridoxine
    B-12 Cobalamin
    Folic Acid
    Pantothenic Acid
    Biotin
    Choline*
    Inositol*
    PABA (Para-aminobenzoic Acid)*

When you perspire, take diuretic drugs, or have diarrhea, you lose an abnormal amount of these water-soluble vitamins. Stress and exertion also deplete the body of these valuable nutrients. Actually, our supply of these vitamins is constantly being diminished by the activity of our own bodies. Therefore, if we are to maintain even reasonably good health, these vitamins have to be replaced.

Those Magic Minerals

Never underestimate the importance of minerals to our total well-being. About 5 percent of your total body weight is mineral matter. Minerals are to be found in your bones, teeth, nerve cells, muscles, soft tissue, and blood. Everyone thinks of minerals as having to do with the teeth and bones, but minerals also preserve the vigor of the heart and brain, as well as the muscle and nervous systems. Not only do minerals strengthen the skeletal structure, but they are important in the production of hor-

---

* These substances, while not officially recognized as vitamins, are sometimes given these vitamin designations.

mones and enzymes, in the creation of antibodies, and in keeping
the blood and tissue fluids from becoming too acid or too alkaline.[2]

These are the essential major minerals (sometimes called macronutrients—needed in large amounts) found in your body, listed
in the order of the most prevalent to the least prevalent: calcium,
phosphorus, potassium, sodium, and magnesium. Other essential
minerals (sometimes called micronutrients—or trace elements)
are found in the body in only minute amounts. The more important trace elements are: iron, zinc, copper, manganese, chromium, iodine, and selenium. There are other essential trace
elements such as sulfur, chloride, vanadium, molybdenum, fluoride and silicon, but generally it is no problem to get enough of
these in your diet.

CALCIUM AND ITS CO-WORKERS   Calcium is the most abundant mineral found in the body. The body of an average adult
contains approximately 2.5 pounds of calcium.[3] Cramps are the
classic symptom of a calcium deficiency. Other symptoms may
include weak-feeling muscles and nervous spasms.

For the calcium in your body to be effectively utilized, you
ideally need to take in equal amounts of calcium and phosphorus. If the diet is equal in calcium and phosphorus, the *blood*
calcium will be two and a half times higher than phosphorus,
which is optimal. (The normal blood test analysis should read
Calcium 10, Phosphorus 4. It is interesting to note that mother's
milk is also two and a half times higher in calcium than phosphorus (the same as our *blood* calcium ratio)—another important
reason for nursing a baby.

Why should we be concerned about all this? Because the average American diet, including many of the foods nutritionists
recommend, is very high in phosphorus in proportion to calcium.
Here are two charts demonstrating this point. Remember, *your
intake of the two nutrients should be approximately equal.* The
following information is from the *United States Government
Composition of Foods Handbook.* One hundred grams is the unit
of measure for each food listed (28 grams = one ounce, so 100
grams is a little less than half a cup).

Remember, if you don't have enough calcium in your diet, or if
you have too much phosphorus, then your body will pull calcium
right out of your bones. The calcium:phosphorus ratio in the

High Phosphorus Foods	Ca	Phos	High Calcium Foods	Ca	Phos
Beef and most red meat	11	207	Milk (whole, nonfat,	118	93
Brewer's yeast	210	1783	dry, skim)	1308	1016
Wheat germ	72	1118	Blackstrap molasses	684	84
Cracked wheat bread	88	128	Cheddar cheese	750	478
Flours (soybean,	119	558	Dark greens (turnip,		
whole grain-wheat,	45	423	kale, collard, broccoli,		
light rye)	22	185	mustard, watercress)	184	37
Bran (wheat)	119	1276	Cottage cheese*	94	152
Bran (rice)	76	1386	Parmesan cheese	1140	781
Beef liver, cooked	11	476	Buttermilk	121	95
Eggs, uncooked	54	205	Sesame seeds (whole,	1160	616
Pumpkin & squash seeds	51	1144	hulled)	110	592
			Kelp	1093	240

*Cottage cheese, generally thought to be high in calcium, is actually low, because the minerals remain in the whey. Parmesan cheese has the highest calcium content of any cheese.

blood must stay constant, even at the expense of your bones. This depletion of calcium may go on for years before the calcium loss will show up on X rays, and by then 30 percent of your calcium may be gone.[4] The calcium:magnesium ratio is also important; it should be approximately 2:1.[5] Magnesium is necessary for efficient calcium utilization. It combines with calcium and phosphorus in forming bones and teeth and is credited with giving them their hardness.[6] Vitamin D is also an important vitamin in bone strength since it enhances the absorption of calcium and phosphorus.

POTASSIUM AND SODIUM   Two of the questions most often asked of nutritionists are "Should I salt my food? Do I really need salt?" Our answer is always yes and no. You see, to discuss salt (sodium chloride) we also need to talk about potassium: your intake of the two should be approximately equal. You can imagine these two minerals on either side of a teeter-totter. Too much sodium causes you to lose potassium and retain water. Too much potassium causes you to lose sodium and lose water.

Briefly, potassium is found in most fresh fruits (especially apricots and bananas) and vegetables, kelp powder, and salt substitutes, while sodium is found in almost all foods, especially those that have been canned and processed.

Sodium triggers the adrenal glands to stimulate production of hydrochloric acid, used to help digest food, so people who have low adrenal function or have exhausted their adrenals from stress also need salt.[7] If you are hypoglycemic, then you lose salt from your body when your blood sugar level drops. This salt needs to be replaced. A low salt intake can lead to fatigue, drowsiness, and depression.[8] So if you are one of those who is swearing off salt, keep in mind the balance we talked about.

Athletes in particular need potassium, especially if they are on a high protein diet, because of their higher excretion rate of potassium.[9]

Many victims of heat prostration or heat exhaustion have been found to have low levels of potassium, and researchers have pointed out the possible relationship between potassium depletion and high incidence of heat stroke among otherwise healthy soldiers in basic training and football players in preseason conditioning.[10]

Fortunately we don't have to count exact milligrams of either of these two minerals, since our kidneys regulate the balance. The kidneys will adjust to a high potassium or sodium intake by increasing excretion in the urine. They even have the ability to spare sodium when intake is inadequate, but not so with potassium. Even after a week or more on a potassium-free diet, potassium will still appear in the urine.[11] Because of this renal control mechanism, a nonathletic or sedentary person does not have to pay too much attention to these two minerals, except to cut back slightly on salt intake.

ZINC AND COPPER   Two other minerals that compete against each other for absorption are zinc and copper. Your zinc intake should be ten to twenty times greater than that of copper. People used to have galvanized pipe (pipe coated with zinc) in their homes, so they got a certain amount of the zinc they needed in their drinking water. Now many homes are fitted with copper pipe, so instead of getting zinc in their water, people are getting copper, throwing off the ratio that they should be receiving. It is much harder to get adequate amounts of zinc in the diet than it is copper. Copper in high doses is considered dangerous; only relatively minute amounts are needed.

Recommended Dietary Allowances (RDA)

People are confused about how much of this vitamin and that mineral they are supposed to take. The RDAs usually stand somewhere in the middle of this confusion. The RDAs were derived by a group of "nutritional" scientists who advise the Food and Nutrition Board, a committee of the National Academy of Sciences–National Research Council. According to this board, the RDAs are "the levels of intake of essential nutrients considered, in the judgment of the Food and Nutrition Board on the basis of available scientific knowledge, to be adequate to meet the known nutritional needs of practically all healthy persons."[12]

The RDAs were first published during World War II, when people were concerned about the nutritional quality of the K-rations provided for our troops. Since then, they have been used as a guideline for the food industry. They should *not* be taken as gospel for each individual (though, unfortunately, that's what generally happens). They have been revised over 70 times since 1968.[13] These guidelines are limited in that they apply only to healthy people: they try to guarantee minimal, not optimal, levels of nutrition, and they take for granted that we are all average. It is interesting to note that no allowance has been made for the loss of vitamins in cooking and storage. Ironically, the RDAs for animals are roughly ten times higher than those for humans![14]

Extra Vitamins and Minerals

"Do I really need extra vitamins and minerals?" That is a question you will hear over and over again in any discussion of the merits of vitamins and minerals. If any subject has generated misunderstanding, misknowledge, and general confusion in recent years, it has to be this one. There is a tremendous amount of true ignorance in this area, and many supposedly reliable sources are in fact woefully uninformed.

Many people feel they can get enough vitamins and minerals in their diet without taking additional supplements. If you are middle aged, then your great-grandparents may have come from the farm, where they performed hard physical labor all day and burned up 4,000 to 6,000 calories a day. These folks got their milk right from the cow, their fruits and vegetables from the garden, and they ate six times a day. They didn't need vitamin or mineral supplements because they got enough nutrients from the large amount of natural and fresh foods that they ate. However, most of us today cannot eat those quantities of food.

Not only that, but the food we now eat varies considerably in the amount of nutrients contained. For example, lettuce grown in poor soil may have only 1 part per million of manganese, 9 of iron, and 3 of copper, whereas in good soil lettuce may have 169 parts permillion of manganese, 516 of iron, and 60 of copper. The same is true for other vegetables, of course.[15]

The process of refining destroys even more vitamins and minerals. The high percentage of minerals lost in the refining of flour is graphically illustrated in the following chart:[16]

Mineral	Percentage Lost
Calcium	60
Phosphorus	70.9
Magnesium	84.7
Potassium	77
Sodium	78.3
Chromium	98
Molybdenum	48
Manganese	85.8
Iron	75.6
Cobalt	88.5
Copper	67.9
Zinc	77.7
Selenium	15.9

There are a variety of other factors that can cause you to expend, excrete, or malabsorb certain vitamins and minerals. Consider these: tobacco, alcohol, salt, sugar, rancid fats, estrogen, cortisone, mineral oil, antibiotics, aspirin, antacids, sleeping pills, tranquilizers, emotional strain, surgery, sickness, accidents, diuretics, laxatives, flourides, polluted air or water, pesticides, food processing, cooking, storage, food additives, extremes of heat or cold, pregnancy, nursing, and oral contraceptives.[17]

"A report published by the Consumer Nutrition Center of the United States Department of Agriculture in January of 1981, reveals that, in general, the "normal diet" does not provide enough calcium, magnesium, iron, vitamin A, and vitamin B-6. That is, about 20 to 25 percent of the households studied were just not consuming adequate amounts of these nutrients.[18] Of course, when they say, "inadequate," they are applying the RDA definition of that word, though the RDAs are considered very low by many nutritionists and apply only to healthy people.

The RDAs are a minimum insurance approach to vitamins and minerals, as we mentioned, and yet perhaps as many as one-fourth of the American population may not get even those amounts. We suggest you take the optimal or maximal nutrition approach rather than the minimal. Strive for the maximum benefits you can derive. Out of ignorance, many are living on the borderline of ill health, just getting by and never knowing the vitality they could have.

When to Take Supplements

When taking vitamin and mineral supplements, be sure to take them all together. Some of the vitamins and minerals will only be of benefit when others are there, and some will be enhanced by the presence of others. Vitamin B-6, for example, cannot be used properly by the body if there is a zinc deficiency.[19] Vitamin E, on the other hand, works fine when taken alone, though its benefits are enhanced with the addition of the trace element selenium.

None of the vitamins and minerals actually cancel each other out, so you needn't worry about taking one certain vitamin in the morning and another one later on. One exception to the rule is that some inorganic iron, which appears in many vitamin-mineral formulas, can destroy vitamin E. Because of this, a good vitamin-mineral formula should contain iron in the form of ferrous gluconate, ferrous fumerate, ferrous citrate, or ferrous peptonate. These forms do not affect vitamin E. (Stay away from the iron in the form of ferrous sulfate, since it can be toxic.)

The Gladys Lindberg Formula

The following is a basic formula to use as the foundation of your supplement program. It has worked for many thousands of Mother's clientele, men, women, and children. (We feel that the only real differences between men's and women's vitamin-mineral needs are in vitamin B-6 and iron, both of which women may need more of than men.) The chart on p. 182 is not to be taken as gospel for everyone's needs, but it is a sample of a well balanced formula. More of certain vitamins and minerals may be added according to individual deficiencies and extra stressors in life.

VITAMINS

Vitamin A (fish liver oil)	25,000 I.U.
Vitamin D (fish liver oil)	400 I.U.
Vitamin E (natural d-Alpha tocopherol)	200 I.U.
Vitamin B-Complex	
B-1 (Thiamine)	20 mg.
B-2 (Riboflavin)	30 mg.
B-6 (Pyridoxine)	20 mg.
Niacinamide (B-3)	100 mg.
Pantothenic Acid	100 mg.
Choline	100 mg.
Inositol	100 mg.
PABA (Para-Aminobenzoic Acid)	50 mg.
Folic Acid	0.4 mg.
Biotin	25 mcg.
B-12 Activity (Cobalamin)	25 mcg.
Vitamin C (Ascorbic Acid)	500 mg.
Bioflavonoids (from lemons, oranges, Hesperidin)	250 mg.

MINERALS

Calcium (eggshell and calcium lactate)	400 mg.
Magnesium (Magnesium Oxide)	200 mg.
Iron (Ferrous Fumarate)	18 mg.
Zinc (Zinc Gluconate)	30 mg.
Copper (Copper Gluconate)	1 mg.
Iodine (Kelp)	0.15 mg.
Manganese (Manganese Gluconate)	5 mg.
Potassium (Potassium Gluconate and Kelp)	25 mg.
Chromium	50 mcg.
Selenium	50 mcg.

This appendix is intended to provide you with a more in-depth analysis of each of the vitamins and minerals mentioned throughout this book. These vitamins and minerals are listed with information relating to:

FACTS.   This section describes the characteristics of each particular vitamin or mineral.

DEFICIENCY SYMPTOMS.   This section describes the common symptoms people suffer from when they are deficient in a particular vitamin or mineral. This information is not meant as a guide for treating disease, but to enhance the reader's awareness of the consequences of a deficiency.

WHAT IT DOES.   This section briefly considers the role a particular vitamin or mineral plays in the body.

WHAT IT MAY DO.   This section suggests what a particular vitamin or mineral may do for some people and what therapeutic benefits some have derived from its use. Other cases show results achieved in animal studies, but not directly related to humans.

TOXICITY. This section tells if it is possible to get too much of a vitamin or mineral and at what intake level the dosage becomes toxic. If toxicity is possible, the symptoms of an overload are described.

BEST SOURCES. This section lists the best possible natural food sources for each particular vitamin or mineral.

SUPPLEMENTS. This section will consider the different forms—synthetic or natural—of each vitamin or mineral. It explains what form is best and why some forms are harmful. Gladys Lindberg's recommendations for intake are also included, but should be used only as a guideline since individual needs may vary.

Intake of vitamins and minerals are measured as follows:

International Units (I.U.) or	Used to measure the activity
United States Pharmacoeia (U.S.P.) =	(potency) of vitamins A, D, & E
Microgram (mcg.) =	1/1,000 of milligram
Milligram (mg.) =	1,000 Micrograms or 1/1,000 of a gram
Gram =	1,000 Milligrams

COMMENTS. This section supplies additional miscellaneous but important information on selected vitamins and minerals.

Vitamins and minerals covered, and the pages on which they appear, are as follows:

Vitamins	Page	Minerals	Page
Vitamin A	184	Calcium	215
Vitamin B-Complex		Chlorine	218
Thiamine (B-1)	186	Chromium	218
Riboflavin (B-2)	188	Cobalt	219
Niacin (B-3)	189	Copper	219
Pyridoxine (B-6)	191	Flourine	221
Folic Acid	194	Iodine	221
Cobalamin (B-12)	195	Magnesium	225
Pantothenic Acid	197	Manganese	228
Biotin	199	Molybdenum	229
PABA	200	Phosphorous	229
Choline	201	Potassium	230
Inositol	202	Selenium	233
Vitamin C	203	Silicon	235
Vitamin D	207	Sodium	236
Vitamin E	208	Sulfur	238
Vitamin K	212	Vanadium	238
Bioflavonoids (vitamin P)	213	Zinc	239

VITAMINS

Vitamin A

FACTS   Fat soluble and can be stored by the body in the liver, which releases it as necessary. It comes from two sources: (1) preformed vitamin A (retinol) is found in foods of animal origin (the body can use preformed vitamin A as it comes), and (2) provitamin of A, called carotene, is found in foods of plant and animal origin. After ingestion by the body, carotene must be converted by the liver and the intestinal wall into useable vitamin A.[1]

Oxidation, not heat, destroys vitamin A. Vitamin A is known as "the growth vitamin."

DEFICIENCY SYMPTOMS   A deficiency of vitamin A may result in night blindness or loss of adaptation to the dark and an increased susceptibility to infection. Some people develop anemia even though they are taking plenty of iron. Other symptoms may be the drying out of the skin and mucous membranes. The skin first starts to look like it has goose bumps that won't go away and then takes on a horny, rough texture. A loss of taste and smell can also accompany a deficiency, and this leads to a loss of appetite. In addition, deficiency may result in loss of vigor, defective teeth and gums, and retarded growth.

Vitamin A deficiency may result in additional problems in the following manner. The skin has four layers of cells and a lack of vitamin A causes the bottom layer of cells to die. The body will then send white blood cells to bring these dead cells to the surface and the result may be a pimple with pus, a sty in the eye, or a carbuncle. In the ear, these dead cells become trapped behind the ear drum and create a fertile environment for infection, which can result in an earache. In vitamin A-deficient people, bits of mucous may accumulate on the eyelashes at night as they sleep and the eyelids will feel stuck together in the morning. The green pus or mucous that runs from the noses of many children denotes a vitamin A deficiency.

WHAT IT DOES   Vitamin A is a specific for cure and prevention of night blindness and day blindness (because it restores visual purple to the eye) and dry eye disease (in which the tear ducts dry up). Vitamin A is essential to the normal structure and behavior of the tissue lining that covers the skin and forms the lining of the nasal, sinus, respiratory tract, mouth, pharynx, entire digestive tract, and the genito-urinary tract. This vitamin prevents the skin and mucous membranes from drying out. It may help you resist infections, but only when you've exhausted your body's resources and there is inadequate intake. Vitamin A is a growth factor.[2]

For the body to absorb protein properly, there must be an adequate supply of vitamin A.[3] The more protein you eat, the more vitamin A you need.[4]

WHAT IT MAY DO   Vitamin A, as well as vitamin E, can be applied topically to help skin wounds or sores heal faster.

Women who suffer abnormally heavy or extended menstrual periods not caused by other factors sometimes have low blood levels of vitamin A. In one study, women who had such menstrual difficulties took 30,000 I.U. of vitamin A twice a day for slightly over a month and almost half of them were restored to normal, with improvement noted in some of the others.[5]

Evidently, vitamin A helps fight cancer in the same way it helps the body resist infection—by building up the immune defense system. A National Cancer Institute study showed that "vitamin A substantially reduced the effects on mice of a potent chemical cause of breast cancer. At "normal" doses of the chemical, none of the vitamin A-protected mice got breast cancer, while twenty-seven percent of the unprotected mice did."[6]

Vitamin A is extremely important during pregnancy. Most research, for ethical reasons we can all appreciate, has been done with animals. "For example, sows give birth to eyeless piglets when their diet is deficient in vitamin A. Cleft palate and lip, extra ears, and kidney defects are also noted. When the same sows are fed adequate vitamin A during subsequent pregnancies, all members of their litters are normal."[7]

TOXICITY   Possible. But you really don't have to worry about taking too much vitamin A. "In one study, doctors administered 150,000 I.U. of Vitamin A daily to a large number of heart patients and observed no toxic symptoms during the study, which went on for six months."[8] About 500,000 I.U. of vitamin A can be absorbed and stored by an adult human liver.[9] "When it comes to a single dose, you would have to take as much as 2,000,000 I.U. to induce acute hypervitaminosis A."[10] Doses of 200,000 or more I.U. daily for prolonged periods of time may induce hypervitaminosis A.[11] Symptoms of toxicity may include loss of hair, nausea, headache, skin peeling, and joint pain which will subside quickly upon lowering the intake of vitamin A.

Note: If you ingest too much carotene (provitamin of A) over a period of time, your skin will take on a yellow tint. This condition is harmless. I've seen this happen to people who drink an excessive amount of carrot juice.

BEST SOURCES   Fish liver oils, liver, milk, cream, cheese, butter, eggs, yellow fruits, green and yellow vegetables. Example: liver (beef, 3 oz., fried)—43,390 I.U.; carrots (1, raw)—7,930 I.U.; eggs (1 large, raw)—590 I.U.[12]

SUPPLEMENTS   Vitamin A supplements are usually available in three forms. The first two forms are from natural fish liver oil, one oil-dispersible and the other water-dispersible. The third form, vitamin A palmitate, is synthetic and water dispersible. The water dispersible or dry form is usually recommended for people who have trouble assimilating oil, especially those people with acne. This assimilation problem, however, can be alleviated by taking digestive aid supplements (hydrochloric acid tablets and pancreatic enzyme tablets with bile).

The most common supplement potencies available are 10,000 to 25,000 I.U. and this is what I recommend you take daily. For diagnosed deficiencies, I recommend 50,000 to 100,000 I.U. of vitamin A a day for several weeks.

A small amount of vitamin E taken with vitamin A helps prevent the vitamin A from oxidizing or becoming rancid. Carlton Fredericks recommends you take 200,000 I.U. of vitamin A a day for two weeks for a cold or for a severe infection, particularly if vitamin C doesn't help with the cold. It is important for diabetics to take vitamin A in the fish liver oil form, since they are not able to fully convert carotene (provitamin A, found in carrots and green leafy vegetables) into completely formed vitamin A.

COMMENTS   It's interesting to note that "one-third of the population of the United States consumes less than the Recommended Daily Allowance of Vitamin A, according to the Congress."[13] The RDA is only 5,000 I.U. for adults and children over four years old, and yet many people can't get even this amount. Remember, the RDA's are the minimum potencies required by the healthy average person.

Thiamine (B-1)

FACTS   Water soluble. Any excess is excreted by the body. Some storage of thiamine is found in the liver, heart, and kidney.[14] High temperatures destroy this vitamin.

Your need for thiamine increases when your carbohydrate intake increases, when antibiotics are used, during pregnancy, lactation, fever, surgery, increased physical activity, other stressful conditions, if you are older, and if you eat sugar, smoke, or drink alcohol.[15] Thiamine is known as "the morale vitamin."

DEFICIENCY SYMPTOMS   A lack of thiamine makes carbohydrates harder to digest and leaves too much pyruvic acid and lactic acid in the body. This condition causes an oxygen deficiency with damaging effects. One of the first symptoms of a thiamine deficiency is loss of appetite. Other symptoms include "easy tiring, weakness, exhaustability, head pressures, poor sleep, feeling of tenseness and irritability, various aches and pains, subjectively poor memory, and difficulty in concentration."[16] Constipation and impaired growth take place in some cases. "As the deficiency gets worse, "pins and needles" begin in the toes and burning sensations begin in the foot."[17] This symptom indicates that nerve pathways are degenerating.

The classic deficiency of thiamine results in beriberi. This is basically a disease of the nervous system and can eventually lead to death. A deficiency of such magnitude can be brought on by a steady diet of polished rice from which the thiamine has been removed.

WHAT IT DOES   Thiamine must be present for pyruvic acid and lactic acid to break down carbohydrates into glucose. The glucose is the form of simple sugar the body uses to produce energy. This vitamin promotes growth, aids digestion, and is essential for normal functioning of the nerve tissues, muscles, and heart. It has been used to cure stubborn cases of constipation. Thiamine plays a role in causing the stomach and intestinal muscles to contract, which gives you an appetite (causes hunger pangs). Thiamine is necessary for your body to manufacture hydrochloric acid, which is required for proper digestion of your food.

WHAT IT MAY DO   In animal studies, the immune response system has been found to be stimulated by thiamine.[18]

Thiamine may help in the fight against multiple sclerosis. Thiamine is a part of the insulation around the body's nerve fibers that degenerate in multiple sclerosis. Some patients have found that their symptoms were eliminated with injections of 150 mg. of thiamine with liver extract every week to ten days. Thiamine taken orally did not work and evidently was not absorbed.[19]

In children, thiamine may help eliminate stuttering. Two- and three-year-olds given 25 to 30 mg. daily improved by 80 percent. Only about 50 percent of the four-year-olds improved and none of the older children improved. The success is attributed to thiamine's effect on the nervous system.[20]

Sudden Infant Death Syndrome (SIDS) has been theorized to be a result of improper thiamine metabolism. Supplements of 30 to 300 mg. per day have been used to relieve the symptoms in infants.[21]

Children aged nine to nineteen were involved in a double-blind study for one year to see if mental ability can be improved with thiamine. With all the tests concluded, the thiamine-supplemented group showed a percentage improvement over the control group from 25 to 3,200 percent.[22]

TOXICITY   No known toxic effects.

BEST SOURCES   Dried yeast, rice husks, whole wheat, oatmeal, peanuts, sunflower seeds, pork, ham, most vegetables, milk, and bran.

SUPPLEMENTS   Thiamine should be taken with all the other B-complex vitamins. For every milligram of thiamine (B-1) taken, you should take roughly 1.5 mg. of B-2 and 1 mg. of B-6. Taking too much B-1 by itself can bring on B-2 and B-6 deficiencies, and high doses can also produce symptoms similar to a manganese deficiency.[23]

I recommend taking no more than 10 to 25 mg. of thiamine at a time. High doses will just cause the excess to be excreted in the urine. It is better to take a lower potency and space it throughout the day. One may of course take more thiamine if treating a deficiency. Your need for thiamine rises as your carbohydrate intake increases.

Riboflavin (B-2)

FACTS   Water soluble. Any excess is excreted and therefore needs to be replaced daily. What little riboflavin is stored in the body is located mainly in the heart, liver, and kidneys. Riboflavin is stable to heat, but disintegrates in the presence of alkali or light. The need for riboflavin increases as protein intake increases. A lack of riboflavin is probably the most common vitamin deficiency.

DEFICIENCY SYMPTOMS   A very common deficiency symptom is cracks and sores in the corners of the mouth. The tongue may be sore and appear purplish- or magenta-colored instead of pink. People deficient in this vitamin may feel as if they have grit and sand on the insides of their eyelids, and the eyes may be bloodshot, watering, itching, burning, and fatigued. The nose, chin, and forehead take on an oily appearance, and fatty deposits accumulate under the skin. A riboflavin deficiency may also be accompanied by trembling, lack of stamina and vigor, retarded growth, digestive disturbances, hair and weight loss, and possibly even personality disturbances. "Laboratory experiments have shown that a deficiency of riboflavin in pregnant mammals causes congenital malformations in their offspring."[24]

WHAT IT DOES   "Riboflavin functions as part of a group of enzymes that are involved in the breakdown and utilization of carbohydrates, fats, and proteins."[25] Riboflavin is necessary for cellular respiration and the maintenance of good vision and healthy skin, nails, and hair. It also promotes growth.[26]

WHAT IT MAY DO   Riboflavin plays a role in preventing visual disturbances such as cataracts.[27] It is reported to increase resistance to fatigue in athletes.[28] Riboflavin helps maintain the immune response, since riboflavin is involved in the production and activity of antibodies.[29] Riboflavin somehow plays a role in detoxifying cancer-causing chemicals.[30]

TOXICITY   No known toxic effects.

BEST SOURCES   Liver, kidney, milk, yeast, cheese, whole grains, eggs, green leafy vegetables.

SUPPLEMENTS   Riboflavin should be taken with all the other B-complex vitamins. I recommend that about 15 to 30 mg. be taken at one time. You should take approximately one and one-half times more B-2 than B-1 or B-6. Any excess riboflavin is readily excreted and can be noticed by the yellow appearance of the urine. When the urine is clear or faintly yellow, you need more riboflavin.

Niacin (B-3, nicotinic acid, niacinamide, nicotinamide)

FACTS   Water soluble. Excess is excreted by the body. Niacin should be taken with the other B-complex vitamins. It is a fairly stable vitamin. The body can produce very small amounts of niacin, if protein intake is adequate.

Niacinamide is a form of niacin that has all the benefits of niacin but does not cause the blood vessels near the skin to dilate and produce a temporary flushing.

DEFICIENCY SYMPTOMS   The classic deficiency of niacin results in pellagra. This disease attacks three major areas of the body: (1) the skin, (2) the gastro-intestinal tract, (3) and the nervous system. The best-known symptoms of pellagra are "the three D's"—dermatitis, diarrhea, and dementia (mental disorder). Although there are few cases of pellagra in the developed countries, many people exhibit pre-pellagra symptoms. The tongue will be a brilliant red instead of a healthy pink color. The tongue and gums can become sore, and the mouth, throat, and esophagus may become inflamed. A niacin or a vitamin C deficiency can also lead to canker sores.

A niacin deficiency may also result in mental illness. Perceptual changes in the five senses are usually a key in determining if the person is deficient in niacin. Some people will say the ground moves when they walk, or they hear voices, or words move when they try to read, or their faces seem to change when they look in the mirror.[31]

Other symptoms of deficiency may be muscle weakness, general fatigue, irritability, recurring headaches, indigestion, nausea, vomiting, bad breath, insomnia, and small ulcers.[32] Many niacin-deficient people have no hydrochloric acid in their stomachs.[33]

WHAT IT DOES   "Niacin assists enzymes in the breakdown and utilization of proteins, fats, and carbohydrates."[34] Niacin improves blood flow by widening the diameter of the blood vessels. It is also necessary for the nervous system to operate properly and for the formation and maintenance of healthy skin, tongue, and digestive system tissues. Along with vitamins A, D, E, and K, niacin plays a role in the production of bile salts, which are needed for the digestion and absorption of fats. Niacin is necessary for the synthesis of hormones, including the sex hormones. Niacin prevents pellagra.

WHAT IT MAY DO   Niacin is used to treat heart disease, mental illness, and arthritis. It is used to reduce high blood cholesterol. Niacin may help in mental illness, including schizophrenia.

(Subclinical pellagra can easily be mistaken for mental illness.) It has proven helpful in the treatment of acne if 100 mg. of niacin are taken three times a day to produce a regular flushing of the skin.[35] Niacin may help with migraine headaches because it acts to widen the diameter of the blood vessels. Canker sores can often be corrected with 100 mg. of niacin or niacinamide.

TOXICITY No real toxic effects are known. When doses of up to 100 mg. of niacin are taken, a harmless, passing side effect manifests itself in the form of an intense flushing of the skin and tingling and itching sensations. This is due to a widening of the blood vessels. The effect usually lasts about a half hour. Very high doses should not be used unless under the care of a doctor.

BEST SOURCES Lean meats, organ meats, fish, brewer's yeast, whole grains, nuts, dried peas and beans, white meat of turkey and chicken, milk and milk products.

SUPPLEMENTS I recommend about 100 to 200 mg. of niacinamide to be included in your daily B-complex supplement. Niacinamide intake should be about ten times higher than that of thiamine (B-1) and pyridoxine (B-6).[36] If you take too much niacin or niacinamide, you may bring on a B-2 deficiency, so watch the ratios between the B-vitamins. Take your niacin with all the other B-complex vitamins.

The niacin form is occasionally recommended to temporarily increase the blood flow throughout the body and open the blood capillaries. The reason I recommend niacinamide over the niacin form is that niacinamide has all the benefits of niacin without the side effect of the flushing of the skin. Niacin, however, is the form generally recommended to those who suffer from migraine headaches and acne.

Pyridoxine (B-6, pyridoxinal, pyridoxamine)

FACTS Water soluble and a member of the B-complex family. Excreted in the urine eight hours after ingestion.[37] Depleted by reducing, fasting, using oral contraceptives, pregnancy, lactation, aging, cardiac failure, exposure to radiation, ingestion of cortisone or the female hormone estrogen.[38]

The more protein you eat, the more pyridoxine you need.

DEFICIENCY SYMPTOMS A deficiency may result in convulsions in babies. "The AMA Journal article recommends that all infants with convulsions be given an immediate large dose of pyridoxine."[39]

The most widely recognized symptom of pyridoxine deficiency is a greasy, scaly dermatitis between the eyebrows, on the sides of the nose, behind the ears, around the mouth, and in areas of the body that rub together. Newborn infants may develop crusty yellow scabs on the scalp called "cradle cap." Other deficiency symptoms may be low blood sugar, numbness and tingling in hands and feet, neuritis, arthritis, trembling in the hands of the aged, edema (water retention) and swelling during pregnancy, nausea, airsickness or seasickness, mental retardation, epilepsy, kidney stones, anemia, excessive fatigue, nervous breakdown, mental illness, and acne (especially during menstruation).[40]

WHAT IT DOES   Pyridoxine, or vitamin B-6, is an essential activator of many enzymes. "B-6 is intricately involved in the metabolism of fats, carbohydrates, potassium, iron, and the formation of hormones such as adrenalin and insulin."[41] Most importantly, protein cannot be absorbed and utilized if pyridoxine is not present.

Pyridoxine is needed to make antibodies and red blood cells, which are part of our immune response capability.[42] It helps convert the amino acid tryptophan into niacin (B-3). It is necessary for the synthesis of RNA and DNA.[43] It helps regulate the fluids in the body by maintaining the balance between sodium and potassium.[44] It is needed for the production of the digestive juice hydrochloric acid. Lack of pyridoxine may cause indigestion.[45]

Pyridoxine aids in the release of glycogen (stored sugar) for energy from the liver and muscles.[46] "Radiologists have found that pyridoxine can prevent the nausea that accompanies x-ray treatment."[47] "Obstetricians use it to control the morning sickness of pregnancy."[48]

WHAT IT MAY DO   Pyridoxine may help some women and girls who suffer outbreaks of acne just before their menstrual periods. "In a recent experiment 72 percent of those taking 50 milligrams of pyridoxine daily for one week before and during their periods had no further problems with acne."[49]

Pyridoxine, along with the mineral magnesium, prevents the formation of kidney stones.[50] Without pyridoxine, the body cannot properly utilize iron to build strong blood cells. The result is anemia, though anemia can also result from a lack of vitamin E, folic acid, B-12, iron, or other nutrients.[51]

Pyridoxine may help prevent hardening of the arteries.[52] It may help prevent tooth decay.[53] It has been shown to control edema (water retention), even when salt intake is not restricted. Most patients responded to 10 mg. of pyridoxine, while those with more severe symptoms, especially swelling of hands and feet, needed 50 to 450 mg. of pyridoxine daily.[54] Intake of 20 mg. of pyridoxine twice a day has been shown to relieve symptoms of depression in women who are deficient as a result of taking oral contraceptives.[55]

Pyridoxine can prevent soreness and puffiness during menstruation, since this vitamin plays a major role in water balance. These results were achieved with an intake of 50 to 100 mg. daily, without diuretics or a limited salt intake.[56]

Rheumatism, though not rheumatoid arthritis, in people found to be deficient in pyridoxine, may respond to 25 mg. of pyridoxine taken morning and night. This treatment relieved pain in finger joints, improved hand-grip strength, reduced stiffness and locking of the finger joints, and eliminated the numbness, tingling, and loss of sensation experienced by most patients.[57]

Women taking oral contraceptives sometimes experience an impairment of the glucose tolerance system similar to diabetes. Pyridoxine helps restore glucose tolerance in such women. Giving 25 mg. of pyridoxine restored glucose tolerance and allowed the body to clear sugar from the bloodstream in a normal fashion.[58]

TOXICITY   No known toxicity. High doses of 600 mg. of pyridoxine a day may suppress lactation in nursing mothers.[59] An oversupply of pyridoxine may stimulate too-vivid dream recall.

BEST SOURCES   The best sources are brewer's yeast, sunflower seeds, wheat germ, and liver and other organ meats. Other sources include bananas, walnuts, roasted peanuts, canned tuna, and salmon.[60]

SUPPLEMENTS   "About twenty-five percent of all people tested between the ages of eighteen and ninety had levels of pyridoxine low enough to indicate a deficiency."[61] "One study of college students found that seventy-five percent of them did not get the RDA for pyridoxine in their diets."[62]

The RDA for pyridoxine is 2 mg. The man who, in 1934, first isolated this vitamin, Dr. Szent-Gyorgyi, says that many individuals "need ten times the RDA as a precaution to prevent possible serious pathological conditions."[63] For adults, I recommend at least 20 mg. daily. Women may need an additional 25 mg. a day.

Always take pyridoxine (B-6) in a B-complex tablet with all the other B vitamins. The ratio of B-1:B-2:B-6 should be 1:1.5:1. If you take too much pyridoxine alone, you may bring on a B-1 deficiency.

Poor dream recall may indicate a shortage of B-6.[64]

Folic Acid (folacin, folate)

FACTS   Given its name "because it was first discovered in green leafy vegetables, or foliage."[65] Water soluble. A member of the B-complex family. Measured in micrograms (mcg.). Folic acid is extremely sensitive; most of it can be destroyed by cooking, canning, processing, and storage.[66] Zinc and vitamin C must be present in the diet for folic acid to be properly utilized.[67]

DEFICIENCY SYMPTOMS   The symptoms of a folic acid deficiency are much the same as those of a B-12 deficiency. They appear very gradually. Anemia resulting from a folic acid deficiency includes the following symptoms: poor growth, weakness, an inflamed and sore tongue that may appear smooth and shiny, numbness or tingling in the hands and feet, indigestion, diarrhea, depression, irritability, pallor, drowsiness, and slow, weakened pulse, graying hair, mental illness, impaired wound healing, and reduced resistance to infection. Birth defects are one of the worst results in a folic acid deficiency in pregnant women. Deficiency also may result in toxemia, premature birth, and after-birth hemorrhaging.[68] During pregnancy, a folic acid deficiency may cause what is called the "restless legs" syndrome, characterized by symptoms of insomnia, leg numbness, and cramps.[69]

WHAT IT DOES   Folic acid is necessary for the synthesis of DNA and RNA, which are proteins required for cell reproduction and division.[70] It is essential to the formation of red blood cells, due to its action on the bone marrow. Folic acid aids in the metabolism of protein and contributes to normal growth. "It also increases the appetite and stimulates the production of hydrochloric acid, which helps prevent intestinal parasites and food poisoning."[71] It is essential for the production of antibodies that fight off infection.[72]

WHAT IT MAY DO   Folic acid may help mental illness, including schizophrenia and senility. It reduces susceptibility to infection. It may help in treating psoriasis. It helps the body maintain a normal blood sugar level. It helps restore the cellular immune system.

BEST SOURCES Deep green, leafy vegetables, liver, brewer's yeast, whole grains, bran, asparagus, lima beans, lentils, orange juice.

TOXICITY Relatively nontoxic. Huge amounts have produced some toxic symptoms, but those dosages were available only by a special prescription.

Note: Folic acid should be given with great caution to epileptic people since it can interfere with epileptic drugs.

SUPPLEMENTS The FDA has set a limit of .8 mg. or 800 mcg. of folic acid to be included in a supplement. Anything over this potency must be purchased by prescription. The FDA's reasoning is that folic acid seems to mask some of the symptoms of a B-12 deficiency anemia, but still allows nerve damage to continue due to the lack of B-12. The FDA is therefore trying to protect those who do not get enough B-12 by restricting the availability of folic acid. A good B-complex formula should contain both B-12 and folic acid for this reason. The most often-used potencies, and what I recommend, are between 400 and 800 mcg. (or .4 to .8 mg.).

B-12 (Cobalamin or cyanocobalamin)

FACTS Water soluble. The only vitamin to contain the essential mineral cobalt. Needed in small amounts and measured in micrograms (mcg.). Found primarily in animal products, so a strict vegetarian diet must usually be supplemented by this vitamin. Older people find it harder to absorb. To be absorbed, B-12 needs calcium, a properly functioning thyroid gland, and the presence of hydrochloric acid and a substance called "the intrinsic factor."

DEFICIENCY SYMPTOMS It may take five or six years for a B-12 deficiency to show up. Deficiencies can result even if plenty is taken. An intrinsic factor made from proteins must be secreted by a normal healthy stomach for the body to absorb B-12.

A deficiency results in pernicious anemia. Symptoms of pernicious anemia include weakness, a sore and inflamed tongue that may appear smooth and shiny, "numbness and tingling in the extremities, pallor, weak pulse, stiffness, drowsiness, irritability, depression, and diarrhea," poor appetite, growth failure in children, and tingling sensations (a feeling of "pins and needles" in the hands and feet).[73]

A deficiency impairs the formation of red blood cells. The structure and function of the nervous system also deteriorates.[74] The function of the small intestine is impaired thereby reducing absorption of essential nutrients.[75] Blood clotting takes longer in the presence of a B-12 deficiency. A deficiency can also hide an ". . . iron deficiency by keeping blood levels of iron deceptively high."[76]

A B-12 deficiency can "cause visual difficulty and reduced color perception."[77] Mental disturbances may also be a sign of a deficiency and include changes in mood, mental slowness, and even severe psychotic symptoms.[78] "If a B-12 deficiency is not spotted in its early stages, it may result in permanent mental deterioration and paralysis."[79]

Another B-vitamin—folic acid—works closely with B-12. Folic acid works so closely that it can cure the blood symptoms of pernicious anemia, but not the nerve symptoms. As a result, possible nerve damage may progress unsuspected.

WHAT IT DOES   B-12 is necessary for normal metabolism of nerve tissue and is involved in protein, fat, and carbohydrate metabolism.[80] "It also helps iron function better in the body and aids folic acid in the synthesis of choline."[81] It is necessary for the synthesis of nucleic acid (RNA and DNA).[82]

WHAT IT MAY DO   B-12 stimulates growth and increases appetite in children.[83] It enhances resistance to infections. Mental illness has been successfully treated with B-12 and folic acid. I've seen many people rid themselves of bursitis when their doctors injected them with a 1,000 mcg. shot of B-12 every day until the pain was gone. It helps three types of herpes.

TOXICITY   Nontoxic, even in doses 5 to 10,000 times greater than the normal therapeutic dose.

BEST SOURCES   Organ meats, liver, beef, pork, eggs, milk, cheese.

SUPPLEMENTS   I recommend 25 mcg. or more to be taken daily with the B-complex vitamins. The RDA for adults and children over four years of age is 6 mcg. Since deficiencies are usually a result of improper absorption, rather than a lack of the vitamin, doctors will give injections of cobalamin (B-12) to bypass the absorption process until the problem with absorption can be corrected. You may also dissolve B-12 tablets under your tongue to bypass the absorption problem.

Pantothenic Acid (calcium pantothenate, panthenol)

FACTS Water soluble. A member of the B-complex family. Found in all living cells. Sometimes known as "the antistress vitamin." A certain amount of this vitamin can be synthesized by your intestinal bacteria. The name *pantothenic* was derived from a Greek word meaning "from everywhere."[84]

DEFICIENCY SYMPTOMS One common symptom of deficiency is a burning sensation in the feet. Other symptoms include an enlarged, beefy, furrowed tongue; skin disorders—eczemas on hands, face, ears, and genitalia; duodenal ulcers; inflammation of the intestines and stomach; decreased antibody formation; upper respiratory infections; vomiting; restlessness; muscle cramps; constipation; and sensitivity to insulin.[85]

A deficiency may lead to adrenal exhaustion, physical and mental depression, overwhelming fatigue, reduced production of hydrochloric acid in the stomach, allergies, some forms of arthritis, nerve degeneration, spinal curvature, disturbed pulse rate, and gout.[86] Furry animals such as rats and dogs, when fed a diet deficient in pantothenic acid, seem to age faster, and their hair turns coarse and gray.

WHAT IT DOES Pantothenic acid protects the adrenal cortex from damage and stimulates the adrenal glands to "increase production of cortisone and other adrenal hormones important for healthy skin and nerves." The adrenals stimulate the body's reaction to stress.[87]

Pantothenic acid is a coenzyme that plays a role in the release of energy from carbohydrates, fats, and proteins.[88] It "is essential for the synthesis of cholesterol, steroids (fat-soluble organic compounds) and fatty acids." (Remember, your body makes cholesterol whether or not you eat it.)[89]

Pantothenic acid helps maintain a healthy digestive tract. It is "absolutely essential to the production of antibodies which help fight off infection." You must have three B-vitamins—pantothenic acid, pyridoxine (B-6), and folic acid to make antibodies.[90] Pantothenic acid reduces the toxic effects of many antibiotics. It may protect against radiation. A Hungarian study showed that pantothenic acid supplements increased by 200 percent the survival rate of mice exposed to radiation.[91]

WHAT IT MAY DO   Dr. Roger Williams says that pantothenic acid consistently brought relief to sufferers of rheumatoid arthritis, but improvement only went so far. Pantothenic acid is just one of the essential elements in the fight against arthritis.[92]

Animal studies show that pantothenic acid plays a vital role in reproduction. A deficiency may produce reproductive failures, including stillbirths, premature births, malformed babies, and mentally retarded babies.[93]

Pantothenic acid was found to be a factor in restoring gray hair to its normal color in experimental animals, although this function has not been substantiated in humans.[94] Pantothenic acid, when combined with calcium may stop people from grinding their teeth at night.[95] "It helps surgical patients recover quicker."[96]

It may help prolong life. Dr. Williams found that mice fed extra pantothenic acid lived 19 percent longer than those fed adequate amounts of pantothenic acid.[97]

It may help allergies by reducing the amount of histamine your body produces. Skin reactions to allergens have been reduced from 20 to 50 percent with the administration of pantothenic acid either orally or by injection.[98]

It may help with gout, since it works on the adrenals to change the harmful uric acid into urea, which can then be harmlessly passed out of the body.

TOXICITY   Relatively nontoxic. No one has ever produced toxic symptoms in humans. Researchers have produced toxic effects in animals by giving them 2,000 to 3,000 mg. per kilogram of body weight (kilogram = 2.2 pounds).

BEST SOURCES   Brewer's yeast, liver, kidney, wheat bran, crude molasses, whole grains, egg yolk, peanuts, peas, sunflower seeds, beef, chicken, turkey, milk.

SUPPLEMENTS   I recommend between 100 and 200 mg. daily in a B-complex supplement. Since pantothenic acid is very closely associated with riboflavin (B-2) supply: a relatively constant proportion should be kept between the two of about 5 or 10:1 (pantothenic acid : riboflavin). In other words, take 5 or 10 mg. of pantothenic acid for every 1 mg. of riboflavin.

Biotin (previously called vitamin H)

FACTS   Water soluble. A member of the B-complex family. Measured in micrograms (mcg.). Manufactured, to a certain extent, in the intestines. Avidin, a protein found in the white part of a raw egg, keeps the body from absorbing biotin. Sulfa drugs and antibiotics can also destroy biotin and are often the causes of a deficiency.

DEFICIENCY SYMPTOMS   The first symptom to appear in a biotin deficiency is usually scaly dermatitis. Symptoms of deficiency in humans include "dermatitis, inflamed and sore tongue, loss of appetite, nausea, depression, muscle pain, sitophobia (morbid dread of food), pallor, anemia, abnormalities of heart function, burning or prickling sensations, increased sensitivity of the skin, insomnia, extreme lassitude, increased blood levels of cholesterol, and depression of the immune system."[99] Full-fledged deficiencies are rare, but a moderate decrease in supply will cause some reduction in health.

WHAT IT DOES   "Biotin is an essential coenzyme in many enzyme reactions."[100] The thyroid, adrenal glands, reproductive tract, nervous system, and skin need an adequate supply of biotin. Biotin is "involved in the metabolism of carbohydrates, proteins, and fats, especially the unsaturated fatty acids."[101] It is needed for normal growth and the "maintenance of the skin, hair, sebaceous glands [sweat glands], nerves, bone marrow, and the sex glands."[102]

WHAT IT MAY DO   Biotin may help in the treatment of seborrheic dermatitis in infants.[103]

TOXICITY   No known toxic effects.

BEST SOURCES   Yeast, liver, organ meats, egg yolk, and a variety of grains, nuts, and fish. It is found in almost every food in very minute quantities.

SUPPLEMENTS   Usually found in doses from 25 to 300 mcg. It is an expensive vitamin, so many manufacturers try to leave it out. Be sure and check the label. I recommend taking 25 to 50 mcg. a day to give your body a strong base for this vitamin. Remember, you'll get more biotin from almost everything you eat and your body also produces very small quantities.

PABA (para-aminobenzoic acid)

FACTS   Water soluble. A member of the B-complex family. Some people question its status as a true vitamin, even though it meets all the requirements.[104] PABA can be synthesized by friendly bacteria in the intestine, if conditions are favorable.

DEFICIENCY SYMPTOMS   A PABA deficiency in rats produces gray hair as do deficiencies of pantothenic acid, biotin, and folic acid.[105] Deficiency symptoms may be similar to symptoms caused by a folic acid or pantothenic acid deficiency, since PABA works intricately with these other B-vitamins. A PABA deficiency may be a contributing factor in the painless disease vitiligo (which is characterized by light blotches on the skin surrounded by a dark border).[106] Other possible "symptoms include fatigue, irritability, depression, nervousness, headache, constipation, and other digestive disorders."[107]

WHAT IT DOES   "PABA stimulates the intestinal bacteria, enabling them to produce folic acid, which in turn aids in the production of pantothenic acid."[108] PABA acts as a coenzyme in the making of blood cells and the metabolizing of proteins.[109] "PABA plays an important role in determining skin health, hair pigmentation, and health of the intestines."[110]

It can be applied to the skin as a sunscreen and can block the harmful portions of ultraviolet light that cause sunburn and skin cancer. (Each year, 300,000 cases of skin cancer develop—this is the most common form of cancer.)[111] PABA competes with sulfa drugs for absorption in the body. Whichever one is ingested first will render the other ineffective.

WHAT IT MAY DO   PABA protects the body from the effects of ozone—most likely because of its antioxidant properties.[112] It is used in treating vitiligo and some parasitic diseases, including Rocky Mountain spotted fever. It may help restore gray hair to its natural color and protect against further graying, although there has been no conclusive evidence to this effect in humans. Large doses have been used to treat many skin diseases.[113]

TOXICITY   No known toxic effects. Symptoms of an oversupply are usually nausea and vomiting.[114] Long-term programs with dosages in the thousands of milligrams are not recommended.

BEST SOURCES   Liver, brewer's yeast, wheat germ, molasses, eggs, organ meats, yogurt, green leafy vegetables.

SUPPLEMENTS   I recommend between 50 and 100 mg. a day to be included in a B-complex formula.

Choline

FACTS   Water soluble. A member of the B-complex family. Found in all living cells.[115] Choline is a lipotropic or fat emulsifier. It can be synthesized in the body to a certain extent by the amino acid methionine.[116] However, all cells need methionine, and they receive first priority. Only leftover methionine not directly engaged by the cells is used to make choline, and therefore it is easy to become choline-deficient.

DEFICIENCY SYMPTOMS   A choline deficiency may result not only from too little choline in the diet, but from too little protein in the diet.[117] There are no clinically official signs of choline deficiency, but it is possible to identify some symptoms that may be attributable to a choline deficiency.

A deficiency may cause a rise in blood pressure.[118] A deficiency may also cause fatty deposits to build up in the liver, blocking hundreds of its functions. Soon the whole body becomes diseased by poisons that the liver cannot detoxify as they enter the bloodstream.

A deficiency may result in "bleeding stomach ulcers; heart trouble; and blocking of the tubes of the kidneys."[119] Other results of a deficiency may be hemorrhaging of the kidneys, "hardening of the arteries, and atherosclerosis."[120]

"Such symptoms as headaches, dizziness, ear noises, palpitation, and constipation improved or disappeared completely five to ten days after this vitamin was started" in patients studied with dangerous hypertension.[121] "A severe deficiency can result in paralysis, cardiac arrest, and death."[122]

WHAT IT DOES   Choline is needed for the proper functioning of the nervous system. Choline is part of the nerve fluid that fills the gap between nerve cells that allow nerve impulses to be transmitted. Without choline to help make this process possible, even the heart would stop beating.

As a component of lecithin, choline helps emulsify cholesterol. It prevents fats from depositing in the liver and helps direct fats into the cells.[123] "It is essential for the health of the liver and kidneys."[124] It strengthens capillary walls, accelerates blood flow, thereby lowering blood pressure by decreasing the work the heart has to do.[125] Choline "aids in the prevention of gallstones."[126] It combines with inositol and other substances to form lecithin. ("It is very important to note that human breast milk also contains lecithin, while cow's milk is lacking in it.")[127] Choline "is one of the few nutrients which are taken by the blood directly to the brain." There it helps manufacture a nerve signal transmitter called acetylcholine, which may aid memory function.[128]

WHAT IT MAY DO   Choline, B-12, folic acid, and the amino acid methionine, are considered vital nutrients in the proper functioning of the immune system. "It only takes a slight deficiency of these nutrients in pregnant animals to shortchange the immune system of their offspring," which leaves the young more susceptible to infections.[129]

Research has found choline injections effective in treating depressive diseases with such symptoms as hypochondria, depression, sleeplessness, paranoia, suicidal tendencies, anxiety, and moodiness.[130] Treatment with choline improves the memories of people who suffer from Alzheimer's disease or presenile dementia. Patients are given 5 to 10 grams a day.[131] Choline treatment reverses loss of control over facial muscles in psychotic patients who suffer from Tardive dyskinesia. This disease is doctor-induced and caused by drugs.[132]

TOXICITY   No known toxic effects. Massive doses over a long period of time may induce a B-6 deficiency.[133] A bodily fishy odor may result from massive doses.

BEST SOURCES   The best source of choline is lecithin. Other sources are brewer's yeast, fish, soybeans, peanuts, beef liver, eggs, and wheat germ.

SUPPLEMENTS   Lecithin granules or capsules are a very good source of choline and inositol. One tablespoonful of the granules contains about 250 mg. of each. A good daily diet contains between 500 and 900 mg. of choline.[134] I recommend 100 to 200 mg. be taken daily in a good B-complex supplement. This regimen will assure that choline will be available for use even if the diet is lacking. As part of the B-complex, choline should be taken with all the other vitamins.

Inositol

FACTS   Water soluble. A member of the B-complex family. Occurs in extremely high concentrations in the brain. Also plentifully contained in the stomach, kidney, spleen, liver, and heart.[135] Inositol, along with choline, is found in lecithin, which breaks down fats. Inositol can be made to a certain extent by the body. "The human body contains more inositol than any other vitamin except Niacin."[136]

DEFICIENCY SYMPTOMS There are no officially recognized deficiency signs, however, an inositol deficiency "may cause constipation, eczema, and abnormalities of the eyes."[137] An inositol deficiency may also contribute to "hair loss and a high blood cholesterol level."[138]

WHAT IT DOES Inositol helps promote the body's own production of lecithin. It aids in the metabolism of fats and helps reduce blood cholesterol.[139] "Inositol is needed for the growth and cell survival in bone marrow, eye membranes and intestines."[140]

WHAT IT MAY DO It may have a "mild inhibitory effect on cancer."[141] It is "used with vitamin E to treat nerve damage in certain forms of muscular dystrophy."[142] Inositol has a greater power to break up fat when combined with choline. It may "prevent thinning hair and baldness."[143] It may be especially valuable in brain cell nutrition.[144]

TOXICITY No known toxic effects.

BEST SOURCES Lecithin, "beef brain, beef heart, wheat germ, bulgar wheat, brown rice, brewer's yeast, molasses, nuts, citrus fruits."[145]

SUPPLEMENTS Available in lecithin granules or capsules. One tablespoonful of lecithin granules provides about 250 mg. of inositol and 250 mg. of choline. Inositol is also found in B-complex formulas. I recommend 100 to 200 mg. daily in a good B-complex formula. You should take approximately equal amounts of choline and inositol daily. (That's why lecithin is such a good food supplement.) Most people get about 1,000 mg. a day in their diet.

Vitamin C (ascorbic acid)

FACTS Water soluble. Most animals can make their own vitamin C, but human beings, apes, guinea pigs, and certain bats must get vitamin C from their diet. "The level of ascorbic acid in the blood reaches a maximum in 2 or 3 hours after ingestion of a moderate quantity, and then gradually decreases, as the ascorbic acid is eliminated in the urine."[146] When the human body is saturated, it will contain about 5,000 milligrams of vitamin C.[147] The words *vitamin C* and *ascorbic acid* are used interchangeably.

DEFICIENCY SYMPTOMS   Deficiency symptoms may include bruising easily, bleeding gums, tooth decay, nose bleeds, swollen or painful joints, anemia, poor wound healing, lowered resistance to infection, and a general weakening of connective tissue (skin, tendons, walls of blood vessels).[148]

An extreme deficiency results in scurvy. The bones fracture easily, weakened arteries rupture and hemorrhage, extreme muscle weakness is experienced, joints are too painful to move, gums are spongy and bleed, teeth fall out, and wounds and sores never heal.[149]

WHAT IT DOES   One of vitamin C's most important functions is the "synthesis, formation, and maintenance of a protein-like substance called collagen." Collagen is the "cement that supports and holds the tissues and organs together.... It is the substance that strengthens the arteries and veins, supports the muscles, toughens the ligaments and bones, supplies the scar tissue for healing wounds and keeps the youthful skin tissues soft, firm, supple and wrinkle free."[150] Vitamin C is necessary for healthy teeth and gums.

"Vitamin C protects thiamine, riboflavin, folic acid, pantothenic acid, and vitamin A and E against oxidation."[151] It helps in the metabolizing of a few amino acids.[152] It helps convert the B-vitamin folic acid into its active form, folinic acid. Taking vitamin C increases the absorption of iron. It also enhances the absorption of calcium and certain essential amino acids.[153]

Vitamin C has an activating effect on insulin, which keeps the blood sugar from going too high during the digestion of carbohydrates.[154] "It is essential to the proper functioning of the nervous system."[155]

Vitamin C "is a potent detoxicant which counteracts and neutralizes the harmful effect of many poisons in the body," such as mercury, arsenic, drugs, bacteria, animal toxins, air pollutants such as carbon monoxide and sulfur dioxide, and carcinogens (cancer-causing substances).[156] "Ascorbic acid in large dosages is a good nontoxic diuretic."[157]

Your body defends itself against harmful bacteria by sending white blood cells to devour and digest the invading bacteria. This process is partially controlled by the level of ascorbic acid in the tissues and blood. If the level is too low, the white blood cells will not attack the invading bacteria. This shows why a low level of ascorbic acid in the body decreases your resistance to infectious diseases.[158] Vitamin C also enhances the therapeutic effect of certain drugs so that less of those drugs is required.[159]

WHAT IT MAY DO   Vitamin C, in doses of 250 mg. up to 5,000 mg. or more, may be needed to prevent the common cold. It has been recommended that at the first sign of a cold, such as a scratchy throat, one should immediately take 500 to 1,000 mg. of vitamin C. This regimen is continued every hour until you have taken up to 10 grams a day and until a day or two after the cold is gone.[160]

Vitamin C may help with fertility, due to the high concentration of ascorbic acid in the ovaries.[161] It may help lower back pain by helping the disc connective tissue strengthen and heal.[162] It "enhances wound healing following surgery."[163] Vitamin C has lowered cholesterol and triglycerides levels.[164] It also helps protect against cardiovascular disease by its role in prolonging the process of blood clotting.[165] (A blood clot that reaches the heart results in a heart attack; a clot that reaches the brain results in a stroke.)

"Vitamin C also boosts the body's production of a natural antibacterial, antiviral substance called interferon."[166] "Vitamin C may also help increase the body's resistance to cancer by allowing the tumor to be 'encapsulated' by a tough wall of collagen."[167] Vitamin C, along with many other nutrients, is important in mental health.

Vitamin C helps protect us against the industrial pollutant cadmium, lead poisoning, and nitrites in processed foods.[168] Vitamin C, in dosages of 1,000 to 2,250 mg., has been given to hay fever and allergy sufferers with moderate success.[169] Vitamin C may help in the prevention of senile cataracts.[170]

TOXICITY   Nontoxic. Intravenous doses in humans, ranging from a few thousand mg. to 200,000 mg. of ascorbic acid, produced no serious side effects.[171]

Individuals hypersensitive to high doses of vitamin C may have side reactions such as "the appearance of gastric distress, vomiting, diarrhea, headache, or skin rashes, all of which disappear on reducing or eliminating the ascorbic acid."[172] If you are sensitive to large doses of vitamin C, you should start out at lower doses and then gradually build up the dosage.

One doctor, responding to fears that large dosages of vitamin C may cause kidney stones, says, "I have used mega doses of ascorbic acid, 3,000 to 30,000 mg. per day since 1953 on perhaps over 1,000 patients. During this long period I have not seen one case of kidney stone formation, or miscarriage, or dehydration or any other serious toxicity."[173] Vitamin B-6, in conjunction with the mineral magnesium, has been shown to prevent kidney stones from forming.[174]

BEST SOURCES   Rose hips, citrus fruits and their juices, strawberries, blueberries, cantaloupes, and raw vegetables. The vitamin C in these sources is easily destroyed by storage, steaming, washing, soaking, and canning.

SUPPLEMENTS   A wide variety of supplements are available from vitamin pills, to powders, to vitamin C breath mints. Ascorbic acid is the form of vitamin C that most people take. Natural vitamin C from rose hips and acerola berries is very expensive and can only be produced in low potencies. Some formulas combine this natural form with ascorbic acid.

I recommend taking from 250 mg. to 10,000 mg. a day, depending on your particular need. It is better to take lower potencies— say, 250 to 500 mg.—spaced throughout the day than to take 5,000 mg. at one time. Vitamin C taken with citrus bioflavonoids is the best way to take vitamin C, since this most closely approximates the way vitamin C is found in nature. It is also more expensive.

I also suggest a calcium-magnesium tablet with every 1,000 mg. of vitamin C you take. This will buffer the vitamin C. It is wise to increase your vitamin C intake gradually over a period of time. This permits your body to become used to higher levels.

COMMENTS   Vitamin C is highly concentrated in the adrenal glands. Under stress, the body uses up vitamin C very rapidly.

The mouse and the goat, both of which manufacture their own vitamin C, have been reported to produce levels of vitamin C that would be equivalent to 19,000 mg. and 13,000 mg. daily in a man weighing 154 pounds.[175] The guinea pig and the monkey are like man in that they do not manufacture their own vitamin C. The recommended diets for them contain 1,100 mg. and 1,250 mg. respectively, corresponding to the intake of a 154-pound man.[176] These animal studies suggest that for humans a few thousand milligrams per day is probably closer to the optimal dosage, compared to the RDA of just 60 mg.

Vitamin D

FACTS   Fat-soluble vitamin stored mainly in the liver. It is commonly called "the sunshine vitamin" because when the ultraviolet rays from sunlight hit the skin, a form of cholesterol in the body is converted into vitamin D. Smoggy or polluted air reduces the amount of vitamin D-producing ultraviolet rays that reach the skin. Black people do not produce their own vitamin D as efficiently, since the dark pigment of their skin screens out much of the ultraviolet rays. Vitamin D is also a pro-hormone.[177]

DEFICIENCY SYMPTOMS   In adults, a vitamin D deficiency robs the bones of minerals and results in osteomalacia (softening of the bones) or osteoporosis (brittle and porous bones). The bones of many older people become soft or brittle and then fracture from the stress of gravity. When such a person falls and breaks a bone, the fracture is not the result of the fall; actually, the bone breaks spontaneously and then the person falls.

In children, rickets can result from insufficient vitamin D. Early signs are irritability, restlessness, fitful sleeping, and frequent crying. Babies will perspire heavily behind the neck so that their hair becomes wet. The teeth are often late in erupting and tooth enamel may be thin and irregular. The first real sign, though, is a soft, yielding skull. Bones become swollen at the ends and soft in the middle, and the results are bowed legs, knock knees, depressions in the chest, and a pigeon-chest deformity of the rib cage. The lower part of the ribs may flare out. The backbone may curve inward, causing swayback (lordosis), and the eyes may appear sunken due to an overly prominent forehead. Walking is usually delayed.[178]

WHAT IT DOES   Vitamin D enhances the absorption of two minerals necessary for bone strength—calcium and phosphorus. It also increases plasma levels of calcium and phosphorus so that these minerals can be laid down properly in the bones. Vitamin D is necessary for the proper functioning of the thyroid and pituitary glands.

WHAT IT MAY DO   Vitamin D, along with calcium and other nutrients, may prevent osteoporosis and osteomalacia in adults and rickets in children.

TOXICITY   Toxicity symptoms of vitamin D have been produced with as little as 50,000 units a day taken for a few weeks. Some people would need to take ten times that amount to produce toxic symptoms.[179] Symptoms of toxicity include loss of appetite, unusual thirst, urinary urgency, vomiting, and diarrhea. In more severe cases, calcium and phosphorus are taken from the bones and then redeposited in the soft tissues of the body, such as the blood vessels, heart, kidneys, and lungs.[180]

Vitamin D produced in the body from the effect of the sun's rays on the skin has never produced toxicity.

BEST SOURCES   The best external source of vitamin D (besides the sun) is the natural form, vitamin D-3, found in fish liver oils such as cod liver oil. Besides this, vitamin D is usually hard to get in the diet. Most sources of vitamin D are foods fortified with synthetic vitamin D (vitamin D-2), called calciferol. The synthetic form of vitamin D, however, binds with magnesium to render that mineral useless. I recommend that you drink whole milk instead of vitamin D enriched milk for that reason.

SUPPLEMENTS   I recommend you take 400 to 800 I.U. of the fish liver oil form of vitamin D daily. One tablespoonful of cod liver oil is just as good since it provides about 400 I.U. daily. Stay away from the synthetic form of vitamin D (called calciferol or D-2).

It is extremely important that all children get plenty of this vitamin. Furthermore, if you work at night, stay out of the sun, live in the northern part of the country, or do not drink vitamin D milk, then you should definitely take a vitamin D supplement. Winter is also a good time to take vitamin D supplements. Cases of osteomalacia with bone fractures seem to be heavily clustered from February to June, when stockpiles of vitamin D tend to run out.

Vitamin E (Tocopherol)

FACTS   Vitamin E is fat soluble and is stored mainly in the liver, while lower quantities are also stored in the fatty tissues, heart, muscles, testes, uterus, blood, and adrenal and pituitary glands. The assimilation of vitamin E is less than 50 percent in healthy persons. The bowel excretes any excess much as it does with the water-soluble vitamins.[181]

Vitamin E is composed of seven factors: the alpha, beta, gamma, delta, epsilon, eta, and zeta tocopherols.[182] "Alpha tocopherol is the most potent form of vitamin E and has the greatest nutritional and biological value."[183] Alpha tocopherol also "constitutes 90 percent of the total tocopherols in the human body."[184]

Vitamin E is measured in International Units (I.U.). An I.U. is the amount needed to produce a specific biological effect. For vitamin E, it is the ability of the vitamin to stimulate proper reproduction in rats.

Vitamin E increases the effect of vitamin A and keeps it from oxidizing. That's why good vitamin A supplements contain a small amount of vitamin E. Vitamin E works synergistically with selenium—that is, they work better together than each does by itself. The synergistic equation is: $1 + 1 = 3$.

Rancid oil or fat, mineral oil, chlorine in drinking water, polyunsaturated fats or oils, oral contraceptives, menopausal drugs, and inorganic iron (iron supplements that start with the word *ferric*) interfere with the activity of vitamin E. The more polyunsaturated oils in your diet, the more vitamin E you need.

DEFICIENCY SYMPTOMS   There are no clear-cut symptoms of vitamin E deficiency, though many health problems are affected by a deficiency of this vitamin.

One effect of vitamin E deficiency in humans is the decreased survival time of red blood cells in humans.[185] Other effects of deficiency include faulty fat absorption, anemia in premature infants, and "a tendency toward muscular wasting or abnormal fat deposits in the muscles and an increased demand for oxygen."[186] "Degeneration of the brain and spinal cord have also been reported in vitamin E–deficient children."[187] In pregnant women, a severe deficiency may cause premature births and can even result in miscarriage.[188]

"Unless vitamin E is adequate, the testicles of all varieties of laboratory and farm animals degenerate; and there is a decrease in both the sex hormones and the pituitary hormone gonadotropin, which stimulate the sex glands."[189]

A severe vitamin E deficiency usually produces irreversible harm no matter how much vitamin E is administered later on.

WHAT IT DOES/WHAT IT MAY DO   Vitamin E reduces the amount of oxygen required by the tissues. Because of this property, it may be useful in "gangrene, coronary and cerebral thrombosis (clots), diabetes mellitus, congenital heart disease, arteriosclerosis, Raynaud's syndrome (characterized by spasm of vessels of the fingers), phlebitis, intermittent claudication, systremma, and other leg problems due to poor circulation, athletics, mountain climbing, aviation, abruptio placentae, threatened miscarriage."[190]

The primary role of vitamin E is as an antioxidant. In this role, vitamin E protects the polyunsaturated fats and oils from breaking down into free radicals that damage and destroy cells. If such a breakdown process is left unchecked, the destruction of cells may cause premature aging and may lead to many diseases.[191]

Vitamin E has been shown to melt fresh blood clots by fibrinolysis, a process that is the opposite of coagulation or blood clotting.[192] "Vitamin E may play a role in the synthesis and function of prostaglandins, which are hormones that regulate many organ systems, including the muscles."[193]

Vitamin E is essential for the proper functioning of the sex glands.[194] It protects the sex hormones from being destroyed by oxygen and the "motility and fertility of sperm are in proportion to the amount of vitamin E in a man's semen."[195]

Vitamin E plays a role in helping the body protect itself against air pollution. Two pollutants, ozone and nitrous oxide, "exert their toxic effect by oxidizing the unsaturated fats in the cells and membranes of the lungs." The vitamin prevents much of this damage to the lungs.[196]

Vitamin E may protect against the damage of radiation. "A National Cancer Institute study found that vitamin E supplements increased both median and overall survival of mice exposed to lethal radiation."[197]

Vitamin E may help with noncancerous breast cysts when patients are given 600 I.U. per day. This is important since women with breast cysts have a much higher incidence of breast cancer.[198] Vitamin E may also help relieve pain in osteoarthritis because it has an anti-inflammatory, stabilizing effect on the membranes of the cells.[199] It may counteract some of the adverse side effects of oral contraceptives, such as thrombosis (blood clots).[200] "Vitamin E supplementation has been shown to promote significant repair of muscles damaged by nutritional muscular dystrophy in animals."[201]

Vitamin E may help relieve menopause pains.[202] Many studies have shown that stamina can be increased in athletes and laboratory animals by giving them vitamin E.[203] Supplementation has been shown to raise vitamin E concentrations to normal in people with sickle cell anemia, and also to "cut to less than half the number of irreversibly sickled cells in their blood."[204] "Vitamin E has shown effectiveness in reducing tartar on the teeth and inflammation of the gums."[205]

Vitamin E may help varicose veins by opening up detours around the sites of venous obstruction. In two months' time, one should be able to tell if vitamin E is helping.[206]

Vitamin E aids in healing wounds or burns. People burned by scalding water or hot irons all responded to vitamin E treatment. Vitamin E was given orally as well as topically (a vitamin E ointment). Quick relief of pain was noticed, the wounds did not contract upon healing, leaving complete flexibility, scarring was minimized, and in many cases where skin grafts had been recommended or performed but refused to take hold, the vitamin E treatment was successful in complete healing.[207]

TOXICITY   Vitamin E does not appear to be toxic in large amounts, though it is stored by the body to a certain extent.

Note: You should be under a doctor's supervision when taking vitamin E if any of the following conditions apply to you.

About one-quarter of insulin-dependent diabetics will require less insulin when given adequate doses of vitamin E. Insulin requirements should be checked carefully for a few months and possible changes noted within two or three days.

People with chronic rheumatic hearts must begin with low levels of vitamin E (90 I.U. daily) and then gradually increase their intake. People with hypertensive heart disease should start out with low doses of vitamin E (75 I.U. daily) and then, after a month, gradually increase their intake. Because blood pressure may increase, the doses are kept low. A prescription of digitalis (a heart-tonic medication) is often reduced after a patient starts to take vitamin E.

The female hormone estrogen should rarely be given at the same time as vitamin E.

People taking anticoagulant drugs should be aware that taking vitamin E may thin the blood too much. The amount of anticoagulant drugs given may have to be reduced.

Anyone with an underactive thyroid who is taking thyroid hormone should take vitamin E at a different time of the day since vitamin E reduces the effectiveness of the thyroid hormone.[208]

BEST SOURCES   Wheat germ oil, soybean oil, safflower oil, and peanuts; whole grains—wheat, rice, and oats; green, leafy vegetables—cabbage, spinach, asparagus, and broccoli.[209]

SUPPLEMENTS   Vitamin E can be taken in the natural or synthetic form. The natural form is labeled "d-alpha-tocopherol," "d-alpha-acetate," or "d-alpha-succinate." The synthetic form of vitamin E is labeled with the letter *l* after the *d* ("dl-alpha tocopherol"). Other possible labels for the synthetic vitamin E are "E-tocopherol," "vitamin E," and "vitamin E acetate."

Watch out for formulas labeled "natural vitamin E" that in reality contain only a trace of the natural vitamin while the rest is synthetic. This is legal, so read your labels. Natural vitamin E is more expensive than the synthetic form.

The synthetic form of vitamin E does not appear in nature. The body treats it as it would any other chemical antioxidant. It is absorbed, but not generally laid down in the tissue. The natural supplement form of vitamin E, however, has the exact same chemical composition as vitamin E found in nature. The natural form is absorbed and generally laid down in the fatty tissue of the liver and other places where it is not given up easily according to a major manufacturer of natural vitamin E.

I recommend 200 to 400 I.U. of vitamin E in the natural form taken daily. One may take up to between 1,000 and 1,600 I.U. of vitamin E, if you can afford it, and it has been prescribed for its therapeutic effects.

Vitamin K

FACTS   A fat-soluble vitamin. There are three major types of K vitamins. Vitamins K-1 and K-2 are manufactured in your intestinal tract "in the presence of certain intestinal flora (bacteria)."[210] K-3 is synthetically produced for those people who cannot make K-1 or K-2.

Antibiotics kill all the friendly and unfriendly bacteria in the intestines and thereby halt the production of vitamin K. Deficiency may also result if the liver fails to secrete bile, which is necessary for the absorption of all fat-soluble vitamins. (Vitamins A, D, and E will not be absorbed either.)

Anticoagulant and sulfa drugs, the ingestion of mineral oil, and conditions such as sprue (malabsorption in adulthood), colitis, celiac disease (intestinal malabsorption), and pancreatic dysfunction all interfere with vitamin K production.[211]

DEFICIENCY SYMPTOMS   Deficiency is relatively rare since the body can usually produce vitamin K and it is available in many foods. In a deficiency, a condition called *hypoprothrombinemia* can occur, in which the time it takes for the blood to clot is prolonged.[212] Hemorrhages can occur in any part of the body with a deficiency. Sometimes blood will appear in the urine and stools.[213] Nosebleeds and miscarriages can also result.[214]

In newborn babies, vitamin K deficiency is fairly common since newborns have no intestinal bacteria. If the deficiency is severe enough, bloody stools or vomiting may occur in the first week or so of life. Some doctors recommend giving a very small dose of vitamin K to infants shortly after birth. The best way to administer the dose, of course, is to have a nursing mother eat plenty of food with vitamin K in it and avoid aspirin or sedatives, which reduce the production of vitamin K.[215]

WHAT IT DOES   Vitamin K is essential to blood clotting (or coagulation). Without it, we would all bleed to death from the slightest wound. "Animal studies have shown it [vitamin K] is required for proper bone mineralization."[216]

WHAT IT MAY DO   "Vitamin K has been used successfully to offset the risks of anticoagulants."[217]

TOXICITY   There is no danger of getting too much vitamin K from food. Stay away from any vitamin K in supplement form. It can be toxic, and it can induce faster-than-average clotting, which is dangerous and can lead to internal blood clots.

BEST SOURCES   When yogurt, kefir (a preparation of curdled milk), or acidophilus milk (fermented milk containing millions of friendly bacteria) are added to the diet, you should be able to manufacture enough vitamin K since your bacteria will feed on these three things. The next best sources of vitamin K are spinach, cabbage, cauliflower, tomatoes, pork liver, lean meat, peas, carrots, soybeans, potatoes, alfalfa, and egg yolks.

SUPPLEMENTS   I do not recommend supplements. If you feel you need vitamin K, it should be administered only under the direction of a doctor.

Bioflavonoids (vitamin P)

FACTS   Water soluble. Not considered a vitamin, although in nature bioflavonoids are found along with vitamin C. "The components of the bioflavonoids are citrin, hesperidin, rutin, flavones, and flavonals."[218]

DEFICIENCY SYMPTOMS   Like vitamin C, bioflavonoids are involved in capillary strength. "Edema, or the accumulation of fluid in the tissue, and bleeding into the tissue (noticeable as red spots and splotches when it occurs close under the skin) both can be the result of fragile faulty capillaries."[219]

WHAT IT DOES   "The principal effect of bioflavonoids is to decrease the permeability and fragility of the blood vessels, and to constrict the capillaries."[220] Bioflavonoids protect vitamin C from oxidation and can actually reverse oxidized vitamin C, making it available to the tissue. They decrease the tendency of blood cells to clump together. Clumping increases the chance of a dangerous blood clot.[221]

They increase the absorption and utilization of vitamin A.[222] They prevent the oxidation of an adrenal hormone that stimulates the cardiovascular system.[223] "The bioflavonoids act as normalizers of blood flow in the capillaries and veins."[224]

WHAT IT MAY DO   Bioflavonoids may help women with a painful or irregular menstrual flow because they protect against abnormal bleeding.[225] They may also help prevent the bleeding that usually follows the insertion of an interuterine contraceptive device (IUD). Improvement was most noted by the third menstrual cycle.[226]

They have been shown to help relieve the painful throbbing and swelling of mild cases of varicose veins.[227] They have been used to treat certain types of hemorrhoids by relieving the pain and hemorrhaging after two to five days.[228]

Bioflavonoids help prevent bruising since bruises "are nothing but a mass of broken or damaged capillaries."[229] Bioflavonoids have been found to halt severe nosebleeds in older people.[230] They may alleviate and prevent recurrence of retinitis, which is an inflammation of the retina along with hemorrhaging.[231] In animals, bioflavonoids have proved effective against frostbite and increased resistance to viral infection.[232]

TOXICITY   None known.

BEST SOURCES   The white part of lemons, oranges, and other citrus fruits including the center part of the fruit, is the richest source of bioflavonoids. Frozen juices are a poor source, since the bioflavonoids are usually separated out with the pulp to preserve the taste of the juice. The pulp of citrus fruits is a good source of bioflavonoids, and other good sources are apricots, cherries, grapes, green peppers, tomatoes, papayas, broccoli, and cantaloupes.[233]

SUPPLEMENTS   Bioflavonoids are usually added to vitamin C supplements to approximate the form of vitamin C obtained in nature. Supplements of bioflavonoids usually range in potencies from 100 to 1,000 mg. When taken for therapeutic purposes, these supplements should be taken three times a day.

I recommend between 250 and 1,000 mg. be taken daily along with your vitamin C.

Since the U.S. federal government has yet to establish any regulations for bioflavonoids, a 100 mg. tablet may contain 1 percent or 50 percent bioflavonoids. Most formulas contain 15 to 25 percent, and most companies will include the lower percentage to save money. The milligram count doesn't tell you a whole lot; it's the percentage that counts.

I recommend that your bioflavonoid supplement be at least a 25-percent concentration. Since this information does not usually appear on the label, we recommend you buy supplements from a highly reputable firm that emphasizes quality.

MINERALS AND TRACE ELEMENTS

Calcium

FACTS   "About 99 percent of your calcium is found in your bones and teeth."[1] The other 1 percent is found in your blood, tissues, and body fluids. There is more calcium than any other mineral in your body. The average adult body contains about two and one-half pounds of calcium.[2] In a child, the skeleton undergoes a complete renewal almost every year. In an adult, renewal takes place about once a decade.[3]

About three-fourths of all calcium eaten in the diet fails to be absorbed. The excess is excreted in the feces and urine.[4] Calcium needs vitamin D, phosphorus, magnesium, vitamin A, and vitamin C in order to perform properly in the body.[5] Calcium and phosphorus intake in the diet should be about equal (a 1:1 ratio). Then, in the blood, the calcium-phosphorus levels will balance at the proper ratio of 2.5:1, which is needed to build healthy bones. It is interesting to note that mother's milk contains the same calcium-phosphorus ratio—2.5:1—as that found in the blood.

Bed rest causes a loss of calcium from the bones and blood. No matter how hard you exercise while lying on your back, your calcium balance will not return to normal until you are able to stand up quietly for a few hours a day. This restoration of calcium balance is due to the action of gravity. Astronauts had difficulty with their calcium balance, and the danger of calcium loss is also one of the many reasons why doctors encourage their patients to get up out of bed as soon as possible after an operation.

DEFICIENCY SYMPTOMS   Symptoms of calcium deficiency include nervous spasms, facial twitching, weak-feeling muscles, cramps, and other muscle-nerve effects.[6]

A lack of calcium slows the growth in children and can result in an extreme case of rickets. A deficiency may lead to osteoporosis (porous and brittle bones) and osteomalacia (a type of bone-softening disease). Both conditions leave people susceptible to bone fractures. Unfortunately, bone demineralizing diseases cannot be detected by X rays until 30 percent or more of the bone mineral has already been lost.[7]

"Heart palpitations and slow pulse rate are also traced to low calcium intake."[8] Calcium deficiency can cause height reduction when unnoticed fractures of the vertebrae are sustained under pressure.[9] Low levels of calcium in the diet can cause high blood and tissue levels of two poisonous metals, lead and cadmium.[10]

WHAT IT DOES   The 1 percent of calcium in our blood has certain functions. It is needed for blood to clot, it activates enzymes (digestive juices), it helps transport impulses of nerves from one part of the body to another, and it helps control the passage of fluids through the cell walls.[11]

Calcium also helps to maintain the delicate acid-alkaline balance of the body.[12] It "works to normalize the contraction and relaxation of the heart muscles"[13] and is necessary for strong bones and teeth.

WHAT IT MAY DO   Along with vitamin D and regular physical exercise, calcium plays a role in the treatment of rickets, osteoporosis and osteomalacia. "Current estimates are that more than 14,000,000 women are visibly affected by osteoporosis in the United States."[14]

Calcium also plays a role in periodontal disease, reducing or eliminating such symptoms as bleeding gums, gingivitis, and loose teeth.[15] Calcium has been found to help lower blood cholesterol and triglycerides.[16] Calcium and the B vitamin, pantothenic acid, can reduce bruxism (tooth-grinding).[17] Calcium may help you sleep better at night. It also may help with backaches, menstrual cramps, and the "growing pains" that teenagers suffer.

Vitamin A and calcium have been used to give protection against the damaging effects of the sun, including redness and peeling.[18]

TOXICITY   Very rarely ever seen. Doses over 2,000 mg. could lead to hypercalcemia (elevated blood calcium level that can lead to calcification of the soft tissue).

BEST SOURCES   Milk is considered the best source of calcium; one cup contains approximately 300 mg. of calcium.

Other sources include egg yolks, fish (eaten with the bones), soybeans, green leafy vegetables (such as turnip greens, mustard greens, broccoli, and kale), roots, tubers, and seeds, as well as soups and stews made from bones.[19] Molasses, almonds, figs, and beans are also good sources.[20]

SUPPLEMENTS   Calcium supplements commonly taken are calcium carbonate, calcium gluconate, calcium lactate, and bone meal. In my opinion, calcium gluconate powder is the easiest supplement form to take, since it is virtually tasteless when mixed with milk. Dolomite is another good source because it combines magnesium with calcium naturally. The most expensive supplement form is chelated calcium, which is readily absorbed by the body.

I recommend 400 to 800 mg. of calcium to be taken daily in a supplement with 200 to 400 mg. of magnesium. (You need to take twice as much calcium as magnesium.) The rest of the calcium your body needs should come from milk and other food sources. Growing boys and girls, pregnant and lactating women, and the elderly need slightly more calcium. The RDA for calcium is 800 to 1200 mg. for any person over the age of one.

COMMENTS   The most common reason for improper utilization of calcium is the presence of too much phosphorus. When there is too much phosphorus in the diet, the phosphorus pulls calcium out of the bones and lowers the calcium level of the blood by flushing it out of the body. The ratio of calcium to phosphorus in the diet should be at least 1:1, or slightly more calcium than phosphorus.

Unfortunately, the American diet has an average ratio more

like 1:2.8 (calcium:phosphorus), which means we are eating almost three times more phosphorus than calcium.[21]

The high phosphorus content of bran, the extremely high phosphorus content of soft drinks, and the fact that meat contains about twenty times more phosphorus than calcium all contribute to the calcium-phosphorus imbalance of the American diet.

Chloride

Chloride is found in large amounts in the body. It stimulates the production of hydrochloric acid needed for digestion. Most people get plenty of chloride in their diets, especially from salt (sodium chloride) or from a salt substitute (potassium chloride).

Chromium

FACTS As a trace element, chromium appears in very minute quantities throughout the body. Studies have shown that "a sizeable portion of the American subjects sampled had a low or negligible quantity of chromium in their tissues, compared to foreigners."[22] Most crop soil is very depleted of chromium and other trace minerals.

DEFICIENCY SYMPTOMS Heavy sugar intake can lower the body's chromium supply because chromium, as well as insulin, is released in the body to reduce high blood-sugar levels. Dr. Henry Schroeder, who has conducted extensive research on chromium, feels that most Americans are chromium-deficient, mainly because chromium is removed from foods during refining.[23]

"Very severe deficiencies will hinder growth, shorten the life span, raise cholesterol levels and produce a whole array of symptoms related to hypo- and hyper-glycemia" (low and high blood sugar).[24]

WHAT IT DOES Chromium "plays an important role in the synthesis of fatty acids and cholesterol in the liver."[25] It has been found that, in animals, chromium is related to optimal glucose (blood sugar) utilization.[26] Chromium works with insulin and makes the release of insulin more effective.[27]

WHAT IT MAY DO In laboratory animals, it was found that chromium may play a role in establishing proper cholesterol levels. Chromium may also inhibit the depositing of cholesterol plaques.[28] In animals, chromium may prevent a form of blindness.[29]

By administering regulated amounts of chromium, scientists

have been able to restore proper blood-sugar regulation and thereby prevent diabetes.[30] In male laboratory animals, chromium has been found to be essential to growth and longevity.[31] The body's chromium levels are more reliable than cholesterol, triglycerides, and blood pressure as a predictor of atherosclerosis.[32]

TOXICITY   Chromium is non-toxic in its trivalent form or GTF (glucose tolerance factor) form.[33] The body can easily eliminate any excess chromium.[34]

BEST SOURCES   Brewer's yeast (by far, the best source), sugar beets, molasses, black pepper, liver, beef, whole wheat bread, beets, and mushrooms.

SUPPLEMENTS   At this time, there is no definitive measurement of the amount of active chromium in most foods. Therefore, it is difficult to say how much chromium an average diet contains and how much chromium the body requires.[35]

Good supplements are available in the form of GTF (glucose tolerance factor) chromium from brewer's yeast. Chelated chromium is found in some vitamin-mineral supplements. The National Research Assembly of Life Science in Washington, D.C., says the safe and adequate amounts of intake of chromium range from 50 to 200 mcg. If you feel you may be lacking in chromium or if you do not eat many foods containing it, I recommend you take from between 25 and 100 mcg. daily.

Cobalt

Cobalt is a part of the vitamin B-12 molecule. This trace element is essential for life. However, we don't need to worry about getting enough cobalt since very little is needed and we get plenty from animal sources. A cobalt insufficiency has never been observed in humans.

Copper

FACTS   The adult body contains between 75 and 150 mg. of copper. About 50 percent of that copper is found in the muscles and bones.[36] Copper is a trace mineral. It is absolutely essential in small amounts, but can be poisonous in large amounts.

DEFICIENCY SYMPTOMS   A copper deficiency may lead to loss of hair. Loss of taste has also been linked to copper and zinc deficiencies. Other symptoms of copper deficiency may include general weakness, impaired respiration,[37] brittleness of bones, chronic or recurrent diarrhea, hair depigmentation, and a low white blood cell count, which leads to reduced resistance to infection.[38] "The more severe symptoms include retarded growth, anemia, edema (retention of water), and nervous irritability."[39]

WHAT IT DOES   Copper must be present with iron and protein to make hemoglobin, the oxygen-carrying pigment of blood.[40] "It is also necessary for the efficient absorption of iron from food."[41] Copper is also involved in the process that forms melanin, a dark pigment that colors the hair and skin.[42] However, this does not mean that taking extra copper will keep your hair from turning gray.

Copper is needed by enzymes for the formation of connective tissues, such as collagen and elastin.[43] A copper-containing enzyme helps to detoxify the body by protecting it against damaging oxidizing agents.[44] "The myelin sheath which covers nerve fibers also depends on copper as a structural element."[45]

WHAT IT MAY DO   Copper may play a role in preventing a heart attack from a ruptured aorta due to its importance "to the tensile strength of the coronary blood vessels."[46]

TOXICITY   Potentially toxic. "Excess copper may compete with other minerals such as zinc, manganese, and magnesium, and cause insomnia, elevated blood pressure, and restlessness."[47] Never use pots or pans, tea kettles, or kitchen utensils made of copper. Use stainless steel, glass, porcelain, or cast iron instead. Most water heaters are lined with copper and the hot water tends to dissolve the copper. For this reason, you should use only cold water for drinking and cooking.[48]

BEST SOURCES   The richest sources of copper are nuts, organ meats, seafood, mushrooms, and legumes.[49]

SUPPLEMENTS   It is estimated that an adult needs about 2 to 3 mg. of copper each day. Some of this copper comes directly from food, while additional amounts come from the copper that is used in the storage and processing of food. Copper pipes in your home are a source of copper. Soft water will leach more copper out of copper pipes than will hard water.

Copper is usually found in vitamin-mineral supplements in potencies of .5 to 5 mg. Except in infants, very few cases of copper deficiency have been observed. I recommend no more than .5 to 1 mg. a day in a supplement. This will provide the necessary minimum amount, guarantee that all the required vitamins and minerals are present at the same time, and enhance the absorption of iron in the body. Copper gluconate and chelated copper are the two most popular forms of copper.

Along with copper in a supplement, you must have zinc. To prevent an accumulation of copper in the body, one may need about fourteen times more zinc than copper.[50] That is why I recommend about 1 mg. of copper to 30 mg. of zinc in a supplement. This does not represent the 14:1 ratio (zinc:copper), but you will get the extra milligram or so of copper in your diet, since copper is found in most every food. Zinc, on the other hand, is very hard to obtain from the food you eat.

Fluoride

This trace element is usually found in nature in the solid form of calcium fluoride. In the ocean, it is found in the form of sodium fluoride. Some studies have shown fluoride necessary for the formation of strong, hard bones and teeth. Controversy surrounds the issue of whether or not we should continue to add this mineral to our drinking water. I am not in favor of the fluoridation of our water system. There are no known fluoride deficiency symptoms.

Iodine

FACTS Iodine is a trace element. The adult body contains about 20 to 50 mg., 8 mg. of which are contained in the thyroid gland.[51]

DEFICIENCY SYMPTOMS An iodine deficiency in certain susceptible people may result in goiter. This condition is characterized by an enlarged thyroid gland, which may visibly thicken the neck and, in extreme cases, restrict breathing and cause bulging of the eyes.[52] As the iodine deficient thyroid gland slows down (hypothyroidism), the following symptoms or effects may occur: physical and mental sluggishness, poor circulation and low vitality, dry hair and skin, cold hands and feet, a tendency to wear excessively heavy clothing, and obesity (the individual gains weight too easily).[53]

"An iodine deficiency may also result in cretinism, which is a congenital disease characterized by physical and mental retardation in children born to mothers who have had a limited iodine intake during adolescence and pregnancy."[54]

WHAT IT DOES   Iodine stimulates the thyroid gland to secrete the hormone thyroxine, which regulates metabolism (the rate at which you burn your food) and energy level.[55] Iodine is "indirectly but closely connected with more than a hundred enzyme systems controlled by the thyroid hormones including energy production, growth, reproduction, nerve function in the muscles, skin and hair growth."[56] "Iodine acts as a catalyst to stimulate conversion of body fat to energy."[57]

WHAT IT MAY DO   Iodine is used in the prevention and treatment of simple goiter. Administering thyroid hormone is the most effective way to obtain regression of a nontoxic goiter.[58] A properly functioning thyroid gland (which is dependent on iodine) is very important in preventing and delaying artery hardening.[59]

Iodine can regulate the basal metabolic rate. In pregnant women, the basal metabolic rate has been found to be higher than average. "Giving iodine to pregnant women kept the metabolic rate within normal bounds. If it was high, the iodine lowered it; if it was low, the iodine raised it."[60]

TOXICITY   No known toxicity from nutritional amounts.

BEST SOURCES   Seaweed, especially kelp, is probably the best source of iodine. Seafood, iodized salt, and sea salt are other good sources. Most other foods are unreliable sources, since the iodine content depends on the soil of the area in which the food was produced.

SUPPLEMENTS   Kelp granules, used in the place of salt, are probably the best way to supplement your diet. A good multivitamin-mineral supplement should contain between 50 and 150 mcg. of iodine. To treat a diagnosed deficiency as severe as goiter, one should take the natural whole thyroid hormone in tablet form. It is available by prescription only. Don't take the synthetic forms of thyroid, such as "Synthroid" or "Cytamel."

COMMENTS   Mother grew up in a small town in Idaho where there was no iodine in the soil. They ate fish, but the fish came from a fresh-water lake and contained no iodine. This was before they even had iodized salt. Mother's two sisters and her mother had goiters as a result of their iodine deficiency. The oldest sister had two daughters who also developed goiter. And they grew to be over six feet tall. Excessive height is fairly common in iodine-deficient people because the underactive thyroid gland is slow to close the ends of the long bones such as those in the legs.

Iron

FACTS Found in red blood cells. "An adult's body contains from 3 to 5 grams of iron."[61] Less than 10 percent of the iron found in vegetables and only about 20 percent of animal protein iron can be absorbed.

To function properly, iron needs many, many nutrients. Nineteen different amino acids are also needed to make hemoglobin (oxygen carrying pigment of the red blood cells), which shows the importance of complete proteins to the diet.[62] New red blood cells are made every day, and they last 120 days before they die.[63]

DEFICIENCY SYMPTOMS Anemia is usually the result of an iron deficiency. "The general symptoms are pallor, weakness, easy fatigability, labored breathing on exertion, headache, palpitation, and persistent tiredness."[64] "Preschool children have been found to suffer diminished coordination, balance, attention span, intelligence quotient, and memory when anemic."[65] Anemia in older children has caused poor learning, reading, and problem solving skills.[66]

The body's immune system may be depressed in an iron-deficiency anemia.[67] In the absence of iron, the body cannot produce white blood cells to fight off infection.[68]

Anemia is not always a result of just an iron deficiency but may be attributable to subtle deficiencies, existing simultaneously, of vitamins B-1, B-2, B-6, and B-12, C, E, niacin, pantothenic acid, folic acid, choline, copper, magnesium and other nutrients.[69]

An iron deficiency may be revealed by the appearance of the fingernails. The normal red flare that spreads out from the halfmoons of the nails may be absent,[70] and the fingernails and toenails may be concave or have a spoonlike shape. "Skin lesions such as pimples, boils and the like are far more likely to occur in individuals lacking body iron."[71]

WHAT IT DOES Iron is needed to form the red-colored substance in red blood cells called hemoglobin. This hemoglobin carries oxygen from the lungs to the individual cells and carbon dioxide from the cells to the lungs. "Iron is found in the enzyme system that works to produce energy and it appears in the mus-

cles as a part of the protein that absorbs and reserves oxygen."[72]
Some iron is found in the bone marrow, and it is used to make
more hemoglobin and form more enzymes.

WHAT IT MAY DO   From animal experiments, researchers have
concluded that "lead absorption and toxicity can be diminished
or prevented by iron in the diet."[73]

TOXICITY   Since the body usually excretes any excess iron, it is
normally very hard to produce iron toxicity from the diet or from
supplements. When the body's vitamin B-6 supply is inadequate,
excessive iron can be absorbed and can cause tissue damage.[74]
Toxicity symptoms of an iron overload, which occurs mostly in
men over 40, may include headache, shortness of breath, fatigue,
dizziness, and loss of weight. The skin may even take on a gray
hue because iron is being deposited in the tissues.[75]

BEST SOURCES   "Liver, heart, kidney, lean meats, shellfish,
dried beans and fruits, nuts, green leafy vegetables, whole grains
and blackstrap molasses."[76]

SUPPLEMENTS   Rumor has it that iron destroys vitamin E.
This is true—*if* the iron is taken in the "ferric" form. However,
most good vitamin-mineral supplements found in health food
stores use iron in the "ferrous" form. The ferrous form does not
destroy vitamin E. Chelated iron is the most preferred form because the body can more readily absorb it. Ferrous *sulfate* is a
form of iron you should stay away from. Check your label. Many
drugstores carry this form. I recommend iron in the form of ferrous *gluconate,* ferrous *fumarate,* ferrous *citrate,* or ferrous *peptonate.*

A man loses about 1 mg. a day of iron through sweat, hair, lost
skin, bleeding, and excretion. A woman loses from 1 to 2 mg. a
day. Women lose more iron through menstruation, in which
some 13.5 mg. are lost with the blood. Remember, for every milligram of iron you lose, you need to take at least 10 mg. to make
up the loss. This is because the body can absorb only about 10
percent of the iron it ingests. "The average American diet provides 6 milligrams of iron per 1,000 calories."[77] A man needs at
least 10 mg. of iron daily, while a woman needs at least 18 mg.
daily. A woman's need for iron increases especially during pregnancy.

You lose about 250 mg. of iron every time you donate 500

milliliters of blood.[78] Taking the 10 percent absorption factor into consideration, you would need to ingest an extra 13.5 to 14 mg. of iron a day for six months to make up for this loss.

The American Medical Association (AMA) conducted a study and "found scant to absent iron stores in 66 of 114 menstruating women."[79] The AMA stated that required amounts for iron are beyond what is available in the diet. According to the AMA, infants from three months to twenty-four months of age especially need iron, since they grow faster at that time than they ever will again. Adolescent girls, too, need iron because the onset of the menstrual cycle can quickly use up the body's store of this mineral.[80] During the last half of pregnancy, and especially during lactation, women vitally need iron.

Since anemia can result from a lack of so many other nutrients besides iron, I always recommend you take a good vitamin-mineral supplement rather than iron alone. Remember, they all work together.

Magnesium

FACTS All human cells contain magnesium, totaling about 25,000 mg. in an adult.[81] About 60 to 70 percent of the body's magnesium is found in the bones.[82] "The rest is located in the soft tissues and blood."[83] To balance this mineral, you should take twice as much calcium as magnesium. Alcohol causes a very high urinary loss of magnesium.[84] The more protein you eat, the more magnesium you need.

DEFICIENCY SYMPTOMS Symptoms of magnesium deficiency were not identified until recently because they overlap heavily with the symptoms of calcium and potassium deficiency. The first symptoms of a magnesium deficiency are usually apathy, depression, apprehensiveness, confusion, disorientation, vertigo (a condition in which the room seems to spin around), muscular weakness and twitching, and over-excitability of the nervous system, which may lead to muscle spasms or cramps. Other possible symptoms of magnesium deficiency may include insomnia, jumpiness, sensitivity to noise,[85] irritability, and a poor memory.[86] More serious deficiencies result in tremors or convulsions.[87]

WHAT IT DOES Magnesium plays a role in the "storage of sugar as glycogen in the liver and in its release into the blood for energy."[88] Magnesium is necessary for the contraction of the muscles and is considered a key element in the regulation of the heartbeat.[89] As a nerve soother, magnesium is necessary for the sending of nerve impulses, for normal brain function, and for sleeping.[90] The body requires magnesium to manufacture protein, fat, and other essentials for the normal structure of cells and growing tissues.[91]

Magnesium participates with calcium and phosphorus in the formation of bones in children.[92] "Magnesium acts as starter or catalyzer for some of the chemical reactions within the body."[93] "The structure of RNA (ribonucleic acid), the genetic substance that synthesizes protein, is built upon magnesium. RNA is believed to control thought and memory and the structure of all organs."[94] Magnesium phosphates regulate the acid-alkaline (pH) balance in the blood and other fluids.

WHAT IT MAY DO   In alcoholics, magnesium therapy often helps to control delirium tremens ("the uncontrollable hallucinations and shaking that develop after long-term excessive drinking").[95] Magnesium protects against the accumulation of calcium deposits in the urinary tract. Such deposits may otherwise lead to bladder or kidney stones.[96] Magnesium seems to be important in "controlling the manner in which electrical charges are utilized to induce the passage of minerals in and out of cells."[97] It may be associated with the regulation of body temperature.[98]

Magnesium has been used to relax the muscles surrounding the walls of the arteries. This has decreased hypertension or lowered blood pressure.[99] Menstrual cramps may be alleviated by increasing magnesium in the diet.[100]

Magnesium operates through the pituitary gland, which regulates all other glands. A magnesium deficiency may occur due to a pituitary malfunction. One doctor believes a pituitary malfunction is a prime cause of epilepsy.[101]

Magnesium is used as a preventative treatment for high altitude sickness. The magnesium helps to keep the blood vessels of the lungs from constricting and from limiting the "amount of blood and in effect the amount of oxygen that can be pumped through the lungs."[102] "It is magnesium, not calcium, that forms the kind of hard [tooth] enamel that resists decay."[103]

Magnesium may play a role in the prevention and treatment of osteoporosis (wherein bones demineralize and become porous and brittle). The following list offers the approximate percentages of magnesium that Dr. Lewis E. Barnet found in various bone materials. These percentages reveal the vital role magnesium plays in bone hardness.

Bones of patients with osteoporosis	.62 percent
Bones of healthy people	1.26 percent
Teeth of healthy people	1.5 percent
Elephant tusks (from which almost indestructible billiard balls are made)	2.0 percent
Teeth of carnivorous animals (which crush and grind the bones of their prey)	5.0 percent[104]

Magnesium may also contain body-deodorizing properties.[105] A magnesium-deficient diet has induced tumors in rats (which very rarely develop cancer spontaneously). Magnesium deficiency could be one of the many causes of cancer.[106]

TOXICITY Magnesium is basically nontoxic, unless a doctor administers large doses directly into the bloodstream. Excess magnesium has a laxative effect. The intestines regulate magnesium absorption. If blood levels of magnesium are already high, then the intestines will allow less of this mineral to pass into the blood stream. More magnesium is absorbed through the intestines when blood levels are low.

BEST SOURCES Magnesium is present in the chlorophyll of all plants. Other sources of magnesium include figs, lemons, grapefruit, green leafy vegetables, alfalfa, yellow corn, soya flour, whole wheat, peas, beans, brown rice, almonds, oil-rich nuts and seeds, and apples.[107]

SUPPLEMENTS Dolomite is a good, balanced source of magnesium. It contains twice as much calcium as magnesium. I recommend between 200 and 400 mg. of magnesium taken daily in supplement form. This regimen provides a strong base for your body's requirements of magnesium, and the rest will come from your diet. Be sure to take twice as much calcium as magnesium. The chelated form of magnesium is used for better absorption. This mineral is most commonly taken in the form of magnesium oxide. The U.S. RDA for magnesium is 400 mg.

COMMENTS Cortisone, diuretics, alcohol, X rays, and sugar deplete the body's supply of magnesium. Synthetic vitamin D (D-2), found in pasteurized milk, binds with magnesium to render it useless. For this reason, doctors usually eliminate milk from the diets of magnesium-deficient children. I recommend you switch to certified raw milk, if possible, and avoid the synthetic vitamin D. The antibiotic tetracycline prescribed by doctors to young people for the treatment of acne also interferes with magnesium metabolism.[108]

Manganese

FACTS   Manganese is a trace mineral. The adult human body contains a total of about 20 mg. of manganese.[109]

DEFICIENCY SYMPTOMS   The only known case of a human manganese deficiency was discovered by accident. This individual "experienced weight loss, dermatitis, nausea, slow growth of hair and beard with color changes, and uncommonly low blood levels of cholesterol."[110] In mammals, a manganese deficiency is characterized by poor growth, defects in bone formation and in the central nervous system, reproductive dysfunction, and disturbances in fat metabolism and glucose tolerance.[111]

A deficiency is also suspected in diabetes, since diabetic patients studied had only half the amount of manganese of normal control subjects.[112] A manganese deficiency during pregnancy may be a factor in epilepsy in the offspring.[113] A severe deficiency may result in myasthenia gravis, characterized by severe loss of muscle strength.

WHAT IT DOES   Manganese is required for many vital enzyme reactions, such as those involved in the utilization of vitamin C, choline, biotin, and thiamine (B-1).[114] Manganese is essential for the normal functioning of the pancreas and for carbohydrate metabolism. The body needs it to make collagen (connective tissue-gristle). Manganese, along with iodine, plays an important part in the formation of thyroxin, one of the hormones secreted by the thyroid gland.[115] Manganese is very important for the proper functioning of the thymus gland, much as iodine is for the thyroid gland.[116]

WHAT IT MAY DO   Manganese may play a role in the metabolism of fatty acids, cholesterol synthesis, and protein synthesis.[117] Superoxide dismutate (S.O.D.) is a manganese enzyme that protects cell membranes from free-radical damage. Vitamin E and manganese (30 mg.) taken daily have been successfully used to treat myasthenia gravis, a disease characterized by severe loss of muscle strength.[118] "The high copper level of many schizophrenics can be reduced by dietary intake of zinc and manganese" (in a ratio of 20:1), since these two minerals increase urinary copper excretion.[119]

TOXICITY   Toxicity is rare, but has been reported in miners who breathe high levels of manganese dust for prolonged periods.[120]

BEST SOURCES   Whole grains, wheat germ, bran, peas, teas, nuts, green leafy vegetables, beets, egg yolks, bananas, and liver.[121]

SUPPLEMENTS   The average daily intake of manganese has been estimated to be between 3 and 9 mg. Only about 40 percent of that amount is absorbed.[122] I recommend that 5 to 10 mg. be taken daily in a vitamin-mineral supplement. This will assure that there is sufficient manganese available in your body for certain enzyme reactions to take place. Manganese gluconate is a very good form of manganese found in many vitamin-mineral preparations. Chelated manganese, although more expensive, can improve absorption. Manganese is also recommended because of its synergistic relationship with chromium, zinc, and other nutrients.

COMMENTS   "In a study comparing trace mineral levels in the diet with death rates from cardiovascular disease, manganese was one of the minerals (along with chromium and selenium) that were found to be high in areas where heart disease deaths were low, and low where heart-disease deaths were high."[123]

Molybdenum

Molybdenum is essential to man and is found in all our tissues. Three important enzymes require molybdenum. Deficiency symptoms have been recognized in animals, but not in human beings. This mineral may play a role in preventing tooth decay. You should be getting plenty of this mineral in your diet. Particularly rich sources of molybdenum are whole grains and wheat germ.

Phosphorus

FACTS   The adult body contains about 1.5–2 lbs. of this mineral.[124] It is found in every body cell. In bone, it is found in a balance with calcium of 2.5 parts calcium to 1 part phosphorus. About 70 percent of phosphorus in the diet is absorbed.[125]

DEFICIENCY SYMPTOMS The typical diet usually makes a phosphorus deficiency very rare in the United States. "The clinical symptoms of a phosphorus deficiency are muscle weakness (to the point of respiratory arrest), anemia and increased susceptibility to infection."[126] Low potassium and magnesium have been associated with a phosphorus deficiency.[127] An upset in the calcium-phosphorus ratio of the body may lead to arthritis, pyorrhea, and tooth decay.[128] "A lack of phosphorus, calcium, or vitamin D can bring about rickets."[129]

WHAT IT DOES Phosphorus is deposited along with calcium to form strong bones and teeth. It combines with fat and protein so that they can be digested and absorbed by the body. Phosphorus is needed for the successful utilization of carbohydrates. It is necessary for the digestion of two B vitamins—niacin and riboflavin. It "stimulates muscular contraction, secretion of glandular hormones, nerve impulses, and kidney functioning."[130] Phosphorus helps maintain the acid-alkaline balance of the blood.[131] It is an essential component of nucleoproteins (RNA and DNA).[132]

TOXICITY No known toxicity. The problem with phosphorus is not quantity, but proportion. For any amount of phosphorus, you need at least the same amount of calcium in the diet.

BEST SOURCES Natural sources usually include high-protein foods such as meat, fish, poultry, eggs, milk, cheese, nuts, and legumes.[133] Many processed foods contain phosphate or phosphoric acid (found in soft drinks) or they contain polyphosphates or emulsifying salts. These processed foods adversely affect the body's calcium-phosphorus balance.

SUPPLEMENTS I do not recommend taking phosphorus in any supplemental form. Your body needs between 800 and 1,200 mg. a day, and you get plenty from your diet.[134]

Potassium

FACTS In a 143-pound person there are about 8.5 gallons of water (weighing 87.5 pounds), with five-eighths of this water located inside the cells and the rest outside the cells.[135] "Potassium is the main element in the water inside the cells, and sodium in the water outside the cells."[136] These two elements are constantly at work in a fluid-balancing act. Most of the body's potassium is found in the water in the muscles. A 154-pound person contains about 9 ounces (300 grams).[137]

DEFICIENCY SYMPTOMS   Most potassium deficiencies are caused by a high sodium chloride (table salt) intake, which causes you to lose potassium in the urine. Deficiency can also result from eating too few fruits and vegetables or too much refined sugar, drinking alcohol or coffee, taking cortisone, prolonged diarrhea, excessive sweating, and the use of diuretics.[138]

Early symptoms of a potassium deficiency are general weakness of muscles and mental confusion. Other symptoms include muscle cramping, poor reflexes, nervous system disruption, soft flabby muscles, and constipation. Muscle tissue can be destroyed if a potassium deficiency continues. In young people, a deficiency may result in acne, while in adults it can cause dry skin.[139] A "severe deficiency leads to failure of heart function—resulting in a heart attack."[140] A deficiency can be detected by an ECG or a direct blood test.

WHAT IT DOES   Potassium does everything in a balancing act with sodium (salt). It's hard to separate the two. Sodium and potassium are necessary to maintain the normal water balance between the insides of the cells (potassium) and the surrounding fluids (sodium). When your body contains too much sodium, you retain water and lose potassium. When there is too much potassium, both sodium and water are lost. The sodium-potassium balance is necessary to preserve the acid-alkali balance of the body.[141] Sodium and potassium, in correct proportion, are needed by the muscles so that they can contract when the nerves have been stimulated.[142] This is especially important to athletes for proper muscle and heart function.

"The red blood cells need potassium to effectively carry carbon dioxide through the blood to the lungs, where it is expelled in exchange for oxygen."[143] Potassium rids the body of poisonous waste materials by stimulating the excretion of water by the kidneys.[144] At least eight enzymes need potassium for normal chemical reactions to take place, particularly the metabolism of carbohydrates.[145] "Potassium is necessary for the proper working of the digestive tract."[146] Potassium is needed for the body to use protein properly. If the body is deficient in potassium, nitrogen is lost and protein will not be assimilated. Potassium assists in converting glucose (blood sugar) to glycogen (the form of sugar that can be stored in the liver). The energy your muscles use comes from glycogen.

WHAT IT MAY DO   Potassium has been used to treat high blood pressure due to an excessive salt intake.[147] Giving potassium to mildly diabetic patients causes the blood pressure and blood sugar to fall.[148] More severe diabetics are found to have high requirements of protein, the B vitamins (pantothenic acid, riboflavin, and niacin), vitamin C, and lecithin.[149] Colic in infants quickly disappeared when they were given injections of 1,000 mg. of potassium chloride. The B vitamin pantothenic acid would probably have worked just as well.[150]

Potassium, along with magnesium, is vital in preventing heart attacks, since a lack of this nutrient may allow clots to form in the heart and brain.[151] Potassium has been used effectively in treating allergies.[152] Potassium chloride prevents blackouts in patients with hypoglycemia (low blood sugar).[153]

TOXICITY   Excess potassium can be toxic. Toxicity may occur by taking 25,000 mg. of potassium chloride per day.[154] Slightly smaller doses could cause diarrhea.[155]

BEST SOURCES   The best sources of potassium usually are bananas, apricots, lettuce, broccoli, potatoes, fresh fruit and fruit juices, sunflower seeds, peanuts (unsalted), nuts, squash, wheat germ, brewer's yeast, desiccated liver, fish, bone meal, watercress, blackstrap molasses, and unsulphured figs found in health food stores. During processing, potassium is actually removed from many foods and sodium (salt) is added. So stay away from processed food. Remember, salt is the enemy of potassium.

SUPPLEMENTS   The average American diet contains between 1.5 and 6.5 grams of potassium a day. You need nearly equal amounts of sodium and potassium each day—say, about 2,600 mg. of each.[156]

"Potassium tablets that are enteric coated to bypass the stomach and liberate the potassium in the intestine may stay in one place too long and produce an ulcer of the intestine which perforates."[157] Encapsulated potassium salts may cause severe stomach pain. To minimize these side effects, most potassium supplements are given in the form of effervescent tablets or powder to be absorbed in the mouth or mixed with water.

Most vitamin-mineral preparations contain a small amount of potassium (5 to 99 mg.) to ensure that nothing will be lacking and that all necessary chemical processes will take place between the different vitamins and minerals. Athletes may need more potassium (3,000 to 6,000 mg. per day) because they sweat profusely. This additional potassium will protect against the destruction of muscle tissue.[158]

The best way to get potassium is from fresh fruits and vegetables that contain this mineral. Another popular and inexpensive way to obtain potassium is to mix equal parts of salt substitute (potassium chloride) and sea salt in your salt shaker. This way you get a timed-release effect and provide your body with a balance of sodium and potassium. Some of the world's communities salt their food entirely with potassium chloride and limit their salt intake to that found naturally in foods. Unfortunately, to the American palate, such salt substitutes do not taste good.

Selenium

FACTS   A trace element needed only in small amounts. People who do not get enough selenium are likely to be those on low-protein diets (since selenium is associated with protein foods) and those eating foods grown in a low soil-selenium area.[159] The acid rains that fall in the eastern United States, which are caused by coal-burning plants, and which have already killed fish in hundreds of lakes, may greatly inhibit the uptake of selenium by plants.[160]

DEFICIENCY SYMPTOMS   The only symptom that has been tied absolutely to a selenium deficiency is dandruff.[161] "Of the thirty-five thousand infant deaths per year in the United States, about one quarter are associated with selenium and/or vitamin E deficiency. Almost none of these babies are breast fed, and it is significant that human milk contains up to six times as much selenium as cow's milk and twice as much vitamin E."[162] "Selenium deficiency also enhances the damaging effects of ozone on the lungs."[163]

"FDA estimated that about 70 percent of the domestic corn and soybeans do not contain adequate selenium. Such a deficiency can lead to decreased growth, disease, and death of animals feeding on such crops."[164] Additionally, selenium-deficient animals are usually infertile.[165]

WHAT IT DOES   "Selenium is necessary for protein synthesis."[166] "It increases the effectiveness of vitamin E."[167] Selenium is part of the first line of defense at the cell membrane, where it is a constituent of an antioxidant enzyme.[168] Like vitamin E, selenium protects the cells against the damaging effects of oxygen exposure.

Selenium is necessary for sexual reproduction. A normal sperm cell contains high levels of selenium, as do the male and female sex organs.

WHAT IT MAY DO   Selenium protects you against the toxic effects of such pollutants as cadmium, mercury in tuna, and possibly even lead.[169]

Although the data are not considered conclusive, selenium may reduce the chances of all types of cancer.[170] "Studies have shown that in communities where selenium intake is low, the cancer rate is high."[171] Selenium added to the drinking water of mice reduced from 82 percent to 10 percent the incidence of spontaneous breast cancer in susceptible females.[172]

Selenium may be very helpful in building a healthy heart. In response to the heart destruction in livestock brought on by selenium-deficient poultry and swine feeds, both Canada and the United States have approved the addition of selenium to animal feed.[173]

One form of heart disease, which strikes children and women of childbearing age living in a low selenium-soil belt in China, has responded tremendously to selenium supplementation. The Chinese, in fact, are seriously considering the addition of selenium to table salt (just as we have added iodine to salt to prevent goiter).[174] Heart disease rates have been shown to be higher in low-selenium intake areas.[175]

Selenium has been shown to increase animal life spans and reduce the free-radical damage that can accelerate aging. Although selenium will not stop you from aging, it will allow you to age at your basic genetic rate.[176]

Selenium has been added to shampoos to treat seborrheic dermatitis, or dandruff.[177]

TOXICITY   Selenium is vital in small amounts, but toxic in larger amounts. "Several adults have taken up to 1000 micrograms (daily) in the organic form for several months and had no ill effects."[178] One of the first signs of excessive selenium is garlicky breath.[179] Toxic symptoms "include loss of hair, nails, and teeth; dermatitis; lassitude, and progressive paralysis."[180]

Although selenium toxicity appears in animals fed on selenium-rich soil in South Dakota and Nebraska, there seems to be very little demonstrable evidence of selenium toxicity in man.[181]

For fifteen years, men were observed in the selenium-exposed environments of the electronics, glass, and paint industries. These men were not statistically affected.[182] The Food and Nutrition Board of the National Research Council has stated that "chronic selenium toxicity would be expected in human beings after long-term consumption of 2,400 to 3,000 micrograms daily."[183]

BEST SOURCES Organ meats, tuna, and other seafood; brewer's yeast, fresh garlic, mushrooms, and whole grains (if grown in selenium-rich soil).

SUPPLEMENTS In 1976, the Food and Nutrition Board of the National Research Council said that "a well balanced diet furnishes about 60 to 120 micrograms of selenium daily."[184] But few people eat a well-balanced diet, and even those who do may not get enough selenium. An FDA survey found that in five samples of a well-balanced diet for nineteen-year-old boys there was no selenium.[185]

In 1980, the National Academy of Sciences offered a range rather than a specific number for the RDA of selenium. The range of 50 to 200 micrograms is considered safe and adequate for adults.[186]

For Americans living in low-selenium areas (roughly, the western one-third and the eastern one-third of the United States) or for people on vegetarian diets, the Nutrition Board recommends that "a daily supplement of 50 to 100 micrograms could probably be taken safely."[187] An interesting bit of information is that Japanese fisherman safely consume about 500 micrograms daily in the large amounts of seafood they eat.[188]

By far the best form of selenium supplementation is the natural and organically bound selenium found in brewer's yeast. It is the most easily assimilated and is of low toxicity.[189] The best quantities to take would be between 25 and 100 mcg. daily, in addition to that which is already in our diet. Supplements should be taken along with other minerals. The research on this mineral is still relatively new. The FDA approved selenium supplements in 1978, and it shouldn't be too long before the RDA for selenium is incorporated into the official U.S. RDA.[190]

Silicon

Silicon makes up over one-quarter of the earth's crust. Silica, a form of silicon, is the chief ingredient in sand. In 1973, it was discovered that silicon is essential for good health. Silicon acts as a ground substance in the body by helping build connective tissue. New evidence suggests that silicon in hard water helps protect against heart disease.[191] Silicon may also help to keep liquids from penetrating the skin. The diet usually supplies all the silicon that the body needs. Alfalfa, fresh fruit, brewer's yeast, and dietary fiber are the best sources of silicon.

Sodium (sodium chloride, salt)

FACTS   Used in processed food to add taste. Sodium chloride contains chloride, an essential mineral. Salt requirements go up as water intake goes up. The fluid outside your body's cells contains most of your sodium. A 154-pound man has about four ounces (150 grams) of sodium in his body.[192]

DEFICIENCY SYMPTOMS   Deficiency is very rare, since most foods contain sodium. However, a deficiency may result from extreme sweating from heat or exercise. You may lose as much as "4 grams of salt in 3 hours of strenuous activity in the sun."[193]

Normally, a sodium intake of about 3 grams is sufficient, though during strenuous activity the body requires greater amounts of sodium. Symptoms of sodium deficiency include headaches, muscular cramps, weakness, collapse of the blood vessels,[194] stomach and intestinal gas, and weight loss.[195] The Lancet says that kidney failure is an inevitable result of sodium starvation.[196] A sodium deficiency may result in tuberculosis of the kidneys or streptococcic infections.[197]

WHAT IT DOES   Sodium functions with potassium to maintain the proper acid-alkaline balance in the blood, and to regulate the water balance within the body. Sodium and potassium are involved in nerve stimulation, which in turn stimulates muscle contraction and expansion. "It also helps keep calcium in solution which is necessary for nerve strength."[198]

"Its main purpose is to render other blood minerals more soluble and prevent them from becoming clogged or deposited in the blood distribution system."[199] Sodium allows for the "free-flow of saliva, gastric juices and enzymes and other intestinal secretions."[200] It is necessary to maintain the fluids of the blood and lymph, helps in digestion, and helps take carbon dioxide out of the body.[201]

WHAT IT MAY DO   Since hypertension (high blood pressure) is associated with retention of salt and water, most authorities feel this condition is caused mainly by a high salt intake.[202] Dropsy, a disease in which the body hoards water, may be due to too much sodium.[203]

A teaspoonful of salt and one and one-half teaspoonsful of baking soda mixed in a quart of water should be given to a patient suffering shock from severe burns and other injuries. This treatment is almost as effective as administering blood plasma. The patient should drink several quarts a day. This will keep the body's water balance between sodium and potassium.[204]

Under severe stress, the adrenals become exhausted and are unable to adequately produce the salt-retaining hormone aldosterone. Salt is needed to alleviate muscle weakness, to stimulate the adrenals, and to bring the potassium level into check.[205]

TOXICITY   Excessive intake of sodium results in abnormal fluid retention. Dizziness and swelling around the legs and face are experienced.[206] Intake of 14 to 28 grams of sodium daily would be considered excessive.[207]

BEST SOURCES   The best sources of sodium are foods from animal sources, including meat, fish (particularly seafoods), poultry, milk, and cheese. Almost all other foods contain certain amounts of sodium.

Sea salt is another fine source for sodium, as well as other minerals, for the following reasons:

(1) Soil fertilizers add to depleted soil minerals that are only necessary for plant growth, not human health.
(2) Recently, table salt has been refined so it will not "cake" or "clump" in damp weather. This process has stripped it of many of the trace minerals essential to health.
(3) The composition of sea water is strikingly similar to the composition of minerals in human blood.
(4) Sea water is extremely rich in minerals and trace elements —some nearly fifty chemicals in all. Many of these trace elements may yet be found to be needed by the body for health, even in extremely minute quantities.[208]

Kelp powder, or powdered seaweed, is another good source of sodium. It contains about 15 percent sodium, compared to about 75 percent found in sea salt.

SUPPLEMENTS   An ordinary diet will provide plenty of sodium and chloride for the body's needs without supplementation. The

National Research Council says you need about 1,100 to 3,000 milligrams of sodium per day. One teaspoon of salt contains about 2,000 milligrams of sodium. Current estimates show, however, that our sodium intake is from 2,300 to 6,900 milligrams, which is much higher than recommended.

Although most people eat too much salt, some people do not get enough, especially if they are vegetarians eating only fruits and vegetables, which are high in potassium. It is interesting to note that herbivors (cattle, rodents, horses, etc.) need salt because of the high potassium, low sodium they get from their vegetable foods.[209] Carnivorous animals like ourselves, however, disregard salt and evidently do not need it, probably because of the levels of sodium found in meat.[210]

I recommend you stay away from table salt as much as possible. If you must salt your food, combine sea salt and a salt substitute (potassium chloride) in your salt shaker to balance out the body's sodium and potassium levels.

People with low blood pressure need salt, while people with high blood pressure need to restrict their intake. Athletes or workers exposed to extreme or prolonged heat should not be afraid to use sea salt on their food. They are losing both sodium and potassium as they perspire. As you become accustomed to hot weather, you will retain more salt and your perspiration will become less salty.[211] Your sodium requirement goes up as you drink more water. The National Research Council suggests you need about half a teaspoon of salt for every quart of water you drink (1,000 mg. per kilogram).[212] Salt tablets should be used only by those persons for whom they were intended: for example, men working all day in a hot boiler room or in front of a hot furnace.

Sulfur

This element is found in every cell of your body and is particularly necessary for beautiful hair, skin, and nails. Sulfur is needed for many reactions within the body, but the likelihood of a deficiency is rare because it is found in so many foods. Protein foods are the richest source of sulfur.

Vanadium

Vanadium is now believed to be essential to man, since deficiency symptoms can be produced in animals by giving them food that lacks this element. However, no deficiency symptoms have yet been recognized in man, and no one really knows how much vanadium we need.

Zinc

FACTS   A trace mineral needed in small amounts. An adult man contains approximately 2,000 to 3,000 milligrams of zinc.[213] Absorption of zinc may be inhibited by phytic acid, which is found in certain grains and breads such as unleavened bread.[214] Alcohol causes you to lose zinc right out of the liver into the urine.[215] Most of the body's zinc is found in the muscles, liver, kidneys, pancreas, and skin, with high concentrations located in the sex glands and organs—particularly the prostate gland in men.

DEFICIENCY SYMPTOMS   You may have a zinc deficiency if there are white spots or bands on your fingernails or if your fingernails appear opaquely white. Once the deficiency is corrected, these white spots will stay in the nails and be eliminated as the nails grow out and are trimmed—but new spots should not appear.[216] A zinc deficiency may result in loss of taste, smell, and appetite.

Boys and girls may suffer delayed sexual development due to a zinc deficiency. A boy's penis may not develop to full size and his beard and auxiliary hair may be less full than normal. "The zinc-deficient girl may not have a regularly established menstrual cycle until age fourteen to seventeen, or the menses may start at thirteen, only to skip for months or even a year."[217] Adults may become infertile, with their sexual function impaired.[218] Other symptoms of deficiency include poor wound healing, loss of hair, increased susceptibility to infection, reduced salivation, skin lesions, stretch marks, and reduced absorption of nutrients.[219]

Since zinc is required for cell growth, impaired development of bones, muscles, and nervous system, as well as deformed offspring, may result from a deficiency.[220] A severe deficiency may cause dwarfism in humans.[221]

WHAT IT DOES   Zinc is a cofactor in over forty different enzyme systems.[222] It plays a major role in the synthesis of protein, RNA, and DNA.[223]

Stress depletes zinc levels, so burn patients are given zinc supplementation to promote normal healing.[224] One study revealed that patients who received no zinc supplements required an average of eighty days for their wounds to heal, while a group that received zinc supplements (three times a day) healed in an average of forty-five days, even though their wounds were larger.[225]

Without the presence of B-6 and other nutrients, zinc cannot function properly.[226] "Zinc is a component of insulin, and it is part of the enzyme that is needed to break down alcohol."[227]

WHAT IT MAY DO   Zinc has been shown to reduce skin eruption and possibly reduce acne. Zinc may do this by stimulating the formation of hormonelike substances called prostaglandins, a lack of which may cause acne.[228] Or zinc may relieve acne because it is involved in increasing the availability of vitamin A to the tissues. Significant improvements were obtained with 45 mg. of zinc.[229]

"With impotent young males who are zinc deficient, a return of sex function may take as long as four to five months of daily zinc supplementation."[230] Zinc can increase testosterone (the male hormone) levels and sperm count.[231] Pregnant women have been treated for nausea with B-6. Success was uneven. When zinc was added, however, many found their difficulty eliminated.[232]

Zinc helps protect against lead poisoning and the toxic effects of cadmium. It can even lower blood levels of these two harmful metals. Elevated blood pressure is a toxic effect of cadmium.[233]

Adequate supplementation of zinc may help prevent the male growth lag that usually occurs during the junior high school years.[234]

TOXICITY   The body will take from the intestines the amount of zinc that is needed and the rest will not be absorbed.[235] "A single oral dose of zinc in excess of 250 mg. may cause vomiting, which itself is another protective mechanism."[236] "Symptoms of a zinc toxicity include dehydration, abdominal pain, nausea, lethargy, vomiting, dizziness, and muscular incoordination."[237] In general, zinc is very safe and is even used by doctors in large quantities to induce vomiting.

BEST SOURCES   By far the best source of zinc is fresh oysters. A one-ounce portion contains approximately 21 mg. of zinc. This may be why oysters have always been used as an aphrodisiac. Other sources of zinc include wheat germ, milk, steamed crab, lobster, chicken, pork chops, turkey, lean ground beef, liver, and eggs.

SUPPLEMENTS There is an antagonism between the minerals zinc and copper. Too much copper will reduce the amount of zinc in the body, while taking too much zinc will cause you to lose copper. Certain animal studies have shown that we might need about fourteen times more zinc in our diet than copper to prevent a harmful accumulation of copper in the liver.[238]

I recommend that you take about 20 to 30 mg. of zinc each day and about 1 mg. or less of copper a day. While these amounts do not represent the 14:1 ratio, I recommend them because it is very easy to get an extra milligram or two of copper from the air, various foods, and drinking water. Zinc, on the other hand, is much harder to obtain from your diet.

Watch out for the many popular vitamin-mineral formulas that are advertised extensively as benefiting iron-poor blood. These formulas usually have a sufficient amount of iron, 2 mg. of copper, and an equal amount or less of zinc. The relatively low amount of zinc in such formulas promotes copper storage, which has been shown to be harmful.

The RDA for zinc is 15 mg. for adults, 20 mg. for pregnant women, and 25 mg. for lactating women.[239] Only the best diets contain 8 to 11 mg. of zinc.[240] Usually B-6 is given along with zinc since both these nutrients must be present in the body for each to work properly. In fact, some deficiency symptoms for these two nutrients overlap each other. Zinc sulfate, zinc gluconate, and chelated zinc are the most popular forms of zinc used. To counteract a zinc deficiency, a 25 to 50 mg. supplement should be taken three times a day. You should not take doses of over 150 mg. a day.

NOTES

1. Marjorie Holmes, *God and Vitamins* (Garden City, N.Y.: Doubleday, 1980), p. 15.
2. Nutrition Search, Inc., *Nutrition Almanac* (New York: McGraw-Hill, 1973, p. 12.
3. Miriam Polunin, *Minerals: What They Are and Why We Need Them* (Willingborough, England: Thorsons Publishers, 1979), p. 23.
4. Carl C. Pfeiffer, *Zinc and Other Micronutrients* (New Canaan, Conn: Keats Publishing, 1978), pp. 90–91.
5. Frank Murray and Ruth Adams, *Minerals: Kill or Cure?* (New York: Larchmont Books, 1980), pp. 77–79.
6. J. I. Rodale and staff, *The Complete Book of Minerals for Health* (Emmaus, Pa: Rodale Press, 1977), pp. 73, 112, 113.
7. Frances S. Goulart, *Eating to Win* (Briarcliff Manor, N.Y.: Stein and Day, 1978), p. 33.
8. Ibid.
9. Pfeiffer, *Zinc and Other Micronutrients*, p. 113.
10. Rodale, *The Complete Book of Minerals*, p. 137.

11. Len Mervyn, Ph.D., *Minerals and Your Health* (New Canaan, Conn: Keats Publishing, 1980), p. 82.
12. Alan R. Gayly, M.D., "Supplementing for Optimal Health," *Prevention*, April 1981, p. 52.
13. Holmes, *God and Vitamins*, p. 92.
14. Ibid.
15. Mervyn, *Minerals and Your Health*, p. 12.
16. Ibid., p. 18.
17. Holmes, *God and Vitamins*, p. 88.
18. Jay R. Reiss, M.S., "Why We Must Take Vitamin Supplements," *Let's Live*, September 1981.
19. Carl C. Pfeiffer, Ph.D., M.D., *Mental and Elemental Nutrients* (New Canaan, Conn: Keats Publishing, 1975), p. 213.

VITAMINS

To simplify and shorten the notes in the Vitamins and Minerals sections, each source reference gives the author's last name, a short form of the title, and the page number(s). Full bibliographic information for each source cited below, as well as other relevant sources, can be found in the Bibliography.

1. Gerras, ed., *Complete Book of Vitamins*, p. 100.
2. Eddy, *Vitaminology*, p. 4.
3. Gerras, ed., *Complete Book of Vitamins*, p. 119.
4. Ibid., p. 121.
5. Bosco, *People's Guide*, p. 26.
6. Ibid., p. 27.
7. Ibid., p. 29.
8. Ibid., p. 32.
9. Gerras, ed., *Complete Book of Vitamins*, p. 101.
10. Ibid., p. 102.
11. Ibid.
12. Ibid., p. 152.
13. Ibid., p. 106.
14. Eddy, *Vitaminology*, p. 127.
15. Gerras, ed., *Complete Book of Vitamins*, p. 157.
16. Eddy, *Vitaminology*, p. 111.
17. Bosco, *People's Guide*, p. 36.
18. Ibid., p. 38.
19. Ibid., p. 39.
20. Ibid., p. 40.
21. Ibid.
22. Gerras, ed., *Complete Book of Vitamins*, p. 163.
23. Rodale, *Complete Book of Minerals*, p. 232.
24. Gerras, ed., *Complete Book of Vitamins*, p. 176.
25. Nutrition Search, Inc., *Nutrition Almanac*, p. 23.
26. Eddy, *Vitaminology*, p. 131.
27. Nutrition Search, Inc., *Nutrition Almanac*, p. 24.
28. Bosco, *People's Guide*, p. 47.
29. Ibid., p. 48.
30. Ibid.
31. Gerras, ed., *Complete Book of Vitamins*, p. 189.
32. Nutrition Search, Inc., *Nutrition Almanac*, p. 36.
33. Davis, *Vitality*, p. 162.
34. Nutrition Search, Inc., Nutrition Almanac, p. 36.
35. Ibid., p. 37.
36. Eddy, *Vitaminology*, p. 169.
37. Nutrition Search, Inc., *Nutrition Almanac*, p. 25.

38. Ibid.; Gerras, ed., *Complete Book of Vitamins*, p. 203.
39. Adams, *Complete Home Guide*, p. 152.
40. Holmes, *God and Vitamins*, p. 176; Nutrition Search, Inc., *Nutrition Almanac*, p. 25; Ebon, *Which Vitamins*, pp. 52, 53.
41. Gerras, ed., *Complete Book of Vitamins*, p. 194.
42. Nutrition Search, Inc., *Nutrition Almanac*, p. 24.
43. Gerras, ed., *Complete Book of Vitamins*, p. 194.
44. Nutrition Search, Inc., *Nutrition Almanac*, p. 25.
45. Adams, *Vitamin B-6 Book*, p. 9.
46. Nutrition Search, Inc., *Nutrition Almanac*, p. 25.
47. Adams, *Complete Home Guide*, p. 158.
48. Ibid.
49. Adams, *Complete Home Guide*, p. 17.
50. Ibid., p. 16; Adams, *Complete Home Guide*, p. 156.
51. Gerras, ed., *Complete Book of Vitamins*, pp. 195, 196.
52. Adams, *Vitamin B-6 Book*, pp. 27, 28.
53. Gerras, ed., *Complete Book of Vitamins*, pp. 198, 199.
54. Ibid., p. 210.
55. Ibid., p. 212.
56. Ibid., pp. 212, 213.
57. Ibid., pp. 520, 529, 530.
58. Bosco, *People's Guide*, p. 65.
59. Ibid., p. 77.
60. Gerras, ed., *Complete Book of Vitamins*, p. 214.
61. Bosco, *People's Guide*, p. 76.
62. Ibid.
63. Gerras, ed., *Complete Book of Vitamins*, pp. 200, 201; Ebon, *Which Vitamins*, p. 5.
64. Mindell, *Vitamin Bible*, p. 33.
65. Gerras, ed., *Complete Book of Vitamins*, p. 90.
66. Bosco, *People's Guide*, p. 90.
67. Ibid., p. 89.
68. Gerras, ed., *Complete Book of Vitamins*, p. 231.
69. Bosco, *People's Guide*, p. 86.
70. Ibid., p. 79.
71. Nutrition Search, Inc., *Nutrition Almanac*, p. 32.
72. Gerras, ed., *Complete Book of Vitamins*, p. 244.
73. Bosco, *People's Guide*, p. 94.
74. Ibid., pp. 92, 93.
75. Ibid., p. 93.
76. Ibid.
77. Ibid.
78. Nutrition Search, Inc., *Nutrition Almanac*, p. 28.
79. Gerras, ed., *Complete Book of Vitamins*, p. 221.
80. Nutrition Search, Inc., *Nutrition Almanac*, p. 27.
81. Ibid.
82. Bosco, *People's Guide*, p. 92.
83. Gerras, ed., *Complete Book of Vitamins*, pp. 222, 223.
84. Eddy, *Vitaminology*, p. 194.
85. Davis, *Let's Eat Right*, p. 88.
86. Nutrition Search, Inc., *Nutrition Almanac*, p. 42; Clark, *Know Your Nutrition*, pp. 116, 118.
87. Nutrition Search, Inc., *Nutrition Almanac*, p. 41.
88. Ibid.
89. Ibid.
90. Gerras, ed., *Complete Book of Vitamins*, p. 244.
91. Ibid., p. 245.
92. Williams, *Nutrition Against Disease*, p. 131.

93. Ibid., p. 57.
94. Goodhart and Shills, *Modern Nutrition*, p. 964.
95. Gerras, ed., *Complete Book of Vitamins*, p. 249.
96. Bosco, *People's Guide*, p. 111.
97. Ibid., p. 112.
98. Gerras, ed., *Complete Book of Vitamins*, p. 639.
99. Bosco, *People's Guide*, pp. 101, 102.
100. Ibid., p. 101.
101. Gerras, ed., *Complete Book of Vitamins*, p. 254.
102. Ibid.
103. Goodhart and Shils, *Modern Nutrition*, p. 257.
104. Gerras, ed., *Complete Book of Vitamins*, p. 269; Eddy, *Vitaminology*, p. 219.
105. Bosco, *People's Guide*, p. 123.
106. Gerras, ed., *Complete Book of Vitamins*, pp. 708, 709.
107. Nutrition Search, Inc., *Nutrition Almanac*, p. 38.
108. Nutrition Search, Inc., *Nutrition Almanac*, p. 37.
109. Gerras, ed., *Complete Book of Vitamins*, p. 269.
110. Nutrition Search, Inc., *Nutrition Almanac*, p. 38.
111. Bosco, *People's Guide*, p. 123.
112. Ibid., pp. 123, 124.
113. Ibid., p. 123.
114. Goodhart and Shils, *Modern Nutrition*, p. 947.
115. Nutrition Search, Inc., *Nutrition Almanac*, p. 30.
116. Bosco, *People's Guide*, p. 114.
117. Nutrition Search, Inc., *Nutrition Almanac*, p. 31.
118. Gerras, ed., *Complete Book of Vitamins*, p. 265.
119. Nutrition Search, Inc., *Nutrition Almanac*, p. 31.
120. Ibid.
121. Davis, *Let's Get Well*, p. 263.
122. Gerras, ed., *Complete Book of Vitamins*, p. 263.
123. Nutrition Search, Inc., *Nutrition Almanac*, p. 31.
124. Ibid.
125. Davis, *Let's Get Well*, p. 263.
126. Nutrition Search, Inc., *Nutrition Almanac*, p. 31.
127. Gerras, ed., *Complete Book of Vitamins*, p. 267.
128. Holmes, *God and Vitamins*, pp. 177, 178.
129. Gerras, ed., *Complete Book of Vitamins*, pp. 265, 266.
130. Bosco, *People's Guide*, p. 117.
131. Ibid.
132. Ibid.
133. Nutrition Search, Inc., *Nutrition Almanac*, p. 31.
134. Gerras, ed., *Complete Book of Vitamins*, p. 267.
135. Ibid., p. 258.
136. Nutrition Search, Inc., *Nutrition Almanac*, p. 34.
137. Ibid.
138. Ibid.
139. Gerras, ed., *Complete Book of Vitamins*, pp. 258, 259.
140. Clark, *Know Your Nutrition*, p. 113.
141. Gerras, ed., *Complete Book of Vitamins*, p. 765.
142. Ibid.
143. Nutrition Search, Inc., *Nutrition Almanac*, p. 34.
144. Williams, *Nutrition Against Disease*, p. 164.
145. Gerras, ed., *Complete Book of Vitamins*, p. 261.
146. Pauling, *Vitamin C*, pp. 63, 64.
147. Nutrition Search, Inc., *Nutrition Almanac*, p. 43.
148. Davis, *Let's Get Well*, pp. 147, 199, 327; Nutrition Search, Inc., *Nutrition Almanac*, p. 44; Pauling, *Vitamin C*, p. 18.
149. Stone, *Healing Factor*, pp. 47, 48.

150. Ibid., p. 47.
151. Nutrition Search, Inc., *Nutrition Almanac*, p. 43.
152. Bosco, *People's Guide*, p. 126.
153. Ibid., p. 149.
154. Stone, *Healing Factor*, p. 48.
155. Ibid.
156. Ibid.
157. Ibid.
158. Ibid.
159. Ibid.
160. Pauling, *Vitamin C*, pp. 65–66, 63.
161. Bosco, *People's Guide*, p. 128.
162. Ibid., p. 131.
163. Gerras, ed., *Complete Book of Vitamins*, p. 769.
164. Bosco, *People's Guide*, pp. 132, 133.
165. Ibid., p. 133.
166. Ibid., p. 136.
167. Ibid., p. 139.
168. Ibid., p. 148.
169. Stone, *Healing Factor*, pp. 122–123.
170. Ibid., p. 131.
171. Bosco, *People's Guide*, p. 153.
172. Stone, *Healing Factor*, p. 62.
173. Clark, *Know Your Nutrition*, p. 144.
174. Adams and Murray, *Vitamin B-6 Book*, p. 16; Adams, *Complete Home Guide*, p. 156.
175. Williams and Kalita, *Physician's Handbook*, p. 47.
176. Ibid., p. 48.
177. Bosco, *People's Guide*, p. 155.
178. Bosco, *People's Guide*, pp. 156–157; Davis, *Let's Have Healthy Children*, p. 292.
179. Bosco, *People's Guide*, p. 161.
180. Ibid.
181. Shute, *Heart and Vitamin E*, p. 14.
182. Goodhart and Shils, *Modern Nutrition*, p. 176.
183. Nutrition Search, Inc., *Nutrition Almanac*, p. 50.
184. Shute, *Heart and Vitamin E*, p. 21.
185. Bosco, *People's Guide*, p. 167.
186. Nutrition Search, Inc., *Nutrition Almanac*, p. 52; Gerras, ed., *Complete Book of Vitamins*, p. 769.
187. Bosco, *People's Guide*, p. 167.
188. Shute, *Heart and Vitamin E*, p. 27; Davis, *Let's Get Well*, p. 281.
189. Davis, *Let's Get Well*, p. 339.
190. Shute, *Heart and Vitamin E*, p. 27.
191. Bosco, *People's Guide*, p. 164; Gerras, ed., *Complete Book of Vitamins*, pp. 445–447.
192. Shute, *Heart and Vitamin E*, p. 25.
193. Bosco, *People's Guide*, p. 166.
194. Ibid., p. 168.
195. Davis, *Let's Get Well*, p. 339.
196. Bosco, *People's Guide*, p. 173.
197. Ibid., p. 174.
198. Ibid., p. 176.
199. Ibid., p. 177.
200. Ibid.
201. Ibid., p. 178.
202. Gerras, ed., *Complete Book of Vitamins*, p. 483.
203. Bosco, *People's Guide*, pp. 459–463.
204. Ibid., p. 179.

205. Ibid.
206. Shute, *Heart and Vitamin E,* p. 86.
207. Shute, *Summary,* pp. 17, 18, 19.
208. Ibid., pp. 4, 12.
209. Gerras, ed., *Complete Book of Vitamins,* p. 489.
210. Nutrition Search, Inc., *Nutrition Almanac,* p. 58.
211. Ibid., p. 59; Bosco, *People's Guide,* p. 186.
212. Nutrition Search, Inc., *Nutrition Almanac,* p. 59.
213. Bosco, *People's Guide,* p. 185.
214. Nutrition Search, Inc., *Nutrition Almanac,* p. 59.
215. Gerras, ed., *Complete Book of Vitamins,* pp. 495, 500; Bosco, *People's Guide,* p. 185.
216. Bosco, *People's Guide,* p. 184.
217. Gerras, ed., *Complete Book of Vitamins,* p. 494.
218. Nutrition Search, Inc., *Nutrition Almanac,* p. 59.
219. Gerras, ed., *Complete Book of Vitamins,* pp. 364, 365.
220. Bosco, *People's Guide,* pp. 273, 274.
221. Ibid., p. 274.
222. Ibid., p. 275.
223. Ibid.
224. Gerras, ed., *Complete Book of Vitamins,* p. 373.
225. Ibid., p. 368.
226. Ibid.
227. Ibid., p. 369.
228. Ibid.
229. Ibid., p. 370.
230. Bosco, *People's Guide,* p. 275.
231. Ibid.
232. Ibid., p. 276.
233. Gerras, ed., *Complete Book of Vitamins,* p. 375.

MINERALS

1. Wade, *Magic Minerals,* p. 17.
2. Polunin, *Minerals,* p. 23.
3. Ibid.
4. Ibid., pp. 24–25.
5. Wade, *Magic Minerals,* p. 17.
6. Polunin, *Minerals,* p. 29.
7. Pfeiffer, *Zinc,* pp. 90–91.
8. Wade, *Magic Minerals,* p. 18.
9. Ibid.
10. Bosco, *People's Guide,* p. 192.
11. Wade, *Magic Minerals,* pp. 17–18.
12. Ibid., p. 18.
13. Ibid., p. 17.
14. Bosco, *People's Guide,* p. 193.
15. Ibid., p. 194.
16. Ibid., p. 196.
17. Rodale, *Complete Book of Minerals,* pp. 28–29.
18. Nutrition Search, Inc., *Nutrition Almanac,* p. 64.
19. Bosco, *People's Guide,* p. 200.
20. Rodale, *Complete Book of Minerals,* p. 60.
21. Bosco, *People's Guide,* p. 199.
22. Rodale, *Complete Book of Minerals,* pp. 176–177.
23. Adams and Murray, *Minerals,* p. 166.
24. Rodale, *Complete Book of Minerals,* p. 175.
25. Ibid., p. 172.

26. Ibid.
27. Ibid., p. 176.
28. Ibid., p. 181.
29. Adams and Murray, *Minerals,* p. 160.
30. Ibid., p. 161.
31. Pfeiffer, *Zinc,* p. 131.
32. Bosco, *People's Guide,* p. 205.
33. Ibid., p. 207.
34. Ibid.
35. Ibid., p. 206.
36. Mervyn, *Minerals and Your Health,* p. 55.
37. Wade, *Magic Minerals,* p. 24.
38. Mervyn, *Minerals and Your Health,* p. 102.
39. Ibid.
40. Wade, *Magic Minerals,* p. 24.
41. Mervyn, *Minerals and Your Health,* p. 103.
42. Ibid., p. 102.
43. Ibid.
44. Ibid.
45. Bosco, *People's Guide,* p. 209.
46. Rodale, *Complete Book of Minerals,* p. 197.
47. Bosco, *People's Guide,* p. 210.
48. Mervyn, *Minerals and Your Health,* p. 54.
49. Bosco, *People's Guide,* p. 211.
50. Pfeiffer, *Zinc,* p. 213.
51. Polunin, *Minerals,* p. 45.
52. Ibid., p. 47.
53. Rodale, *Complete Book of Minerals,* p. 204; Polunin, *Minerals,* p. 47; Nutrition Search, Inc., *Nutrition Almanac,* p. 70.
54. Nutrition Search, Inc., *Nutrition Almanac,* p. 70.
55. Wade, *Magic Minerals,* p. 20.
56. Polunin, *Minerals,* pp. 45–46.
57. Mervyn, *Minerals and Your Health,* p. 100.
58. Goodhart and Shils, *Modern Nutrition,* p. 370.
59. Rodale, *Complete Book of Minerals,* pp. 204–205.
60. Ibid., pp. 205–206.
61. Bosco, *People's Guide,* p. 222.
62. Davis, *Let's Get Well,* p. 285.
63. Ibid., p. 279.
64. Bosco, *People's Guide,* p. 222.
65. Ibid., p. 223.
66. Ibid.
67. Bosco, *People's Guide,* p. 222.
68. Mervyn, *Minerals and Your Health* p. 89.
69. Davis, *Let's Get Well,* pp. 280–285.
70. Mervyn, *Minerals and Your Health,* p. 87.
71. Ibid., p. 90.
72. Rodale, *Complete Book of Minerals,* p. 151.
73. Bosco, *People's Guide,* p. 223.
74. Davis, *Let's Get Well,* p. 280.
75. Pfeiffer, *Zinc,* p. 61.
76. Bosco, *People's Guide,* p. 226.
77. Rodale, *Complete Book of Minerals,* p. 147.
78. Ibid.
79. Ibid., pp. 147–148.
80. Ibid., p. 146.
81. Polunin, *Minerals,* p. 77.
82. Ibid.; Nutrition Search, Inc., *Nutrition Almanac,* p. 73.

83. Adams and Murray, *Minerals*, p. 110.
84. Davis, *Let's Get Well*, p. 271.
85. Ibid., pp. 179, 271.
86. Adams and Murray, *Minerals*, p. 110.
87. Polunin, *Minerals*, p. 78; Nutrition Search, Inc., *Nutrition Almanac*, p. 74.
88. Adams and Murray, *Minerals*, p. 109.
89. Ibid., p. 110; Rodale, *Complete Book of Minerals*, p. 84.
90. Adams and Murray, *Minerals*, p. 110.
91. Ibid.
92. Rodale, *Complete Book of Minerals*, p. 73.
93. Adams and Murray, *Minerals*, p. 111.
94. Rodale, *Magnesium*, p. 55.
95. Rodale, *Complete Book of Minerals*, p. 74.
96. Adams and Murray, *Minerals*, p. 110.
97. Rodale, *Complete Book of Minerals*, p. 84.
98. Nutrition Search, Inc., *Nutrition Almanac*, p. 73.
99. Rodale, *Complete Book of Minerals*, p. 85.
100. Polunin, *Minerals*, p. 80.
101. Rodale, *Complete Book of Minerals*, p. 99.
102. Ibid., p. 102.
103. Ibid., p. 105.
104. Ibid., pp. 112–113.
105. Ibid., p. 116.
106. Ibid., pp. 118–119.
107. Wade, *Magic Minerals*, p. 24.
108. Rodale, *Complete Book of Minerals*, p. 82.
109. Goodhart and Shils, *Modern Nutrition*, p. 388.
110. Bosco, *People's Guide*, p. 235.
111. Goodhart and Shils, *Modern Nutrition*, p. 389.
112. Pfeiffer, *Mental and Elemental Nutrients*, p. 254.
113. Bosco, *People's Guide*, p. 235.
114. Pfeiffer, *Mental and Elemental Nutrients*, p. 254; Goodhart and Shils, *Modern Nutrition*, p. 389.
115. Pfeiffer, *Mental and Elemental Nutrients*, p. 253.
116. Josephson, *Thymus, Manganese and Myasthenia Gravis*, p. 6.
117. Goodhart and Shils, *Modern Nutrition*, p. 389.
118. Josephson, *Thymus, Manganese and Myasthenia Gravis*.
119. Pfeiffer, *Mental and Elemental Nutrients*, pp. 253, 339.
120. Goodhart and Shils, *Modern Nutrition*, p. 390.
121. Bosco, *People's Guide*, p. 236.
122. Goodhart and Shils, *Modern Nutrition*, p. 388.
123. Bosco, *People's Guide*, p. 235.
124. Polunin, *Minerals*, p. 83.
125. Nutrition Search, Inc., *Nutrition Almanac*, p. 77.
126. Pfeiffer, *Zinc*, p. 100.
127. Ibid.
128. Rodale, *Complete Book of Minerals*, p. 63.
129. Ibid., p. 65.
130. Wade, *Magic Minerals*, p. 19.
131. Nutrition Search, Inc., *Nutrition Almanac*, p. 77.
132. Ibid.
133. Bosco, *People's Guide*, p. 240.
134. Polunin, *Minerals*, p. 84.
135. Ibid., p. 57.
136. Ibid.
137. Pfeiffer, *Zinc*, p. 110.
138. Nutrition Search, Inc., *Nutrition Almanac*, p. 79.
139. Polunin, *Minerals*, p. 59; Nutrition Search, Inc., *Nutrition Almanac*, p. 79.

140. Polunin, *Minerals*, p. 59.
141. Mervyn, *Minerals and Your Health*, p. 83.
142. Ibid.
143. Rodale, *Complete Book of Minerals*, p. 132.
144. Ibid.
145. Ibid., pp. 132–133.
146. Ibid., p. 122.
147. Nutrition Search, Inc., *Nutrition Almanac*, p. 79.
148. Rodale, *Complete Book of Minerals*, p. 125.
149. Davis, *Let's Get Well*, p. 114.
150. Ibid., p. 172.
151. Ibid., p. 71.
152. Nutrition Search, Inc., *Nutrition Almanac*, p. 79.
153. Davis, *Let's Get Well*, p. 83.
154. Bosco, *Complete Book of Vitamins*, p. 244.
155. Ibid., p. 244.
156. Ibid., p. 243.
157. Pfeiffer, *Zinc*, p. 111.
158. Bosco, *People's Guide*, p. 244.
159. Prasad, *Trace Elements*, p. 118.
160. Passwater, *Selenium*, pp. 162–163.
161. Polunin, *Minerals*, p. 63.
162. Pfeiffer, *Zinc*, p. 86.
163. Bosco, *People's Guide*, p. 247.
164. Passwater, *Selenium*, p. 165.
165. Ibid., pp. 126–127.
166. Pfeiffer, *Zinc*, p. 86.
167. Ibid., p. 85.
168. Passwater, *Selenium*, p. 37.
169. Pfeiffer, *Zinc*, p. 85; Passwater, *Selenium*, pp. 129–130.
170. Prasad, *Trace Elements*, p. 119.
171. Pfeiffer, *Zinc*, p. 85.
172. Passwater, *Selenium*, p. 30.
173. Ibid., pp. 50–51.
174. Ibid., pp. 56–57.
175. Ibid., pp. 52–56.
176. Ibid., p. 79.
177. Prasad, *Trace Elements*, p. 123.
178. Passwater, *Selenium*, p. 137.
179. Prasad, *Trace Elements*, p. 121.
180. Pfeiffer, *Mental and Elemental Nutrients*, p. 85.
181. Prasad, *Trace Elements*, pp. 120, 121.
182. Ibid., p. 121.
183. Passwater, *Selenium*, p. 156.
184. Ibid.
185. Ibid., p. 170.
186. Ibid., p. 157.
187. Ibid., pp. 10, 156.
188. Ibid., p. 157.
189. Ibid., p. 186.
190. Ibid., p. 158.
191. Kunin, *Mega-Nutrition*, p. 192.
192. Pfeiffer, *Mental and Elemental Nutrients*, p. 111.
193. Mervyn, *Minerals and Your Health*, p. 29.
194. Bosco, *People's Guide*, p. 255.
195. Wade, *Magic Minerals*, p. 22.
196. Rodale, *Complete Book of Minerals*, p. 352.
197. Ibid., pp. 350–351.

198. Wade, *Magic Minerals,* p. 22.
199. Ibid., p. 21.
200. Ibid., p. 22.
201. Rodale, *Complete Book of Minerals,* p. 133.
202. Ibid., p. 327.
203. Ibid., p. 319.
204. Ibid., p. 354.
205. Davis, *Let's Get Well,* p. 294.
206. Nutrition Search, Inc., *Nutrition Almanac,* p. 81.
207. Ibid.
208. Rodale, *Complete Book of Minerals,* pp. 339–344.
209. Ibid., p. 288.
210. Ibid., p. 288.
211. Ibid., p. 336.
212. Nutrition Search, Inc., *Nutrition Almanac,* p. 81.
213. Mervyn, *Minerals and Your Health,* p. 50.
214. Nutrition Search, Inc., *Nutrition Almanac,* p. 83; Pfeiffer, *Zinc,* p. 7.
215. Rodale, *Complete Book of Minerals,* p. 266.
216. Polunin, *Minerals,* pp. 72, 73; Pfeiffer, *Zinc,* pp. 18, 19.
217. Pfeiffer, *Zinc,* pp. 11, 12.
218. Bosco, *People's Guide,* p. 259.
219. Ibid., pp. 258–259; Pfeiffer, *Zinc,* p. 11.
220. Bosco, *People's Guide,* p. 258.
221. Nutrition Search, Inc., *Nutrition Almanac,* p. 84.
222. Bosco, *People's Guide,* p. 257.
223. Ibid.
224. Pfeiffer, *Zinc,* p. 13.
225. Bosco, *People's Guide,* p. 260.
226. Pfeiffer, *Zinc,* p. 14.
227. Nutrition Search, Inc., *Nutrition Almanac,* p. 83.
228. Polunin, *Minerals,* p. 74.
229. Bosco, *People's Guide,* p. 261.
230. Pfeiffer, *Zinc,* p. 12.
231. Bosco, *People's Guide,* p. 264.
232. Pfeiffer, *Zinc,* p. 14.
233. Bosco, *People's Guide,* p. 264.
234. Pfeiffer, *Mental and Elemental Nutrients,* p. 229.
235. Pfeiffer, *Zinc,* p. 23.
236. Bosco, *People's Guide,* p. 267.
237. Ibid.
238. Pfeiffer, *Zinc,* p. 213.
239. Bosco, *People's Guide,* p. 265.
240. Pfeiffer, *Zinc,* p. 49.

Bibliography

Abrahamson, E. M., M.D., and Pezet, A. W. *Body, Mind, and Sugar*. New York: Avon Books, 1951.

Adams, Ruth. *The Complete Home Guide to All the Vitamins*. New York: Larchmont Books, 1972, 1976.

Adams, Ruth, and Murray, Frank. *Improving Your Health with Calcium and Phosphorus*. New York: Larchmont Books, 1978.

————. *Minerals: Kill or Cure?* New York: Larchmont Books, 1980.

————. *The Vitamin B-6 Book*. New York: Larchmont Books, 1980.

Atkins, Robert C., M.D. *Dr. Atkins' Nutrition Breakthrough*. New York: William Morrow, 1981.

Bailey, Herbert. *CH3—Will It Keep You Young Longer?* New York: Bantam Books, 1977.

Barnes, Broda O., M.D., and Barnes, Charlotte W. *Hope for Hypoglycemia*. Fort Collins, Colo.: Robinson Press, 1978.

Barnes, Broda O., M.D., and Galton, Lawrence. *Hypothyroidism: The Unsuspected Illness*. New York: Crowell, 1976.

Benowicz, Robert J. *Vitamins and You*. New York: Grosset & Dunlap, 1979.

Bland, Jeffrey. *Your Health Under Siege: Using Nutrition to Fight Back*. Brattleboro, Vt.: The Stephen Greene Press, 1981.

Bosco, Dominick. *The People's Guide to Vitamins and Minerals*. Chicago: Contemporary Books, 1980.

Bradley, Robert A., M.D. *Husband-Coached Childbirth*. New York: Harper & Row, 1965.

Brewer, Gail Sforza, and Brewer, Tom, M.D. *What Every Pregnant Woman Should Know*. Penguin Books, 1977.

Cameron, Ewan, M.B., Ch.B., F.R.C.S. (Glasgow), F.R.C.S. (Edinburgh), and Pauling, Linus, Ph.D. *Cancer and Vitamin C*. Menlo Park, Calif.: Linus Pauling Institute of Science and Medicine, 1979.

Cheraskin, E., M.D., D.M.D., and Ringsdorf, W. M., Jr., D.M.D., M.S. *New Hope for Incurable Diseases*. New York: Arco Publishing, 1971.

————. *Psychodietetics*. New York: Stein & Day, 1974.

Clark, Linda. *Know Your Nutrition*. New Canaan, Conn.: Keats Publishing, 1973.

Cooper, Kenneth H., M.D., M.P.H. *Aerobics*. New York: Bantam Books, 1968.

————. *The Aerobics Way*. New York: Bantam Books, 1977.

Cousins, Norman. *Anatomy of an Illness*. New York: Bantam Books, 1979.

Couture, Gary L., Ph.D., and Gladden, Lee, Ph.D. *How to Win the Aging Game*. Newport Beach: Harbor House, 1979.

Cureton, Thomas Kirk, Ph.D. *The Physiological Effects of Wheat Germ Oil on Humans in Exercise*. Springfield, Ill.: Charles C. Thomas, 1972.

Davis, Adelle, A.B., M.S. *Let's Eat Right to Keep Fit*. New York: Harcourt, Brace & Company, 1954.

_____. *Let's Get Well*. New York: Harcourt, Brace & World, 1965.

_____. *Let's Have Healthy Children*. New York: Harcourt Brace Jovanovich, 1972.

_____. *Let's Stay Healthy*. New York: Harcourt Brace Jovanovich, 1981.

_____. *Vitality Through Planned Nutrition*. New York: Macmillan, 1942, 1949.

Davison, Jaquie. *Cancer Winner*. Pierce City, Mo.: Pacific Press, 1977.

De Kruif, Paul. *Life Among the Doctors*. New York: Harcourt, Brace & Company, 1949.

Douris, Larry, and Timon, Mark. *Dictionary of Health and Nutrition*. New York: Pyramid Publications, 1975.

Ebon, Martin. *Which Vitamins Do You Need?* New York: Bantam Books, 1974.

Eddy, Walter H., Ph.D. *Vitaminology*. New York: Williams & Wilkins, 1949.

Elam, Daniel. *Building Better Babies*. Millbrae, Calif.: Celestial Arts, 1980.

Eugene, E., and Greer, Elaine W. *Daily Guide Toward Fitness*. Nashville, Tenn.: Broadman Press, 1981.

Ford, Frank. *The Simpler Life Cookbook from Arrowhead Mills*. Fort Worth, Tex.: Harvest Press, 1974.

Fredericks, Carlton, Ph.D. *Arthritis: Don't Learn to Live with It*. New York: Grosset & Dunlap, 1981.

_____. *Eating Right for You*. New York: Grosset & Dunlap, 1972.

_____. *High-Fiber Way to Total Health*. New York: Pocket Books, 1976.

_____. *Look Younger, Feel Healthier*. New York: Grosset & Dunlap, 1975.

_____. *Low Blood Sugar and You*. New York: Grosset & Dunlap, 1969.

_____. *The Nutrition Handbook*. Chatsworth, Calif.: Major Books, 1964.

_____. *Psycho-Nutrition*. New York: Grosset & Dunlap, 1976.

_____. *Winning the Fight Against Breast Cancer: The Nutritional Approach*. New York: Grosset & Dunlap, 1977.

Gerras, Charles, ed. *The Complete Book of Vitamins*. Emmaus, Pa.: Rodale Press, 1977.

Gertler, Menard M., M.D. *You Can Predict Your Heart Attack and Prevent It*. New York: Random House, 1963.

Goodhart, Robert S., and Shils, Maurice E. *Modern Nutrition in Health and Disease*. Philadelphia: Lea & Febiger, 1973.

Gorman, Marion, and deAlba, Felipe P. *The Dione Lucas Book of Natural French Cooking*. New York: E. P. Dutton, 1977.

Gots, Ronald E., M.D., Ph.D., and Gots, Barbara A., M.D. *Caring for Your Unborn Child*. New York: Bantam Books, 1977.

Hall, Ross Hume, Ph.D., *Food for Nought*. New York: Harper & Row, 1974.

Hauser, Gayelord. *New Guide to Intelligent Reducing*. Greenwich, Conn.: Fawcett Publications, 1967.

_____. *New Treasury of Secrets*. Greenwich, Conn.: Fawcett Publications, 1951, 1974.

Hoffer, Abram, Ph.D., M.D., and Walker, Morton, D.P.M. *Orthomolecular Nutrition— New Lifestyle for Super Good Health*. New Canaan, Conn.: Keats Publishing, 1978.

Holmes, Marjorie. *God and Vitamins*. Garden City, N.Y.: Doubleday, 1980.

Hromas, R. P. *Passport to the Bible*. Wheaton, Ill.: Tyndale House, 1980.

Hunter, Beatrice Trum. *Whole-Grain Baking Sampler*. New Canaan, Conn.: Keats Publishing, 1972.

Hunton, Richard E., M.D. *Formula for Fitness*. Nashville, Tenn.: Broadman Press, 1966.

Josephson, Emanuel M., M.D. *The Thymus, Manganese and Myasthenia Gravis*. New York: Chedney Press, 1961.

Kerner, Fred. *Stress and Your Heart.* New York: Hawthorn Books, 1961.

Kugler, Hans J., Ph.D. *Dr. Kugler's Seven Keys to a Longer Life.* New York: Stein & Day, 1978.

Kunin, Richard A., M.D. *Mega-Nutrition.* New York: McGraw-Hill, 1980.

Lansky, Vicki. *Feed Me! I'm Yours.* New York: Bantam Books, 1974.

Lappe, Frances Moore. *Diet for a Small Planet.* New York: Ballantine Books, 1971.

Lesser, Michael, M.D. *Nutrition and Vitamin Therapy.* New York: Bantam Books, 1980.

Marsh, Anne C.; Klippstein, Ruth N.; and Kaplan, Sybil D. *The Sodium Content of Your Food.* Washington, D.C.: U.S. Department of Agriculture, 1980.

McCarrison, Sir Robert. *Studies in Deficiency Disease.* London: Henry Frowde and Hodder & Stoughton; reproduced by photo-lithography, 1945, Lee Foundation for Nutritional Research, Milwaukee, Wisconsin.

McGrady, Pat, Sr. *The Persecuted Drug—The Story of DMSO.* New York: Grosset & Dunlap, 1973.

Mervyn, Len, Ph.D. *Minerals and Your Health.* New Canaan, Conn.: Keats Publishing, 1980.

Mindell, Earl. *Vitamin Bible.* New York: Rawson, Wade Publishers, 1979.

Moskowitz, Milton; Katz, Michael; and Levering, Robert. *Everybody's Business.* San Francisco: Harper & Row, 1980.

Murray, Frank. *Program Your Heart for Health.* New York: Larchmont Books, 1977.

Newbold, H. L., M.D. *Mega-Nutrients for Your Nerves.* New York: Peter H. Wyden, 1975.

Nichols, Joe D., M.D. *"Please Doctor, Do Something!"* Atlanta, Tex.: Natural Food Associates, 1972.

Niehans, Paul, M.D. *Introduction to Cellular Therapy.* New York: Pageant Books, 1960.

Nutrition Search, Inc. *Nutrition Almanac.* New York: McGraw-Hill, 1973, 1975, 1979.

Ott, John N. *Health and Light.* Old Greenwich, Conn.: The Devin-Adair Company, 1973.

Passwater, Richard A., Ph.D. *Cancer and Its Nutritional Therapies.* New Canaan, Conn.: Keats Publishing, 1978.

————. *Selenium as Food and Medicine.* New Canaan, Conn.: Keats Publishing, 1980.

————. *Supernutrition.* New York: The Dial Press, 1975.

————. *Super Nutrition for Healthy Hearts.* New York: Harcourt Brace Jovanovich, 1977.

Pauling, Linus. *Vitamin C and the Common Cold.* New York: Bantam Books, 1970.

Pfeiffer, Carl C., Ph.D., M.D. *Mental and Elemental Nutrients.* New Canaan, Conn.: Keats Publishing, 1975.

————. *Zinc and Other Micro-Nutrients.* New Canaan, Conn.: Keats Publishing, 1978.

Pinckney, Edward R., and Pinckney, Cathey. *The Cholesterol Controversy.* Los Angeles: Sherbourne Press, 1973.

Polunin, Miriam. *Minerals: What They Are and Why We Need Them.* Wellingborough, Eng.: Thorsons Publishers, 1979.

Popov, Ivan, M.D. *Stay Young.* New York: Grosset & Dunlap, 1975.

Prasad, Ananda D. *Trace Elements in Human Health and Disease.* Vol. 2. New York: Academic Press, 1976.

Price, Weston A., D.D.S. *Nutrition and Physical Degeneration.* Los Angeles, Calif.: The American Academy of Applied Nutrition, 1939.

Rodale, J. I. *Magnesium: The Nutrient That Could Change Your Life.* New York: Pyramid Publications, 1968.

————. *Natural Health, Sugar and the Criminal Mind.* New York: Pyramid Books, 1968.

Rodale, J. I., and staff. *Cancer: Facts & Fallacies.* Emmaus, Pa.: Rodale Press, 1969.

————. *Complete Book of Minerals for Health.* Emmaus, Pa.: Rodale Press, 1977.

Rohrer, Virginia, and Rohrer, Norman. *How to Eat Right and Feel Great.* Wheaton, Ill.: Tyndale House, 1977.

Sandler, Benjamin P., M.D. *How to Prevent Heart Attacks.* Milwaukee, Wis.: Lee Foundation for Nutritional Research, 1958.

Schmid, K., M.D., and Stein, J., M.D. *Cell Research and Cell Therapy.* Thoune, Switzerland: Ott Publishers, 1967.

Schroeder, Henry A., M.D. *The Trace Elements and Man.* Old Greenwich, Conn.: Devin-Adair Company, 1973.

Selye, Hans, M.D. *The Stress of Life.* New York: McGraw-Hill, 1956, 1976.

Sheehan, George, M.D. *Dr. Sheehan on Running.* New York: Bantam Books, 1975.

Shute, Evan V., F.R.C.S.(C). *The Heart and Vitamin E.* New Canaan, Conn.: Keats Publishing, 1956, 1969, 1976.

Shute, Wilfrid E., M.D. *Your Child and Vitamin E.* New Canaan, Conn.: Keats Publishing, 1979.

Smith, Lendon H., M.D. *Feed Your Kids Right.* New York: McGraw-Hill, 1979.

————. *Improving Your Child's Behavior Chemistry.* New York: Pocket Books, 1976.

————. *The Encyclopedia of Baby and Child Care.* New York: Warner Books, 1972.

Stone, Irwin. *The Healing Factor.* New York: Grosset & Dunlap, 1972.

Thurston, Emory D., Ph.D., Sc.D. *Nutrition for Tots to Teens.* Encino, Calif.: Argold Press, 1976.

Verrett, Jacqueline, and Carper, Jean. *Eating May Be Hazardous to Your Health.* New York: Anchor Press/Doubleday, 1974.

Wade, Carlson. *Magic Minerals.* New York: Arco Publishing Company, 1967.

Williams, Roger J., Ph.D. *Nutrition Against Disease.* New York: Bantam Books, 1971.

————. *The Wonderful World Within You.* New York: Bantam Books, 1977.

————. *You Are Extra-ordinary.* New York: Pyramid Publications, 1971.

Williams, Roger J., and Kalita, Dwight K. *A Physician's Handbook on Orthomolecular Medicine.* New York: Pergamon Press, 1977.

Yudkin, John, M.D. *Sweet and Dangerous.* New York: Peter H. Wyden, 1972.

Index

NOTE: The index contains entries, subentries, and sub-subentries. To avoid confusion, sub-subentries are set in italic type.

A

Acetylcholine, 202

Aches, 4

Acidophilus culture (*lactobacillus acidophilus*), 6, 109–10; as aid to elimination, 107, 112, 151; as relief for bad breath, 108–109; as relief for perspiration odors, 108–109; benefits of, 161–62; effect of, on bacteria, 161; forms of, 109–10; infection related to, 125; nursing related to, 109; recommended dosage, 162

Acne, 191, 192, 240

ACTH, 24

Adenoids, swollen, 121, 122

Adrenal glands: adrenal glandulars as therapy for, 144, 164; allergies and, 105–106; arthritis and, 48; blood sugar levels and, 42, 50–51; cholesterol and, 76; effect of alcohol on, 48; exhaustion of: *as cause of arthritis, 125; as cause of infection, 125; calcium deficiency related to, 51–52; menopause problems as symptom of, 141; pantothenic acid and, 197; salt and, 237; swollen glands as symptom of, 122; ulcers related to, 26;* hypoglycemia related to, 48; linoleic acid and, 156; pantothenic acid and, 34, 106; role of, in digestion, 100; stimulation of, 48, 117; stress and, 24, 25; triggered by sodium, 177–78; vitamin A and, 34; vitamin C and, 26, 35

Adrenal glandulars. *See* Glandulars, adrenal

Adrenaline, stress and, 24

Africans, diets of, 110

Aging, 134–48; alcohol related to, 145; as chronic disease, 147; attitudes toward life and, 147; cell function and, 135–37; effect of exercise on, 146; garlic as therapy for, 20; health and, 3, 134–35; improper diet related to, 139; lecithin as therapy for, 140; lifestyle and, 145; malnutrition and, 134,
147; pantothenic acid as therapy for, 140; premature, mineral deficiencies as cause of, 140; senility and, 134, 143 (*see also* Senility); skin test for, 134; vitamin C as therapy for, 140; vitamin E and, 139. *See also* Elderly

Airsickness, 192

Alcohol: aging related to, 145; as stressor, 24, 125; cell destruction and, 144; effect of, on adrenal glands, 48; emotional and mental problems caused by, 145–46; hypoglycemia related to, 48, 49, 146; magnesium depletion and, 225, 227; zinc depletion and, 239

Alcoholism: magnesium therapy for, 226

Alfalfa: as chelating agent, 97; as remedy for hiatal hernia, 104; benefits of, 6, 162; tablets: as aid to elimination, 107; as heart problem preventive, 143; as relief for bad breath, 108–109; as relief for perspiration odors, 108–109; as source of fiber, 111, 112; as therapy for arthritis, 162; for elimination, 151; recommended dosage, 162; with fortified drink, 156

Alfin-Slater, Roslyn, 85

Alka-Seltzer, 102

Allergies, 105–107; adrenal glands and, 105–106; as stressor, 23; as symptom of hypoglycemia, 49; as symptom of poor digestion, 166; bee pollen for relief of, 162; blood sugar levels related to, 49, 52; eosinophil test for, 106; food, 104, 105; from airborne allergens, 104–105; pantothenic acid and, 34, 106, 197, 198; salt and soda remedy for, 52; vitamin A and, 107; vitamin C and, 107–108, 205; vitamin E and, 107

Alpha tocopherol, 208–09

Altitude sickness, 226

Aluminum: accumulation related to calcium, 140; in antacids, poor effects of, 103

Alzheimer's disease, 202

American Academy of Medical Preventics (AAMP), 95, 96
American Cancer Society, 128
American Heart Association, 79
American Medical Association, 96, 146, 225
Amino acids: as body chemicals, 3; as chelating agents, 97; biological value of, 60; chelation therapy and, 94; deficiency of, in white flour, 47; essential, 59–60; negative nitrogen balance and, 61; nonessential, 60; protein and, 59
Ancestors, diet of, 8, 19–21. *See also* Primitive peoples
Anderson, Terence W., M.D., 123
Anemia: causes of, 6, 184, 192, 194, 199, 204, 209, 220, 223, 230; iron for, 5; liver as therapy for, 13; pernicious, 195–96; protein deficiency related to, 65
Angina, 95
Ankles, swollen, 113
Anitschkow, N., 79
Antacids, 102–103
Antibiotics: as cure for germ and viral diseases, 17; as stressor, 23; bacteria destruction by, 161; biotin and, 199; effects of, 109; given to children, 118; pantothenic acid and, 197; side effects of, 118–19; vitamin K and, 212
Antibodies, 118–19; folic acid and, 194; pantothenic acid and, 197; produced by thymus, 26; production of, 119: *protein and, 118, 122;* protein nature of, 72, 117; pyridoxine and, 192, 197; riboflavin and, 189; salt and soda remedy drink to produce, 117; thymus glandulars as therapy for, 164
Anticoagulant drugs: vitamin E and, 211; vitamin K and, 212, 213
Antihistamines, 107
"Antistress vitamin," 197
Anxiety, 202; as symptom of hypoglycemia, 48–49; effect of, on adrenal glands, 48; tryptophane as therapy for, 62
Apathy, 225
Appendicitis, 110, 111
Appetite, loss of, 184, 187, 199, 239
Arginine, 59–60
Arsenic, 204
Arteries, hardening of, 79, 193, 201, 222
Arteriosclerosis: blood sugar levels related to, 49; chelation therapy and, 94; defined, 19; malnutrition as cause of, 17; stress as cause of, 27; vitamin E to treat, 209
Arthritis: adrenal glands and, 48; alfalfa as therapy for, 162; calcium-phosphorus ratio and, 230; causes of, 125; chelation therapy and, 95; garlic as

therapy for, 20; Gerovital H_3 therapy for, 145; health related to, 2; infection related to, 125; malnutrition as cause of, 17; niacin to treat, 190; pantothenic acid and, 34, 140, 197, 198; prevention of, by silicon, 111; pyridoxine and, 192
Arthritis, rheumatoid, as symptom of hypoglycemia, 49
Arthritis and Folk Medicine (Jarvis), 112
Ascorbic acid. *See* Vitamin C
Ashmead, DeWayne, 140–41
Aslan, Ana, 145
Asthma: adrenal glands and, 48; blood sugar levels related to, 49, 52; remedy for, 52, 106; test for, 51
Atherosclerosis: as choline deficiency sympton, 201; bypass surgery and, 93–94, 96; chelation therapy and, 95; cholesterol and, 76, 79–80; defined, 19; experiments with eggs and, 79–80; fat and, 79–80, 83; lipoproteins and, 87, 90; malnutrition as cause of, 17; nutrition and, 79; predicted by chromium level, 219; prevention of, by silicon, 111; pyridoxine deficiency and, 87–88; sucrose as major cause of, 44, 46, 83; thyroid deficiency and, 92; triglycerides and, 90–91; vitamin C and, 86, 87
Atkins, Robert, 53, 121
Attitudes: aging and, 147; good health and, 3
Avidin, 199

B
Backaches, 64
Bacteria: antibiotics and, 19, 161; antibody deficiency and, 118; growth and acidophilus culture, 109; hydrochloric acid and, 103; intestinal: *effect of hydrochloric acid on, 121; growth related to fiber, 11; importance to health of, 109;* removal by white blood cells, 119; role of, in digestion, 101–102, 103, 109; vitamin A and, 119–20
Barbary root, in remedy, 20
Barnes, Broda, 52, 92
Barnet, Dr. Lewis E., 226
Bee pollen, 162
Beriberi, 187
Bile: lipoproteins and, 90; role of, in digestion, 99–100: *cholesterol and, 76; fats and, 83; salts: effect of lecithin on, 88; food allergies related to deficiency of, 105; production of, 190;* vitamin K deficiency and, 212
Bioflavonoids, 86; as water-soluble vitamin, 175, 213; best sources, 214–15; characteristics, 213; deficiency symptoms, 213–14; supplements to take,

215; toxicity, 214; what it does and
may do, 214
Biotin: as water-soluble vitamin, 175,
199; best sources, 199; characteristics,
199; deficiency symptoms, 199, 200;
manganese and, 228; supplements to
take, 199; toxicity, 199; what it does
and may do, 199
Birth defects, 194
Black tongue, 11
Bladder stones, 226
Bland, Jeffrey, 54, 136
Bleeding gums, 204, 216
Bloating, 100
Blood: clotting: *as cause of heart attacks,
87; liver and, 70; vitamin K and, 213;*
platelets, fats and, 83; sticky: *bioflavonoids and, 86; heart disease and, 87*
Blood pressure, high: garlic as therapy
for, 20; Gerovital H₃ therapy for, 145;
potassium and, 232; smoking related
to, 145; stress as cause of, 27
Blood sugar levels: adrenal glands and,
42; calcium deficiency related to, 51–
52; defined, 41–42; diabetes and, 42,
164; folic acid as treatment, 195; food
selection for proper, 56–58; fortified
drinks for, 149, 154, 156; importance
of breakfast to, 58; insulin and, 41,
42; low (*see* Hypoglycemia); oxygen
deficiency related to, 51–52; protein
and, 41–42; pyridoxine deficiency related to, 192; sugar and, 42–43, 163;
tolerance factor for (GTF), 49, 50, 51,
54. *See also* Glucose
Bone(s): calcium: *removed in, antacids
related to, 102–103; calcium dosage
for, 141;* degeneration of, 21; fractures, protein deficiency related to,
68; tissue: *loss during menopause,
141; loss while dieting, 141. See also*
Osteoporosis
Bone meal, 163
Brain: cholesterol and, 76; damage, high
protein diet as therapy for, 72; function, smoking related to, 145; tumor
related to blood sugar levels, 49
Brain Bio Center (Princeton, N.J.), 37
Bran: as remedy for hiatal hernia, 104;
as remedy for poor elimination, 111;
as source of fiber, 111; as source of
minerals, 54; high phosphorus content
of, 111
Bread, contents of, 118, 158, 167
Breakfast: elimination and, 176; impor-
tance of eating, 55–56; suggestions,
157, 170–71
Breast cysts, 210
Breast milk, 176, 202, 215
Breath, bad, 108–109, 190
Brewer's yeast. *See* Yeast, brewer's

Bricklin, Mark, 117
Briggs, George, 18
Brodribb, A. J. M., 110
Bronchitis, 20
Bruises, 204, 214
Bruxism: calcium and, 217; pantothenic
acid and, 198, 217
Bulgarian people, diet of, 109
Burkitt, Dennis, 110
Burns, 37, 66, 211, 239–40
Bursitis, 64, 196
Butter: as part of Hunza diet, 9; as
saturated fat, 83–84; atherosclerosis
and, 80; calorie, carbohydrate, and
protein guide, 74–75; cholesterol and,
78; contents and qualities of, 8, 83,
84; for lunch, 159; recipe for extend-
ing, 84
B vitamins: added to white flour, 47; as
cancer preventive, 131; as therapy for:
*pellagra, 12–13; poor elimination, 67,
108; swollen glands, 122;* as water-
soluble vitamins, 175; effect of, on immune system, 151; fat metabolism
and, 88, 156; fortified drinks with,
153; good health and, 8, 13; hair
health related to, 68; heart disease
prevention and, 87–88; in brewer's
yeast, 163; in eggs, 20; in liver, 164;
in wheat, 19; liver and, 70, 131; nail
health related to, 68; nervous system
and, 34; stress and, 24, 34, 129, 151;
sources of, 107; storage, 70; sucrose
and, 46, 88; synthesis of, 109. *See also*
Vitamins; specific B vitamins

C
Cadmium, 205, 216, 234, 240
Caffeine: as stressor, 24, 125; effect of,
on adrenal glands, 48
Calcium: aluminum related to removal
of, 140; best sources, 177, 217; bone
fractures related to lack of, 68–69;
characteristics, 215–16; deficiency, 70:
*adrenal exhaustion related to, 51–52;
as cause of stress, 129; during pregnancy, 141; dowager's hump related
to, 141; liver damage related to, 70;
while nursing, 141;* deficiency symptoms, 176, 216, 225; deposits: *antacids
related to, 102; chelation therapy and,
94;* dosage for bone density, 141; in
blackstrap molasses, 43, 162; in bone
meal, 163; in brewer's yeast, 62, 163;
in lecithin, 163; in liver, 163, 164; in
skim milk, 165; in wheat germ, 62;
nail health related to, 68; osteoporosis
related to, 68; removal from bones,
antacids related to, 102; role in heart
activity, 143; supplements to take,
217; taken with magnesium, 177, 217,

225, 226; taken with phosphorus, 176
–77, 207, 208, 215, 217–18, 226, 229,
230; taken with vitamin C, 206; therapy for menopause, 141–42; toxicity,
217; what it does and may do, 216–17
Calcium carbonate, 103
Calcium gluconate, 152, 163
Calcium pantothenate. *See* Pantothenic
acid
California Medical Association, 106
Calories: guide to, 73; in fructose, 163
Cameron, Ewan, 126–27
Cancer, 125–32; acidophilus therapy for,
129; bone, Adelle Davis and, 14; B vitamins as preventive of, 131; causes
of, 117, 227; cells, 119, 137; described,
125–26; effects of sugar on, 129, 130–
31; estrogen therapy related to, 142;
garlic as therapy for, 20; health related to, 2; immune system against,
116–17; immunotherapy for, 126;
inositol and, 203; interferon studies
and, 128; lung, smoking related to,
145; malnutrition as cause of, 17;
mega-vitamin therapy for, 129–30;
mineral therapy for, 129–30; nontoxic
therapy for, 130; of the colon: *aluminum as cause of, 103; fiber deficiency
related to, 110; intestinal bacteria related to, 102;* polyunsaturated fats
and, 85; protein as preventive of, 131;
selenium as preventive of, 130, 131,
234; skin: *PABA as preventive of, 200;*
stress and, 36, 129; thymus therapy
for, 122; vitamin A as preventive of,
205; vitamin C and, 125, 126–27; vitamin C as preventive of, 131, 205; vitamin E as preventive of, 130, 131, 139
Canker sores, 190, 191
Cannon, Walter B., 30
Carbohydrates: blood sugar levels and,
42; cholesterol manufacture and, 77;
complementarity of, with protein, 73;
digestion of, 100; dysfunction and
breast cancer, 131; for lunch, 158;
guide, 73; heart disease and, 80, 90;
lipoproteins and, 90; metabolism of, in
liver, 70; pancreatic enzymes as digestant of, 166; protein intake related
to, 72–73; refined: *content of, in popular foods, 45–46; diet and, 47; effect
of, on diabetes, 55; hypoglycemia related to, 48*
Carbon monoxide, 204
Carcinogens, 204
Cardiac arrest, 201
Cardiovascular disease. *See* Heart disease
Carotene, 184, 185
Caseinate, 165
Castelli, William P., 90

Cataracts, protein deficiency and, 65;
riboflavin as preventive of, 189; vitamin C as preventive of, 205
Celiac disease, 212
Cell(s): destruction and alcohol, 144;
function: *aging and, 135–37; cancer
and, 119, 137; diabetes and, 137; lecithin and, 89;* membranes, cholesterol and, 76; protection, vitamin E
and, 136, 137; white blood: *cancer
and, 126; storage of, in lymph glands,
121; T-lymphocytes, 119;* therapy,
143–44
Cereals: as source of fiber, 111; cholesterol and, 78; for breakfast, 157; use
of freshly ground, 167
Ceroid pigment, 84
Cheese: atherosclerosis and, 80; calorie,
carbohydrate, and protein guide, 73–
74; cottage, 20, 158; for vegetarians,
63–74; meal suggestions, 158, 161.
See also Milk products
Chelation therapy, 94, 95, 97
Chelation Therapy (Halstead), 95
Chemicals: as cause of cancer, 117;
avoidance of, 132; detoxification of, by
liver, 70, 131; effect of, on body, 4; oxidative damage of, 137. *See also* Preservatives
Chemicals (body), 3; deficiencies, research into, 12; degenerative diseases
and, 17
Chemotherapy, as stressor, 24
Cheraskin (M.D.), 49
Chest pain, 145
Children: acidophilus establishment, in
nursing, 109; effects of antibiotics on,
118; flu vaccine responses in, 138; immune systems of, 118, 138; importance of protein to, 71–72; life
expectancy in, 139–40; need for vitamin E in, 137; refined foods for, 160;
rheumatism in, egg yolk remedy
for, 118; vitamin C dosages for,
125
Chittam bark, in remedy, 20
Chloride, 218, 236
Cholesterol: as stressor, 129; atherosclerosis and, 76; biotin and, 199; calcium and, 216–17; choline and, 201;
chromium and, 218; deficiency of, in
skim milk, 88; diet and, 76, 78–79, 80
–81; digestion, alfalfa as therapy for,
162; facts about, 76–77, 79; fat metabolism and, 83, 89; heart disease and,
76, 78–79, 91; in eggs, 20, 61, 76, 78–
80; inositol and, 203; lecithin and, 88,
89, 140, 201; levels, tests for, 91; niacin and, 190; removal by pectin and
lignin, 111; thyroid deficiency and, 92;
vitamin C and, 87

Choline: as chelating agent, 97; as water-soluble vitamin, 175, 201; best sources, 202; characteristics, 201; cirrhosis related to deficiency in, 70; deficiency: *as cause of anemia, 223; symptoms, 201;* in eggs, 79; in lecithin, 164; inositol and, 203; manganese and, 228; supplements to take, 202; toxicity, 202; what it does and may do, 201–202

Chromium: best sources, 219; characteristics, 218; deficiency symptoms, 218; glucose tolerance factor related to, 54; heart disease and, 229; importance of, for diabetes, 53–54; in brewer's yeast, 163; in molasses, 43; supplements to take, 219; toxicity, 219; what it does and may do, 218–19

Cigarettes. *See* Nicotine; Smoking

Circulation (blood), 139, 146

Cirrhosis. *See* Liver cirrhosis

Citrus bioflavonoids. *See* Bioflavonoids

Clark, Linda, 34

Claudication, 95

Cobalamin. *See* Vitamin B-12

Cobalt, 195, 219

Coburn, Al, 118

Cod liver oil, 8

Colds: as symptom of scurvy, 123; garlic as therapy for, 20; salt and soda remedy drink for, 117; stress and, 24, 26, 129; sucrose and, 47; vitamin A therapy for, 120; vitamin C therapy for, 120, 123, 205. *See also* Flu; Viruses

Colic, 232

Colitis, 113, 212

Collagen, 204, 220, 228

Colon: cancer of, fiber deficiency related to, 110; diverticulitis of, 108, 110; effects of antacids on, 103

Color perception, and vitamin B-12, 196

Confusion and disorientation, 225

Constipation, 107–108; aluminum as cause of, 103; choline as cure, 201; effect of laxatives on, 107, 108; enemas and, 108; inositol deficiency and, 203; PABA deficiency and, 200; pantothenic acid deficiency and, 197; potassium deficiency and, 231; relief of, 107, 108; swollen lymph glands as symptom of, 121, 122; thiamine as cure, 187; water in intestine related to, 102

Consumer Nutrition Center, USDA, 180

Convulsions, 191–92, 225

Copper: balance with zinc, 178, 221, 241; best sources, 220; characteristics, 219; deficiency: *as cause of anemia, 6, 223; symptoms, 219–20;* hair health related to, 68; in molasses, 43; supplements to take, 220–21; toxicity, 220; what it does and may do, 220

Coronary disease. *See* Heart disease

Coronary thrombosis, 87

Cortisone: cholesterol and, 76; interferon deficiency related to, 129; magnesium and, 227; pantothenic acid and, 197; therapy for arthritis, 125; vitamin C and, 107

Cousins, Norman, 30–31

"Cradle cap," 192

Cream, 8, 80. *See also* Milk; Milk products

Cretinism, 221

Cureton, Thomas K., 165

Cyanocobalamin. *See* Vitamin B-12

Cybila Laboratory, 144

Cystine, 70, 79

D

Dandruff, 233, 234

Davis, Adelle, 14, 113, 131

Day blindness, 184

Death, from choline deficiency, 201

Delirium tremens, 226

Dementia, as pellagra symptom, 190

Depression: as symptom of hypoglycemia, 48–49; choline to treat, 202; Gerovital H$_3$ therapy for, 145; magnesium deficiency as cause of, 225; methionine deficiency related to, 61; PABA deficiency as cause of, 200; pyridoxine to treat, 193; tryptophane as therapy for, 62

Dermatitis, 190, 192, 199

deVries, Herbert, 32

Diabetes: blood sugar levels and, 42, 49; cell function related to, 137; chromium as preventive, 218–19; defined, 42; effect of vitamin C on, 54–55; glucose tolerance factor and, 54; health related to, 2; importance of minerals for, 53–54; magnesium, 54; malnutrition as cause of, 17; manganese deficiency and, 228; pancreas glandulars as therapy for, 164; potassium and, 232; retinopathy and, 54; sucrose and, 44, 46, 47; vitamin E to treat, 209, 211

Diarrhea: aluminum as cause of, 103; as food allergy symptom, 105; as pellagra symptom, 190; copper deficiency as cause of, 219; garlic as remedy for, 20; gelatin as remedy for, 113; hydrochloric acid tablets for, 103; prevention of, 103

Dieting: as stressor, 125; effects of extremes in, 146; fortified drink for, 155–56; nutrition during, 146; tissue loss as result of, 141; "war on weight" plan, 150, 155–56. *See also* Fasting; Weight

Digestion, 99–114; aids, 166; emotions related to, 104; health and, 3; importance of bacteria to, 109; poor (*see* Indigestion); process of, 99–100; supplements for, 151

Digestive enzymes. See Enzymes, digestive

Dinner suggestions, 160, 172

Diphtheria, 17

Diseases, degenerative: adrenal glands and, 48; chronic, 19; defined, 17; effect of protein on, 117; freedom from, by primitive peoples, 22; malnutrition as cause of, 19; poor health as cause of, 2, 5; poor nutrition and, 3, 9, 18, 115; resistance to, vitamin E and, 137; sugar as contributor to, 19

Diuretics, magnesium and, 227

Dizziness: blood sugar levels related to, 48–49, 50; choline deficiency as cause of, 201; garlic as therapy for, 20; iron toxicity and, 224

DNA, 192, 194, 196, 230, 239

Dr. Wilfred Shute's Vitamin E Book, 93

Dowager's hump, 141

Dream recall, pyridoxine and, 194

Drinks, fortified, 13, 123, 149, 151–55, 158; antistress recipes, 153; brewer's yeast in, 13; digestion of, 166; for meals, 157, 161; fructose as sweetener in, 163; liver powder in, 13, 39; proper eating patterns and, 155; protein in, 153–54. See also Serenity Cocktail

Dropsy, 162

Drugs: as mask of symptoms, 4; as stressor, 125; detoxification of, by liver, 70, 131; effect of, on adrenal glands, 48, 51–52; effect of vitamin C on, 55; hypoglycemia related to, 48

Dry eye disease, 184

Dunn Nutritional Laboratory, 120

E

Ear infection, Vitamin A deficiency and, 184

Eczema, 83, 105, 197, 203

Edema, 67–68, 192, 193, 214, 220

EDTA, 94

Eggs: allergy to, 105; artificial: *experiments with, 79; heart disease and, 78; ingredients in, 78;* as abater of pellagra, 9, 10; as heart disease preventive, 20, 143; as ideal protein, 61; as source of lecithin, 70; as source of tryptophane, 62; atherosclerosis and, 79–80; calorie, carbohydrate, and protein guide, 73–74; cholesterol in, 20, 61, 76, 77, 79; DNA in, 20; experiments with, 79; for breakfast, 56, 157; for vegetarians, 63–64; good health and, 8, 13; in fortified drinks, 117,

118, 154; ingredients in, 20, 79; lecithin in, 61; RNA in, 20; used by our ancestors, 20; yolk: *fat content in, 83; increase in antibodies related to, 66; lecithin in, 164*

Elastin, 220

Elderly: bone density in, 141; dietary needs of, 69; flu vaccine responses in, 138; immune systems of, 138; life expectancy in, 140; osteoporosis in, 68–69, 141; protein needs of, 69; senility in, 143 (*see also* Senility). See also Aging

Elimination, 99–114; breakfast and, 107; fiber related to process of, 111; in children, 107; intestinal transit time of, 110, 111; poor, protein deficiency related to, 66, 67; regularity, 107; remedies for, 111, 112; role of large intestine in, 101–102; skin as primary organ of, 108; supplements for, 151; water conservation and, 102

Emotions: B vitamins and, 34; digestion related to, 104; factor affecting immune system, 117; problems caused by alcohol, 145–46; stress and, 26, 28–31, 125

Emphysema: as symptom of protein deficiency, 65; malnutrition as cause of, 17; smoking related to, 145

Encephalitis, 124

Enemas, recipe for, 108

Environmental Protection Agency, 168

Enzymes, digestive: deficiency of, in elderly, 69; elimination and, 108; food allergies related to deficiency of, 105, 106; for relief of gas, 104; process of, 99–100; protein and, 66, 104, 147; tablets (*see* Hydrochloric acid; Pancreatic enzymes)

Enzymes, pancreatic, 103, 151, 156, 166. See also Enzymes, digestive; Hydrochloric acid

Epilepsy, 49, 192, 195, 226, 228

Ershoff, Benjamin, 38–39

Esophagus, effects of alcohol on, 146

Estrogen, 76, 142, 211

Exercise: aging related to, 145; effects of, 146; for bone density, 141; health and, 32, 81; lipoproteins and, 90; stress and, 24, 26, 32; vitamin E and, 36; weight loss and, 67. See also Muscle(s); Physical

Eyes, 65, 120

F

Faintness, 48–49, 50

Fasting, as stressor, 24, 26. See also Dieting

Fat(s): cholesterol manufacture and, 77; digestion of, 99–100; heart disease and, 81; hydrogenated, 82: *athero-sclerosis and, 83; experiments with, 82; heart disease and, 80;* in meat, 62; metabolism of, 88–89: *heart disease and, 89; in liver, 70; lecithin and, 89;* pancreatic enzymes as digestant of, 166; polyunsaturated, 81–82: *as vitamin sources, 84; cancer and, 85; experiments with, 84; harmful effects of, 84–85; oils containing, 83; oxidation and, 81–82, 84; reproductive functions and, 85;* protein intake related to, 72–73; pyridoxin deficiency and, 156; removal by pectin and lignin, 111; saturated, 81–82: *butter as, 84; lard as, 84; meat fat as, 83–84; reproductive functions and, 83;* unsaturated, 81–82: *as vitamin sources, 84; oils containing, 83; rancidity and, 82; vitamin E added to, 82. See also* Oil(s)

Fatigue: as food allergy symptom, 105; as indicator of poor health, 4; as symptom of poor digestion, 100, 166; blood sugar levels related to, 50; iron toxicity as cause of, 224; mineral deficiency as cause of, 140; protein deficiency related to, 65; vitamin deficiency related to, 190, 192, 200

Fat-soluble vitamins, 174–75

Fatty acids: as body chemicals, 3; unsaturated: *avocado as source of, 159; linoleic acid as, 154; linolenic acid as, 154*

Federal Trade Commission, 78

Federation of the American Society for Experimental Biology, 82

Fertility, vitamin C as therapy for, 205

Fiber, 110–112; as aid to elimination, 107; as arthritis preventive, 111; cellulose in, 112; deficiency as cause of disease, 110–111; deficiency of, in white flour, 47; in alfalfa, 162; intestinal transit time and, 110, 111; process of elimination related to, 111; sources of, 111, 112

Fibrinolysis, 210

Fish, calorie, carbohydrate, and protein guide, 74–75

Flax seed meal, as remedy for elimination, 112

Flour: soy, good health and, 8; wheat, 19, 167; white: *deficiencies of, 46–47, 180; effect of, on immune system, 22; heart disease and, 80*

Flu: garlic as therapy for, 20; sucrose and, 4; vaccines, 137. *See also* Colds; Viruses

Fluoride, 221

Folacin. *See* Folic acid

Folate. *See* Folic acid

Folic acid, 6; as water-soluble vitamin, 175, 194; best sources, 195; characteristics, 194; deficiency: *as cause of anemia, 192, 223; symptoms, 194, 200;* immune system and, 202; in antibody formation, 197; supplements to take, 195; toxicity, 195; vitamin B-12 and, 196; vitamin C and, 204; what it does and may do, 194–95

Folinic acid, 204

Food(s): as cause of cancer, 117; assimilation, 99, 101, 102; cholesterol and, 77; environmental contaminants and, 22; for breakfast, 157; for dinner, 160–61; for lunch, 157–60; for proper blood sugar levels, 56–58; for snacks, 161; intake, effect of exercise on, 146; nonessential, 18; proper eating patterns of, 155; unprocessed, 168

Food and Drug Administration, 96

Food and Nutrition Board, 179, 235

Fredericks, Carlton, 46, 49, 96, 120, 131, 135, 139, 142, 186

Friedman, Meyer, 91

Frostbite, 214

Fructose: as ingredient in fortified drinks, 152, 154; as sweetener, 163, 168; blood sugar levels and, 42; in protein powders, 165

Fruit(s): as abater of pellagra, 10; as part of Hunza diet, 9; as source of fiber, 111; dried, used by our ancestors, 19; for breakfast, 157; for lunch, 158, 159, 160; for snacks, 161; good health and, 13; pesticides removal from, 160, 168; raising fresh, 168; raw: *as remedy for hiatal hernia, 104; as sources of B vitamins, 107*

Fungi, 119–20

G

Galfant, S., 136

Gallstones, 111, 201–202

Gangrene: chelation therapy and, 95; vitamin E to treat, 209

Garlic, 20, 97

Gas: bad breath related to, 108; hiatal hernias related to, 104; lack of bile as source of, 100; pains, alfalfa as therapy for, 162; perspiration odor related to, 108; poor digestion and, 100, 101–102, 166

Gastritis, 100, 166

Gelatin, as remedy for diarrhea, 113

Geriatric Institute (Bucharest), 145

Germs: dislike of, by garlic, 20; factor affecting immune system, 117; vitamin A as defense against, 119–20

Gerovital H_3 therapy, 144–45

Gertler, Menard, 92

Gingivitis, 216

Ginter, Emil, 86–87
Glandulars, 122–23, 144, 163–64; adrenal: *as therapy for adrenal glands, 144, 164; as therapy for arthritis, 125; as therapy for asthma, 106; benefits of, 106, 164;* pancreas, benefits of, 164; thymus, benefits of, 122, 151, 164. *See also* Meats, organ
Glaucoma, 52
Glucose: defined, 41; importance of, 43; levels in blood (*see* Blood sugar levels); liver and, 70; tolerance: *improved by pyridoxine, 193;* tolerance factor (GTF), 54; tolerance tests, 49–50, 51; vitamin C and utilization of, 54
Glycogen, 192
Goiter, 221, 222
Goldberger, Joseph, 9–10
Gout, 197, 198
Grains: allergy to, 105; as part of Hunza diet, 9; as protein food, 63; as source of fiber, 111; cholesterol and, 78; in bread, 158, 167; protein complementary of, 63; use of, 167
Gravity, and calcium balance, 215–16
Gray hair, 197, 198, 200
"Growth vitamin," 184
Gunkel, Herman, 112
Gutterman, Jordan, 128
Guy, Walter, 103
Gyland, Stephen, 48, 49

H
Hair: health, 3: *B vitamins and, 68; copper and, 68; fats and, 83; oil for, 154; protein and, 64, 66, 68; vitamins and, 68; zinc and, 68;* loss, 219; *methionine deficiency related to,* 61
Halstead, Bruce, 95
Harman, Denham, 137
Harrell, Ruth, 72
Harvard Medical School, 10
Hauser, Gaylord, 135
Hayflick, Leonard, 136
Headaches: as symptom of hypoglycemia, 48–49; as symptom of poor digestion, 100, 166; blood sugar levels related to, 50; choline deficiency as cause of, 201; garlic as therapy for, 20; iron toxicity as cause of, 224; niacin deficiency as cause of, 190; PABA deficiency as cause of, 200. *See also* Migraines
Healing Factor, The (Stone), 36, 54, 139
Health, 1–6; comprehensive program for, 149–69; fortified protein drinks for, 151–56; good: *of our ancestors, 19; indicators of, 3; nutrition as insurance for, 15;* meals for, 157–61; poor, 3, 4; proper eating patterns for, 155–56;

rules to live by, 166–69; "shotgun approach" to, 5; supplements for, 161–66
Heart: attacks: *chelation therapy and, 95; confused with hypoglycemia, 52–53; copper as preventive, 220; eggs and, 20; fat metabolism and, 89; lipoproteins and, 89, 90; magnesium as preventive, 232; potassium as preventive, 232; potassium deficiency and, 231; stress related to, 146;* disease, 76–85: *artificial eggs and, 78; bypass surgery and, 93–94, 96; carbohydrates and, 90; cell therapy and, 143–44; chelation therapy and, 95; cholesterol and, 76, 77, 91; chromium as preventive, 229; effect of chlorine on, 21; eggs and, 20, 80; fats and, 81; fiber deficiency related to, 110; garlic as therapy for, 20; heart transplants and, 93; high cholesterol foods and, 88; history of, 93; magnesium as protection against, 37–38; manganese as preventive, 229; margarine and, 78; niacin to treat, 190; nutrition and, 76, 77, 80; potassium as protection against, 37–38; selenium as preventive, 229, 234; stress as cause of, 37–38; sucrose as cause of, 44, 46, 88; thyroid deficiency and, 92; triglycerides and, 90; vitamin B and, 87–88; vitamin C as preventive, 205; vitamin E as protection against, 37, 85–86; vitamin E to treat, 209, 211;* palpitations: *blood sugar levels related to, 50–51; calcium deficiency as cause of, 216; choline deficiency as cause of, 201;* problems: *alcohol and, 146; as symptom of hypoglycemia, 48–49; garlic as therapy for, 20; health related to, 2; lecithin as preventive, 140, 143; potassium as preventive, 143; preventing, after menopause, 142–43; smoking related to, 145; vitamin E dosage for, 139. See also* Angina; Coronary thrombosis; Strokes
Heartburn, 100, 102, 166
Heat stroke, 178
Hemoglobin, 220, 223, 224
Hemorrhaging, 213; stress as cause of, 35; vitamin C loss and, 25–26, 27
Hemorrhoids, 214; fiber deficiency related to, 110–111
Herbs, used by our ancestors, 20
Hernia, 104, 111
Herpes, 196
Hillman Hospital (Birmingham, Alabama), 11, 12
Histamine, food allergies and, 105, 198
Histidine, as essential amino acid, 59–60
Hives, related to blood sugar levels, 49
Holmes, Thomas H., 32–33

Honey: as sweetener, 168; blood sugar levels and, 42–43; used by our ancestors, 19

Hope, Bob, 135

Hormones, 24, 26, 190

Hunzas, diet of, 9

Hydrochloric acid: after drinking fortified drink, 156; as destroyer of infection, 121; deficiency of: *food allergies related to, 105; in elderly, 69;* elimination and, 108; lack of, as cause of hiatal hernias, 103; niacin deficiency and, 190; pantothenic acid deficiency and, 197; protein assimilation and, 66; pyridoxine and, 192; role of, in digestion, 99–100, 103, 104, 177–78, 187, 194; tablets, 104: *as digestion aid, 151, 166; as therapy for protein deficiency, 147; for prevention of diarrhea, 103; recommended dosage, 166;* ulcers, caused by, 103; vitamin B-12 and, 195. *See also* Enzymes, digestive; Enzymes, pancreatic

Hypercalcemia, 217

Hyperglycemia, 218

Hypertension, 201, 226, 236–37

Hypochondria, 202

Hypoglycemia, 41–58; alcohol addiction as cause of, 146; causes of, 47–48; chromium deficiency and, 218; defined, 42; in children, 53; night remedy for, 52; protein deficiency related to, 65–66; related to sucrose, 41, 42, 47; symptoms of, 48–49, 50–53; tests for, 49, 50, 51. *See also* Blood sugar levels; Glucose

Hypoprothrombinemia, 212–13

Hypothyroidism, 221

Hypothyroidism: The Unsuspected Illness (Barnes), 92

I

Immune System, 115–33; antibodies and, 118–19; biotin and, 199; cancer and, 126, 137; choline and, 202; effects of diet on, 115, 138–39; effects of protein on, 71, 117; folic acid and, 195, 202; gland and organ meats and, 122–23; interferon and, 128–29; iron and, 223; methionine and, 202; pyridoxine and, 192; resistance factor of, 116–17; riboflavin and, 189; role of thymus gland in, 119; role of white blood cells in, 119; sucrose and, 47, 130; supplements for, 151; thiamine and, 187; thymus glandulars as therapy for, 164; vitamin A and, 119–21; vitamin B-12 and, 202; vitamin C and, 120; vitamin E and, 137

Indigestion: antacid use for, 102; as symptom of hypoglycemia, 48–49; as symptom of poor digestion, 100, 166; garlic as therapy for, 20; lack of bile as source of, 100; niacin deficiency as cause of, 190: protein deficiency related to, 66. *See also* Digestion

Infection(s): acidophilus culture and, 109; antibiotics and, 109, 118–19; antibody deficiency and, 118; arthritis related to, 125; as symptom of scurvy, 123; bacterial, 70; effect of, related to age, 137; garlic as therapy for, 20; hydrochloric acid as destroyer of, 121; mineral deficiencies as cause of, 140; protein and, 66, 72, 117, 122; remedy drinks against, 117; remedy for urinary tract, 112–13; resistance to, 3, 109; viral, stress related to, 129; vitamin A and, 120; vitamin C and, 120

Influenza. *See* Flu

Inositol: as chelating agent, 97; as water-soluble vitamin, 175, 202; best sources, 203; cancer and, 203; characteristics, 202–203; deficiency symptoms, 203; in eggs, 79; in lecithin, 164, 202; supplements to take, 203; toxicity, 203; what it does and may do, 203

Insomnia. *See* Sleeplessness

Insulin: chromium and, 218; sensitivity to: *pantothenic acid deficiency as cause of, 197;* vitamin C and, 204; vitamin E and, 211; zinc and, 240

Interferon, 128–29, 205

Intestine(s): effect of laxatives on, 107; infection of, 125; large, 101–102; linings of, 119; small, 100–101

"Intrinsic factor," 195

Iodine, 168; best sources, 222; characteristics, 221; deficiency symptoms, 221, 222–23; manganese and, 228; supplements to take, 222; toxicity, 222; what it does and may do, 222

Iron: best sources, 224; characteristics, 223; deficiency: *as cause of anemia, 192; symptoms, 223;* for anemia, 5; in molasses, 43; storage, in liver, 70; supplements to take, 224–25; toxicity, 224; what it does and may do, 223–24

Irritability: as symptom of copper deficiency, 220; as symptom of food allergy, 105; as symptom of hypoglycemia, 48–49; as symptom of magnesium deficiency, 225; as symptom of niacin deficiency, 190; as symptom of PABA deficiency, 200; as symptom of poor digestion, 100, 166; blood sugar levels related to, 50

Isoleucine, 59

J

Jarvis (D.C., M.D.), 112

Johns Hopkins Hospital, 72
Joints, 95, 140; swollen and painful, 204

K
Kalita, Dwight, 4
Kelp: as chelating agent, 97; thyroid deficiency and, 93; use of, 167–68
Kidney(s), 112–113; diet and, 113; disease: *choline deficiency as cause of,* 201; effect of calcium carbonate on, 103; effect of fluids on, 112; failure: *sodium deficiency as cause of, 236;* hardening of, stress as cause of, 27; stones: *magnesium as preventive, 192, 206, 226; pyridoxine as preventive, 192, 206; vitamin C and, 13;* urine alkalinity related to, 112
Kilbourne, Edwin, 129
Klenner, Frederick R., 113, 124, 125
Know Your Nutrition (Clark), 34
Koch, Robert, 11
Kummerow, Fred A., 78, 82
Kunin, Richard, 70

L
Lactic acid, 187
Lactose, 43
Lancet, the, 236
Lard, 82, 83–84
Laxatives, 107, 108
Lead, 94, 111, 205, 216, 224, 234, 240
Lecithin: as chelating agent, 97; as heart problem preventive, 143; as ingredient in fortified drinks, 152, 154; as phosphatide, 89; as source of choline, 70, 201, 202; as source of inositol, 203; as therapy for aging, 140; as therapy for liver regeneration, 131; benefits of, 164; cell functioning and, 89; cholesterol and, 88, 89; dosage, 140; for cholesterol levels, 140; for heart health, 140; in eggs, 61, 79; linoleic acid and, 88; phosphorus-calcium imbalance in, 163; pyridoxine and formation of, 87
Legumes, 63, 97
Leslie, Constance R., 87
Let's Get Well (Davis), 113, 131
Leucine, 59
Lignin, 111
Lindberg Nutritional Service, 1, 15
Lindquist, (M.D.), 120
Linkletter, Art and Lois, 135
Linoleic acid, 88, 154
Linolenic acid, 154
Lipoproteins: atherosclerosis and, 87; cholesterol and, 77; heart attacks related to, 89; lecithin as, 89; tests for, 90
Liver (body): antibody production and, 118; cirrhosis of: *choline deficiency re-*

lated to, 70; dietary cure for, 131; protein deficiency related to, 65, 70; damage, related to protein deficiency, 70; diet for regeneration of, 131; effects of alcohol on, 146; functions of, 70, 131; metabolism related to, 69–70; problems, cell therapy for, 144; stress and, 38–39
Liver (food): as abater of pellagra, 10; as builder of hemoglobin, 39; as therapy for anemia, 13; good health and, 13; powder: *as source of minerals, 54; as therapy for liver regeneration, 131; in fortified drinks, 13, 39;* raw: *benefits of, 164; for immune system, 151; for physical fitness, 150; for stress, 150, 164–65; in fortified drinks, 152, 153; phosphorus-calcium imbalance in, 163; recommended dosage, 165*
Loomis, H., 90
Low Blood Sugar and You (Fredericks), 46
Lunch suggestions, 157, 171
Lungs: as barriers to disease, 119; infections, effect of vitamin A on, 120; ozone-induced damage to, vitamin E as defense against, 137
Lymph glands, swollen, 121–22
Lysine, 59

M
Macronutrients, 176
Magnesium: as heart attack preventive, 232; as kidney stone preventive, 192; best sources, 227; characteristics, 225; deficiency, 70: *as cause of anemia, 223; in American diet, 70; in white flour, 47; phosphorus deficiency and, 230; symptoms, 225;* deodorizing properties of, 109; importance of, for diabetes, 53–54; in molasses, 43; loss through chelation therapy, 94–95; nail health related to, 68; oxide: *as ingredient in fortified drink, 152; benefits of, 165;* ratio with calcium, 177, 215, 217, 225; stress and, 37; supplements to take, 227; therapy for menopause, 141–42; toxicity, 227; what it does and may do, 225–27
Malnutrition: aging and, 134, 147; artificial eggs and, 78–79; as cause of diseases, 3, 9, 17, 18; defined, 115; immune system suppression and, 115; in elderly, 69; swollen glands as symptom of, 122
Maltose, 42
Manganese: as antioxidant, 139; as heart disease preventive, 229; best sources, 229; characteristics, 228; deficiency of, in white flour, 47; deficiency symptoms, 228; importance of, for diabetes, 53–54; loss through chelation

therapy, 94–95; supplements to take, 229; toxicity, 229; what it does and may do, 228–29

Margarine: as health hazard, 82, 84; as hydrogenated fat, 82; cholesterol and, 78; heart disease and, 79

Martin (M.D.), 49

McCarrison, Sir Robert, 9, 101

M. D. Anderson Hospital and Tumor Institute, 128

Meal suggestions, 170–73; breakfast, 170–71; dinner, 172; lunch, 171; snacks, 172–73

Meat(s): additives, 62; as abater of pellagra, 9, 10; calorie, carbohydrate, and protein guide, 74–75; cholesterol and, 78; for lunch, 158, 159; good health and, 13; increase in antibodies related to, 66; lean, as source of niacin, 12; natural, used by our ancestors, 21; organ, 122–23 (*see also* Glandulars)

Meat loaf, recipe for, 172

Melanin, 220

Meniere's Syndrome, 49, 52

Meningitis, 124

Menopause, 49, 141–43, 210

Menstrual disorders: bioflavonoids as treatment, 214; magnesium as treatment, 226; pyridoxine as treatment, 193; vitamin A deficiency and, 185

Menstruation, and iron deficiency, 225

Mental: good health and, 3; health related to, 2; illness: *folic acid as treatment, 194; niacin deficiency as cause of, 190; pyridoxine deficiency as cause of, 192; vitamin B-12 deficiency as cause of, 196;* problems: *alcohol as cause of, 145–46; as symptom of hypoglycemia, 48–49; mineral deficiency as cause of, 140; protein deficiency related to, 71–72;* retardation, 192; state, health and, 2, 3

Mercury, 204, 234

Mertz, Walter, 54

Metabolism: fats and, 83; hypoglycemia related to, 48; liver and, 69–70; stress and, 24; wheat germ oil and, 166

Metchnikoff, Ilya, 109

Methionine: as essential amino acid, 59; choline and, 201; content in protein powders, 165; deficiency, 70: *in soybeans, 62; related to liver damage, 70;* immune system and, 202; in skim milk, 61

Miami Symposium on Theoretical Aspects of Aging, 136

Micronutrients, 176

Migraine(s), 49, 50, 52, 191. *See also* Headaches

Milk, 8; allergy to, 105; as abater of pellagra, 9, 11; as part of Hunza diet, 9; as protein food, 61; as source of tryptophane, 62; atherosclerosis and, 80; calorie, carbohydrate, and protein guide, 73–74; cholesterol and, 78–79; fat content in, 83; for breakfast, 55–56, 157; for lunch, 160; for vegetarians, 63–64; increase in antibodies related to, 66; in fortified drinks, 117, 118, 152–155; mother's, 71, 141; powdered skim (nonfat), 167: *as complement to brewer's yeast, 165; as source of methionine, 61; benefits of, 165; cholesterol deficiency in, 88; formulas for babies, 78; in bread, 158; in fortified drinks, 152, 153, 155; linoleic acid deficiency in, 88; to fortify peanut butter, 159;* protein complementarity of, 63; pyridoxine deficiency and, 87–88; raw and pasteurized compared, 21; used by our ancestors, 20; vitamin D enriched, 208, 227–28

Milk products: as protein foods, 61; calorie, carbohydrate, and protein guide, 73–74; cholesterol and, 78; protein complementarity of, 63. *See also* Cheese; Yogurt

Mineral(s): aging and, 140–41; as body chemicals, 3, 15, 175–76; as chelating agents, 97; as therapy for infection, 125; deficiency: *as kind of stress, 125, 129; in white flour, 47;* digestion of, 70, 140–41; food sources of, 54; Gladys Lindberg formula for taking, 182; good health and, 8; in alfalfa, 162; in brewer's yeast, 163; in eggs, 20; in liver, 164; in sea salt, 167; in skim milk, 165; in wheat, 19; in whey, 166; loss of, in flour refining, 180; loss of, through chelation therapy, 94; nail health related to, 68; need for extra, 179–81; protein deficiency related to, 65; storage, 70; supplements, 54: *dieting and, 155–56; recommended dosage of, 169; weight gain and, 146*

Mineral oil, vitamin K and, 212

Molasses: as sucrose substitute, 168; blackstrap, 5: *as ingredient in fortified drinks, 153; benefits of, 162; in candy, 14; recommended dosage, 162;* blood sugar levels and, 43; mineral content in, 43

Molybdenum, 229

Moore, Thomas, 120

"Morale vitamin," 187

Morning sickness, 192

Morrison, Lester, 88–89

Mount Zion Hospital, 91

Mucous membranes: importance of healthy, 119–20; vitamin A and, 107, 119–20; vitamin E and, 107

Multiple sclerosis, 65, 187
Muscle(s): building, protein intake during, 72; tone: *Gerovital H₃ therapy for, 145; good health and, 3; mineral deficiencies and, 140; protein deficiency and, 67;* weakness, 48–49, 50. *See also* Exercise; Physical
Muscular dystrophy, 203
Myasthenia gravis, 228
Myelin sheath, 220

N
Nail(s), 64, 68
National Academy of Sciences, 179, 235
National Cancer Institute, 142, 210
National Heart, Lung, and Blood Institute, 90
National Research Assembly of Life Science, 219
National Research Council, 123, 179, 235, 238
Nausea and vomiting, 190, 199, 240
Nephrosis, 49, 65
Nerves, degeneration of, 197
Nervousness, 200
Nervous system, 48–49, 77, 201
Neuritis, 13, 64, 192
New England Journal of Medicine, The, 103
New York Medical College, 94
Niacin: as therapy for pellagra, 11–12; as water-soluble vitamin, 175, 189; best sources, 191; characteristics, 189–90; content in body, 203; deficiency: *as cause of anemia, 6, 223; related to senility, 143; symptoms, 190;* phosphorus and, 230; pyridoxine and, 192; supplements to take, 191; toxicity, 191; tryptophane related to, 62; what it does and may do, 190–91
Niacinamide. *See* Niacin
Nicotinamide. *See* Niacin
Nicotine: as poison, 11; as stressor, 24; effect of, on adrenal glands, 48. *See also* Smoking
Nicotinic acid. *See* Niacin
Niehans, Paul, 143–44
Night blindness, 184
Nitrites, 205
Nitrogen, 61
Nitrous oxide, 210
Nosebleeds, 204, 214
Nucleic acid supplements, 145
Nutrition: aging related to, 145; as cure for pellagra, 10–13; as health insurance, 15; as protection against stress, 28, 34–39; cholesterol and, 76; comprehensive program of, 149–69; effect of, on immune system, 9, 115, 117; fortified protein drinks for, 151–56;

meals for, 157–61; proper eating patterns for, 155–56; rules to live by, 166–69; supplements, 61–66. *See also* Malnutrition
Nuts: as source of fiber, 111; as source of tryptophane, 62; for meals, 160, 161; protein and, 63

O
Obesity, 47, 146. *See also* Weight gain
Oil(s): importance of, in diet, 154; peanut, to fortify peanut butter, 159; unhydrogenated, 167. *See also* Fat(s)
Onions, used by our ancestors, 20
Oranges, to prevent sticky blood, 86
Osteoarthritis, 210
Osteomalacia: calcium deficiency and, 216; vitamin D deficiency and, 207
Osteoporosis: calcium deficiency related to, 141, 216; caused by poor diet, 68–69; in elderly, 141; magnesium as preventive, 226–27; vitamin D deficiency related to, 207. *See also* Bone(s)
Overweight. *See* Weight gain
Oxygen, intake of: as symptom of hypoglycemia, 49; blood sugar levels related to, 52; wheat germ oil and, 166
Ozone, PABA as protector against, 200; peroxidation and, 137–38; selenium deficiency and, 233; vitamin E as protector against, 210

P
PABA: as water-soluble vitamin, 175, 200; best sources, 200; characteristics, 200; deficiency symptoms, 200; supplements to take, 201; toxicity, 200; what it does and may do, 200
Pancakes: recipe for, 171; toppings for, 171
Pancreas: dysfunction, vitamin K and, 212; effects of alcohol on, 146; enzymes in, digestion and, 99–100 (*see also* Enzymes, pancreatic); glandulars, benefits of, 164 (*see also* Glandulars); importance of minerals for, 53–54; manganese and, 228
Pancreatin, 105
Pancreatitis, 100, 166
Panthenol. *See* Pantothenic acid
Pantothenic acid: allergies and, 34, 106; as therapy for swollen glands, 122; as water-soluble vitamin, 175, 197; best sources, 198; characteristics, 197; deficiency: *as cause of anemia, 223; symptoms, 197;* effect of, on adrenal glands, 34; eosinophil test for, 106; experiment with deficiency of, 34–35; in antibody formation, 197; sources of, 107; stress and, 24, 34; supplements to take, 198; toxicity, 198; vitamin C

and, 204; what it does and may do, 197–98
Para-aminobenzoic acid. *See* PABA
Paralysis, 201
Paranoia, 202
Parkinson's Syndrome, 49
Passwater, Richard, 77, 88, 130
Pasteur, Louis, 11
Pauling, Linus, 36, 78, 81, 123, 126–27
Peanut butter, 14, 62–63, 159
Peanut butter candy, recipe for, 172–73
Pectin, 111
Pellagra, 9–13, 190
Pepsin, 104, 105
Periodontal disease, 216
Pernicious anemia, 195–96
Perspiration odor, 108–109
Pesticides: as stressors, 24; potential effects of, 168; removal, 160, 168
Pfeiffer, Carl, 37
Phenylalanine, 59, 70
Phlebitis, 209
Phosphorus: best sources, 177, 230; characteristics, 229; deficiencies, 69, 70; deficiency symptoms, 230; foods containing, 20, 62, 163, 164; imbalances in, 163: magnesium and, 226; ratio with calcium, 176–77, 215, 217–18, 229, 230; supplements to take, 230; toxicity, 230; vitamin D and, 207, 208; what it does, 230
Physical: exertion: *of our ancestors, 19; supplements for, 150;* fitness: *bee pollen for, 162; liver dosage for, 165; wheat germ oil and, 166. See also* Exercise; Muscle(s)
Phytic acid, 239
Pinckney, Cathey and Edward, 84
Pinderfields General Hospital (England), 87
Pituitary gland, 36, 207, 226
Pneumonia, 20, 124
Poisons. *See* Toxins
Polio: antibiotic cure for, 17; antibody deficiency and, 118; vitamin C therapy for, 124
Pollution, 22, 116, 117
Potassium: best sources, 177, 232; characteristics, 230–31; chloride, mixed with sea salt, 168; deficiency symptoms, 225, 231; in alfalfa, 156; in molasses, 43, 162; ratio with sodium, 177–78, 192, 230, 231, 236, 237; role of, in heart activity, 143; stress and, 37, 129; supplements to take, 232–33; toxicity, 232; what it does and may do, 231–32
Poultry: calorie, carbohydrate, and protein guide, 74–75; for lunch, 159, 160; natural, used by our ancestors, 21
Prednisone, 129

Pregnancy: as stressor, 24; calcium deficiency during, 141; edema during, 67–68; folic acid deficiency during, 194; iodine deficiency during, 221, 222; iron during, 225; manganese deficiency during, 228; protein during, 67–68, 71; pyridoxine deficiency during, 192; vitamin A deficiency during, 185; vitamin E deficiency during, 209
Presenile dementia, 202
Preservatives, 22; as stressors, 23–24; in bread, 167
Price, Weston, 21
Primitive peoples, diet of, 9, 10, 21–22, 64, 122. *See also* Ancestors
Protein(s), 59–75; animal, 60, 61–62; antibody production and, 118, 122; as cancer preventive, 131; blood sugar levels and, 41–42; carbohydrate complementarity for, 73; cholesterol manufacture and, 77; complete, 60, 61; daily requirements of, 66–67, 168: *guide to, 73;* deficiencies, 64, 147: *anemia related to, 6; mental retardation related to, 71–72; osteoporosis related to, 68;* digestion of, 66, 69, 70, 99–100, 104, 156; drinks, fortified, 149, 168: *benefits of, 151–52; for infection, 117; for protein deficiency, 147; in reference chart, 150–51; recipes for, 152–55;* effect of, on diabetes, 55; effect of, on disease, 117; for lunch, 158; function, 59, 60, 61, 65, 72; hair health related to, 68; hydrochloric acid as digestant of, 166; importance of, at breakfast, 55; in alfalfa, 162; in brewer's yeast, 163; in eggs, 20; in mother's milk, 71; in liver, 164; in protein powders, 165; in skim milk, 165; in soy flour, 167; liver cirrhosis and, 70, 131; nail health related to, 68; needs of, in elderly, 69; powders, 154, 165; reproduction and, 71; stress and, 24, 28, 38; vegetable, 60, 61, 62–63; vitamin C and, 124. *See also* Amino acids
Prunes, 108
Psoriasis, 95, 195
Purdue University, 137
Pyorrhea, 230
Pyridoxamine. *See* Pyridoxine
Pyridoxinal. *See* Pyridoxine
Pyridoxine: as therapy for walking disability, 13; as treatment for nausea, 240; as water-soluble vitamin, 175, 191; atherosclerosis and, 87–88; best sources, 193; characteristics, 191; deficiency: *as cause of anemia, 233; from antibiotics, 119; symptoms, 191–92;* fat energy conversion and, 156; in antibody formation, 197; in eggs, 79;

iron toxicity and, 224; supplements to take, 193–94; toxicity, 193; what it does and may do, 192–93; zinc and, 240, 241

Pyruvic acid, 187

R

Radiation: as cause of cancer, 117; avoidance of, 132; liver as protection from effect of, 39; pantothenic acid as protection against, 197–98; vitamin E as protection against, 210

Rahe, Richard H., 32–33

Raynaud's syndrome, 209

RDA. *See* Recommended Dietary Allowances

Recipes, 170–73

Recommended Dietary Allowances, 178–79

Red blood cells: decreased survival of, with vitamin E deficiency, 209; folic acid in formation of, 194; iron in, 223; potassium used by, 231; pyridoxine in formation of, 192; vitamin B-12 in formation of, 196

Refining: of flour, minerals lost in, 180; of food, chromium removal during, 218

Reproduction, 71; fats and, 83, 85; importance of protein to, 71

Research Institute of Human Nutrition (Czechoslovakia), 86–87

Respiratory tract, 107

"Restless legs" syndrome, 194

Restlessness, 197

Retinitis, 214

Retinol, 184

Rheumatic fever, 20

Rheumatism, 118, 193

Riboflavin, 6, 13–14; as water-soluble vitamin, 175, 188; best sources, 189; characteristics, 188; deficiency: *as cause of anemia, 223; symptoms, 189;* phosphorus and, 230; supplements to take, 189; toxicity, 189; vitamin C and, 204; what it does and may do, 189

Rickets: calcium deficiency as cause of, 216, 230; phosphorus deficiency as cause of, 230; vitamin D deficiency as cause of, 207, 230

RNA, 192, 194, 196, 226, 230, 239

Rocky Mountain spotted fever, 200

Rodale, J. I., 85

Roots, used by our ancestors, 20

Rosenman, Ray, 91

Russek, Henry, 94

Rutin, 97

Ryder, Richard, 4

Rytel, Michael, 129

S

Salt: in remedy drink for cold, 117; loss, blood sugar levels related to, 52; ratio with potassium, 177–78; sea, use of, 167, 237

Salzman (M.D.), 49

Schizophrenia: folic acid to treat, 194; niacin to treat, 190–91; related to blood sugar levels, 49; zinc and manganese to treat, 228–29

Schrauzer, Gerhard N., 130–31

Schroeder, Dr. Henry, 218

Scleroderma, 95

Scurvy, 13, 123, 204

Seasickness, 192

Seeds: as protein food, 63; as source of tryptophane, 62; for meals, 160, 161

Selenium: as antioxidant, 139; as cancer preventive, 130, 131; as heart disease preventive, 229; best sources, 235; characteristics, 233; deficiency symptoms, 233; depletion as cause of stress, 129; effect of, on immune system, 130; in brewer's yeast, 163; sources of, 130; supplements to take, 235; toxicity, 234–35; what it does and may do, 233–34

Selye, Hans, 24–28, 30, 37, 128

Senility: aging and, 134, 143; aluminum accumulation and, 103, 140; blood sugar levels related to, 49; chelation therapy and, 95; deficiencies related to, 65, 143; folic acid to treat, 194; zinc therapy for, 140. *See also* Aging; Elderly

Senna leaves, 108

Serenity Cocktail, 39, 81, 151–52, 157–58, 168; brewer's yeast in, 62; for dieting, 155–56; for strength and energy, 156–57; meal plans with, 156; recipe for, 152–53. *See also* Drinks, fortified

Sex glands, vitamin E and, 210

Sexual: development: *butter and, 84; delayed by zinc deficiency, 239;* problems, as symptom of hypoglycemia, 49

Shock, treatment for, 237

Shumway, Norman, 93

Shute, Evan V., 85–86, 139

Shute, Wilfrid, 85–86, 93

Sickle cell anemia, 210

SIDS. *See* Sudden Infant Death Syndrome

Siegel, Benjamin, 128

Silicon, 111, 235–36

Sitophobia, 199

Skin: aging test for, 134; allergies, pantothenic acid and, 106; as barrier to disease, 119; cracking, riboflavin as therapy for, 13–14; diseases, garlic as therapy for, 20; disorders, blood sugar levels related to, 49; dryness, vitamin

A deficiency as cause of, 184; fats and, 83; good health and, 3; oils and, 154; problems, as symptom of hypoglycemia, 49; tone, mineral deficiencies as cause of, 140; vitamin A and, 107, 120; vitamin E and, 107

Sleeplessness: as symptom of hypoglycemia, 48–49; as symptom of mineral deficiency, 140; as symptom of poor digestion, 100, 166; biotin deficiency as cause of, 199; magnesium deficiency as cause of, 225; niacin deficiency as cause of, 190; tryptophane as therapy for, 62

Smallpox, 17

Smell, loss of, 239

Smith, Lendon, 72

Smoking: aging related to, 145; as stressor, 125; cell destruction and, 144; elimination of, 132; lipoproteins and, 90; poor effects of, 145; strokes related to, 145. *See also* Nicotine

Snacks, suggestions for, 161, 172–73

Soda, in remedy, 117

Sodium: best sources, 177, 237; characteristics, 236; deficiency symptoms, 236; ratio with potassium, 177–78, 192, 230, 231, 236, 237; supplements to take, 237–38; toxicity, 237; what it does and may do, 236–37

Sodium chloride, 106; ratio with potassium, 231

Soy: beans: *as protein food, 62; lecithin in, 164;* flour, 8, 167; oil: *fat content in, 83; in fortified drink,* 154; *linoleic/ linolenic acid content of,* 156; protein, as base of protein powders, 165

Spencer, Herta, 102

Spies, Tom, 10–13, 18

Spinal curvature, 197

Sprue, 212

Stanford Medical Center, 93

Starch, digestion of, 99–100

Stein, Joachim, 143, 144

Sterility, 139

Stimulants, 48, 51–52

Stone, Irwin, 54, 139

Story of the Adaptation Syndrome, The (Selye), 25

Stress: aging related to, 145; as cause of cancer, 36; B vitamins and, 34; bodily reaction to, 24; causes of, 23–24; colds as cause of, 129; crying as therapy for, 31; disease related to, 24, 34, during child-bearing years, 142; during menopause, 142; effect of exercise on, 146; effect of, on adrenal glands, 51–52; emotions as cause of, 28–31; exercise as therapy for, 32; factor affecting immune system, 117; general adaptation syndrome and, 25–28; health re-lated to, 2, 3, 81; heart attacks related to, 146; high cholesterol levels caused by, 129; interferon deficiency related to, 128–29; kinds of, 125; laughter as therapy for, 30–31; liver as protection against, 38–39, 164–65; love as therapy for, 29–30; menopause as form of, 141; mineral depletion caused by, 129; nutrition as protection against, 28, 34–39; pantothenic acid as treatment for, 197; protein and, 38, 72; rating chart, 32–33; supplements for, 150–51; tranquilizers and, 32; tryptophane as therapy for, 62; viral infection as cause of, 129; vitamin A and, 34; vitamin B deficiency caused by, 129; vitamin C and, 30, 35–36, 128; vitamin depletion and, 175; vitamin E and, 36–37; zinc depletion and, 239

Stress of Life, The (Selye), 25, 30

Strokes: artificial eggs and, 78; chelation therapy and, 95; garlic as therapy for, 20; margarine and, 78; smoking related to, 145. *See also* Heart

Studies in Deficiency Disease (McCarrison), 9

Stuttering, 188

Sucrose: as stressor, 24; atherosclerosis and, 44, 46, 83; blood sugar levels and, 42, 43; B vitamin destruction related to, 46; cancer related to, 129, 130–31; diabetes related to, 44, 46, 55; diet and, 43, 44, 47, 168; digestion of, 88, 99–100; effect of, on immune system, 22; heart disease and, 44, 46, 80, 88; hypoglycemia related to, 41, 42; in popular foods, 45–46; triglycerides and, 88

Sudden Infant Death Syndrome, 188

Sugar. *See* Fructose; Glucose; Lactose; Maltose; Sucrose

Sugar intake: and chromium depletion, 218; and magnesium depletion, 227

Suicidal tendencies, 202

Sulfa drugs: biotin and, 199; PABA and, 200; vitamin K and, 212

Sulfur, 238

Sulfur dioxide, 204

"Sunshine vitamin," 207

Sweet and Dangerous (Yudkin), 44, 90

Sweetbreads, 122, 123

Syrup, maple, 43

Systremma, 210

Szent-Gyorgyi, Dr. Albert, 124, 193

T

Tappel, A. L., 85, 137

Tardive dyskinesia, 202

Taste, loss of, 219, 239

Teeth: good health and, 3; degeneration,

21; *vegetarianism and, 64;* decay, 22, 108; infection, 125
Testosterone, 76
Tetracycline, 228
Thiamine: as therapy for neuritis, 13; as water-soluble vitamin, 175, 186; best sources, 188; characteristics, 186–87; deficiency: *as cause of anemia, 223; symptoms, 187;* manganese and, 228; role of, in digestion, 100; sucrose related to destruction of, 46; supplements to take, 188; toxicity, 188; vitamin C and, 204; what it does and may do, 187–88
Threonine, 59
Thrombosis, 209, 210
Thymus, 122–23. *See also* Glandulars, thymus
Thymus gland, 228; as producer of antibodies, 26; role in immunity system, 119
Thyroid deficiency: cholesterol and, 92; kelp to prevent, 93; nail health related to, 68; test for, 92–93
Thyroid gland, 207, 211, 221, 222, 223, 228
Thyroxine, 222, 228
Tocopherol. *See* Vitamin E
Tonsils, swollen, 121, 122
Tooth decay, 193, 204, 230
Tooth-grinding. *See* Bruxism
Toxemia, 194
Toxins: as stressors, 24; detoxification of, by liver, 70, 131; effect of vitamin C on, 54; reabsorption related to fiber, 110
Trace minerals. *See* Minerals
Tranquilizers, 32
Triglyceride(s): atherosclerosis and, 90–91; calcium and, 216–17; heart disease and, 90; levels, 76, 87, 88
Tryptophane: 192; as essential amino acid, 59, 62; deficiency, 70
Tuberculosis: antibiotic cure for, 17; eggs as therapy for, 19–21; garlic as therapy for, 20

U
Ulcers: alfalfa as therapy for, 162; choline deficiency as cause of, 201; hydrochloric acid as cause of, 103; niacin deficiency as cause of, 190; pantothenic acid deficiency as cause of, 197; stress as cause of, 26; zinc as therapy for, 37
Ultraviolet light, blocked by PABA, 200
Underweight. *See* Weight loss
U.S. Public Health Service, 9
United States Government Composition of Foods Handbook, 176

University of California: at Berkeley, 18; at Davis, 85: *Department of Food Science, 137; Section of Infections and Immunologic Diseases, School of Medicine, 138;* at Los Angeles, 85; at San Diego, 130
University of Heidelberg, 144
University of Illinois, 78, 82, 165; Physical Fitness Institute, 165
University of Nebraska, 138
University of Puget Sound, 136
University of Oregon Health Sciences Center, 128
University of Southern California School of Medicine, 32
Urine/urinary tract, 112–13

V
Valine, 59
Vanadium, 238–39
Varicose veins, 110–111, 211, 214
Vegetables: as abater of pellagra, 10; as part of Hunza diet, 9; as source of fiber, 111; for meals, 158, 159, 160, 161; fresh, 8, 168; *eaten by our ancestors, 19;* good health and, 13; pesticide removal from, 168; protein complementarity for, 63; raw, 161: *as remedy for hiatal hernia, 104; as sources of B vitamins, 107*
Vegetarianism, 63–64
Vertigo, 225
Vinegar, apple cider, 112–13
Viruses: antibody deficiency and, 118; as cause of cancer, 117; location of, in bowel, 121; protein deficiency and, 66; removed by white blood cells, 119; vitamin A deficiency and, 120; vitamin C as fighter of, 124. *See also* Colds; Flu
Vision, poor: as symptom of hypoglycemia, 49; mineral deficiencies as cause of, 140; vitamin A therapy for, 13; vitamin B-12 and, 196
Vitality Through Planned Nutrition (Davis), 14
Vitamin(s): as body chemicals, 3, 15; as therapy for infection, 125; as therapy for liver cirrhosis, 131; daily intake of, 169: deficiency: *as stressor, 125; caused by alcohol, 146; in white flour, 47;* Gladys Lindberg formula for taking, 182; good health and, 8; in alfalfa, 162; in whey, 166; mineral assimilation and, 140–41; need for extra, 179–81; pancreatic enzymes as digestant of, 166; supplements: *dieting and, 155–56; weight gain and, 146.* *See also* B vitamins; specific vitamins
Vitamin A: allergies and, 105, 107; antibiotics and, 212; as antioxidant, 139;

as fat-soluble vitamin, 174; as healing agent, 184; as therapy for cold, 120; as therapy for poor vision, 13; as therapy for swollen glands, 122; best sources, 186; bioflavonoids and, 214; calcium and, 215, 217; characteristics, 184; deficiency symptoms, 184; effect of, on adrenal glands, 34; elimination and, 108; fats as source of, 84; immune system and, 34, 119–20; in bile salt production, 190; in butter, 84; in eggs, 20; in liver, 164; mucous membranes and, 119–20; nail health related to, 68; storage of, in liver, 70; stress and, 24, 34; supplements to take, 186; toxicity, 121, 185–86; vitamin C and, 204; vitamin E and, 209; what it does and may do, 184–85

Vitamin B. *See* B vitamins
Vitamin B-1, 6
Vitamin B-2, 6
Vitamin B-3. *See* Niacin
Vitamin B-5. *See* Pantothenic acid
Vitamin B-6. *See* Pyridoxin
Vitamin B-12: as supplement for vegetarians, 64; as water-soluble vitamin, 175, 195; best sources, 196; characteristics, 195; deficiency: *as cause of anemia, 6, 192, 223; in brewer's yeast, 163; symptoms, 194, 195–96;* immune system and, 202; supplements to take, 196–97; toxicity, 196; what it does and may do, 196

Vitamin C, 123–25; aging and, 139–40; allergies and, 105, 106–107; as antioxidant, 137, 163; as chelating agent, 97; as therapy for: *colds, 120, 123; liver regeneration, 131; scurvy, 13, 123; swollen glands, 122;* as water-soluble vitamin, 175, 203–204; atherosclerosis and, 86, 87; best sources, 206; bioflavonoids and, 213, 214, 215; blood sugar utilization and, 54; cancer and, 126, 127, 131; characteristics, 203–204; deficiency: *as cause of anemia, 223; symptoms, 190, 204;* dosage, 125; effect of, on adrenal glands, 26, 35; effect of, on drugs, 55; effect of, on toxins, 54; folic acid and, 194; hemorrhaging from loss of, 25–26, 27; immune system and, 151; in fortified drinks, 152; kidney stones and, 113; manganese and, 228; nail health related to, 68; production of interferon by, 128; protein and, 66, 124; senility and, 143; sources of, 35; storage, 26, 124; stress and, 24, 28, 30, 35–36, 129, 151; studies, 124; supplements to take, 206; toxicity, 205–206; what it does and may do, 204–205

Vitamin D: antibiotics and, 212; as fat-soluble vitamin, 174, 207; best sources, 208; calcium and, 215; characteristics, 207; cholesterol and, 76–77; deficiency symptoms, 207, 230; fats as sources of, 84; in bile salt production, 190; in butter, 84; in eggs, 20; for bone strength, 177; osteoporosis related to, 69; storage, 70; supplements to take, 208; toxicity, 121, 208; what it does and may do, 207

Vitamin E: adding to unsaturated fats, 82; aging and, 137–39; antibiotics and, 212; atherosclerosis and, 85–86; as antioxidant, 36–37, 137, 139, 167, 210; as cancer preventive, 130, 131, 139; as chelating agent, 97; as fat-soluble vitamin, 174, 208; as healing agent, 185, 211; as protection against heart disease, 37; as remedy for allergies, 105, 107; as therapy for: *aging, 137, 139; liver, 70, 131; menopause, 142;* best sources, 211; cell protection and, 137; characteristics, 208–209; deficiency: *as cause of anemia, 192, 223; symptoms, 209;* dosage, 139; effects of, 70, 85–86; exercise and, 36; fat as source of, 84; for first aid, 36; heart disease and, 85–86; immune system and, 139; in bile salt production, 190; in butter, 84; inositol and, 203; in wheat, 19; iron and, 224; polyunsaturates and, 84; red blood cell destruction and, 136; selenium and, 233, 234; storage, 36, 70; stress and, 24, 36–37; supplements to take, 212; toxicity, 211; to treat myasthenia gravis, 228; vitamin A and, 186, 209; vitamin C and, 204; what it does and may do, 209–11

Vitamin H. *See* Biotin
Vitamin K: and antibiotics, 212; best sources, 213; in bile salt production, 190; blood coagulation and, 109; characteristics, 212; deficiency symptoms, 212–13; as fat-soluble vitamin, 174, 212; storage, 70; supplements to take, 213; synthesis of, 109; types of, 212; what it does and may do, 213

Vitamin P. *See* Bioflavonoids
Vitiligo, 200
Vomiting, 197

W
Warshauer, D., 137
Water: chlorine in, 21; conservation, 102; fresh, used by our ancestors, 21; importance of drinking, 102; pollution, 22
Water-soluble vitamins, 175
Watson, Ronald R., 137

Weg, Ruth, 69
Weight: gain: *aging related to, 145; as symptom of poor digestion, 166;* mortality rates from, 146; vitamin and mineral supplements and, 146 (see also Obesity); loss: *as symptom of poor digestion, 100; edema related to, 68; poor digestion and, 166; protein deficiency related to, 67* (see also Dieting)
Weller (M.D.), 49
Wheat germ: as abater of pellagra, 11; as protein food, 62; as source of minerals, 54; calcium content in, 62; good health and, 5, 8; in bread, 158; in candy, 13–14; oil: *benefits of, 165–66; for physical fitness, 150; recommended dosage, 166;* phosphorus content in, 62
Wheat germ candy, recipe, 173
Whey, 152, 166
Williams, Dr. Roger J., 3, 87, 127–28, 140, 198
Winning the Fight Against Breast Cancer (Fredericks), 131, 142
Wisdom of the Body, The (Cannon), 30
Worms, garlic as therapy for, 20
Worry. *See* Anxiety
Wounds: garlic as therapy for, 20; healing related to: *protein, 66; vitamin C, 123; vitamin E, 185, 211; zinc, 239–40*

X
X rays, and magnesium depletion, 227

Y
Yeast, brewer's, 5; antibody increase related to, 66; as abater of pellagra, 10; as protein food, 62; as source of minerals, 54; as therapy for liver cirrhosis, 131; B-12 deficiency in, 163; benefits of, 163; calcium and, 62, 163; elimination and, 108; good health and, 6, 8, 13; in fortified drinks, 13, 152, 153; skim milk as complement to, 165
Yogurt: as aid to elimination, 107; as source of tryptophane, 62; calorie, carbohydrate, and protein guide, 74–75; for lunch, 159, 160; good health of Bulgarian people and, 109
You Can Predict Your Heart Attack and Prevent It (Gertler), 92
Yudkin, John, 44, 91

Z
Zinc: aluminum related to removal of, 140; as antioxidant, 139; as treatment for burn patients, 37; best sources, 240; characteristics, 239; deficiency of, in white flour, 47; deficiency symptoms, 239; effect of, on immune system, 130; folic acid and, 194; importance of, for diabetes, 53–54; in molasses, 43; loss through chelation therapy, 94–95; ratio with copper, 178, 221, 241; stress and, 37, 129; supplements to take, 241; therapy for senility, 140; toxicity, 240; what it does and may do, 239–40